STUDY GUIDE
FOR THE
PSYCHIATRY BOARD
EXAMINATION

STUDY GUIDE FOR THE PSYCHIATRY BOARD EXAMINATION

Edited by

Philip R. Muskin, M.D.

Professor of Psychiatry, Columbia University Medical Center;
Chief, Consultation-Liaison Psychiatry at New York-Presbyterian
Hospital/Columbia Campus;
Faculty, Columbia University Center for Psychoanalytic Training
and Research, New York, New York

Anna L. Dickerman, M.D.

Assistant Professor of Clinical Psychiatry,
Department of Psychiatry, Weill Cornell Medical College;
Assistant Attending Psychiatrist, Psychiatry Consultation-Liaison
Service, New York-Presbyterian Hospital/Weill Cornell Medical
Center, New York, New York

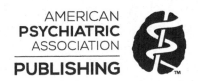

AMERICAN
PSYCHIATRIC
ASSOCIATION
PUBLISHING

Note: The authors have worked to ensure that all information in this book is accurate at the time of publication and consistent with general psychiatric and medical standards, and that information concerning drug dosages, schedules, and routes of administration is accurate at the time of publication and consistent with standards set by the U.S. Food and Drug Administration and the general medical community. As medical research and practice continue to advance, however, therapeutic standards may change. Moreover, specific situations may require a specific therapeutic response not included in this book. For these reasons and because human and mechanical errors sometimes occur, we recommend that readers follow the advice of physicians directly involved in their care or the care of a member of their family.

If you wish to buy 50 or more copies of the same title, please go to www.appi.org/special discounts for more information.

Manufactured in the United States of America on acid-free paper

20 19 18 17 16   5 4 3 2 1

ISBN 978-1-61537-033-7
First Edition

Typeset in Palatino LT Std and Helvetica Neue LT Std

American Psychiatric Association Publishing
1000 Wilson Boulevard
Arlington, VA 22209-3901
www.appi.org

Contents

Contributors xi

Preface xv

Part I: Questions

CHAPTER 1
Anthropology/Sociology/Ethology/Psychology 3

CHAPTER 2
Anxiety Disorders 7

CHAPTER 3
Bipolar Disorders 11

CHAPTER 4
Dangerousness 13

CHAPTER 5
Depressive Disorders 15

CHAPTER 6
Development: Adulthood 17

CHAPTER 7
Development: Infancy Through Adolescence 21

CHAPTER 8
Developmental Issues in Older Adults 25

CHAPTER 9
Diagnostic Procedures 29

CHAPTER 10
Disruptive Behavior Disorders 33

CHAPTER 11
Dissociative Disorders 35

CHAPTER 12
Elimination Disorders 37

CHAPTER 13
Epidemiology and Public Policy:
Health Care Economics/Public Policy Issues 39

CHAPTER 14
Feeding and Eating Disorders 43

CHAPTER 15
Law 47

CHAPTER 16
Mental Status 49

CHAPTER 17
Neurocognitive Disorders. 51

CHAPTER 18
Neurodevelopmental Disorders 57

CHAPTER 19
Nonpharmacological Somatic Treatments 63

CHAPTER 20
Obsessive-Compulsive and Related Disorders 69

CHAPTER 21
Paraphilic Disorders. 73

CHAPTER 22
Personality Disorders. 75

CHAPTER 23
Principles of Psychopharmacology. 77

CHAPTER 24
Professionalism 85

CHAPTER 25
Psychiatric Consultation 87

CHAPTER 26
Psychiatric Interview 91

CHAPTER 27
Psychoanalysis. 93

CHAPTER 28
Psychological Testing 95

CHAPTER 29
Psychopharmacology. 97

CHAPTER 30
Psychosocial Interventions 103

CHAPTER 31
Psychotherapies. 107

CHAPTER 32
Research/Biostatistics. 115

CHAPTER 33
Schizophrenia Spectrum and Other Psychotic Disorders 117

CHAPTER 34
Sexual Dysfunction/Gender Dysphoria 121

CHAPTER 35
Sleep-Wake Disorders 125

CHAPTER 36
Somatic Symptom and Related Disorders 127

CHAPTER 37
Special Topics: Seclusion/Risk Management/
Abuse and Neglect 131

CHAPTER 38
Spirituality. 135

CHAPTER 39
Substance-Related and Addictive Disorders .137

CHAPTER 40
Suicidality 141

CHAPTER 41
Trauma- and Stressor-Related Disorders 145

Part II: Answer Guide

CHAPTER 1
Anthropology/Sociology/Ethology/Psychology 149

CHAPTER 2
Anxiety Disorders 159

C H A P T E R 3
Bipolar Disorders 165

C H A P T E R 4
Dangerousness. 171

C H A P T E R 5
Depressive Disorders 177

C H A P T E R 6
Development: Adulthood 183

C H A P T E R 7
Development: Infancy Through Adolescence 191

C H A P T E R 8
Developmental Issues in Older Adults. 201

C H A P T E R 9
Diagnostic Procedures. 211

C H A P T E R 1 0
Disruptive Behavior Disorders 223

C H A P T E R 1 1
Dissociative Disorders 229

C H A P T E R 1 2
Elimination Disorders 235

C H A P T E R 1 3
Epidemiology and Public Policy:
Health Care Economics/Public Policy Issues 237

C H A P T E R 1 4
Feeding and Eating Disorders 245

C H A P T E R 1 5
Law 253

C H A P T E R 1 6
Mental Status 257

C H A P T E R 1 7
Neurocognitive Disorders. 261

C H A P T E R 1 8
Neurodevelopmental Disorders 273

CHAPTER 19
Nonpharmacological Somatic Treatments 285

CHAPTER 20
Obsessive-Compulsive and Related Disorders. 301

CHAPTER 21
Paraphilic Disorders 307

CHAPTER 22
Personality Disorders 311

CHAPTER 23
Principles of Psychopharmacology 317

CHAPTER 24
Professionalism 335

CHAPTER 25
Psychiatric Consultation 341

CHAPTER 26
Psychiatric Interview 349

CHAPTER 27
Psychoanalysis 353

CHAPTER 28
Psychological Testing 357

CHAPTER 29
Psychopharmacology 363

CHAPTER 30
Psychosocial Interventions 377

CHAPTER 31
Psychotherapies 387

CHAPTER 32
Research/Biostatistics 405

CHAPTER 33
Schizophrenia Spectrum and Other Psychotic Disorders 411

CHAPTER 34
Sexual Dysfunction/Gender Dysphoria 417

CHAPTER 35
Sleep-Wake Disorders 427

CHAPTER 36
Somatic Symptom and Related Disorders 431

CHAPTER 37
Special Topics: Seclusion/Risk Management/
Abuse and Neglect 441

CHAPTER 38
Spirituality 451

CHAPTER 39
Substance-Related and Addictive Disorders 457

CHAPTER 40
Suicidality . . . . , ...465

CHAPTER 41
Trauma- and Stressor-Related Disorders 475

Bibliography 481

Contributors

Iqbal "Ike" Ahmed, M.D., FRCPsych
Faculty Psychiatrist, Tripler Army Medical Center; Clinical Professor of Psychiatry, Uniformed Services University of Health Sciences; Clinical Professor of Psychiatry and Geriatric Medicine, Department of Geriatric Medicine, University of Hawaii, Honolulu, Hawaii

Rachel Caravella, M.D.
Instructor of Clinical Psychiatry and Assistant Attending Inpatient Psychiatry, Department of Psychiatry, Columbia University Medical Center/New York-Presbyterian Hospital, New York, New York

Alanna Chait, M.D.
Resident Physician, Department of Psychiatry, New York-Presbyterian Hospital/Weill Cornell Medical Center, New York, New York

Stephanie Cheung, M.D.
Assistant Professor of Psychiatry and Assistant Attending, Department of Psychiatry/Consultation-Liaison Psychiatry, Columbia University Medical Center, New York, New York

Adam Critchfield, M.D.
Fellow in Psychosomatic Medicine, Columbia University Medical Center and New York State Psychiatric Institute, New York, New York

Catherine Daniels-Brady, M.D.
Assistant Clinical Professor of Psychiatry and Attending Psychiatrist, Division of Consultation-Liaison Psychiatry, New York Medical College at Westchester Medical Center, Valhalla, New York

Meena Dasari, Ph.D.
Clinical Psychologist and Assistant Professor, Department of Psychiatry, New York University School of Medicine, New York, New York

Anna L. Dickerman, M.D.
Assistant Professor of Clinical Psychiatry, Department of Psychiatry, Weill Cornell Medical College; Assistant Attending Psychiatrist, Psychiatry Consultation-Liaison Service, New York-Presbyterian Hospital/Weill Cornell Medical Center, New York, New York

Elizabeth Evans, M.D.
Clinical and Research Fellow, Division on Substance Abuse, Department of Psychiatry, Columbia University/New York State Psychiatric Institute, New York, New York

Christina Kitt Garza, M.D.
Instructor of Psychiatry and Assistant Attending, Department of Psychiatry/Consultation-Liaison Psychiatry, Columbia University Medical Center, New York, New York

Liliya Gershengoren, M.D.
Fellow in Psychosomatic Medicine, Columbia University Medical Center and New York State Psychiatric Institute, New York, New York

Jennifer S. Harrington-Knopf, B.A.
Medical Student, Columbia University College of Physicians and Surgeons, New York, New York

Yael Holoshitz, M.D.
Psychiatrist, OnTrackNY/Washington Heights Community Service; Assistant Attending Psychiatrist, Columbia University Medical Center, New York, New York

Sarah Richards Kim, M.D.
Chief Resident, Child and Adolescent Psychiatry at New York-Presbyterian Hospital/Columbia and Cornell; Fellow in Child and Adolescent Public Psychiatry, New York City Children's Center-Queens, Bellerose, New York

Daniel Knoepflmacher, M.D., M.F.A.
Chief Resident, Payne Whitney-Weill Cornell Department of Psychiatry, New York-Presbyterian Hospital, New York, New York

John Luo, M.D.
Director of Psychiatry Residency Training and Clinical Professor of Psychiatry, Department of Psychiatry, University of California Riverside School of Medicine, Riverside, California

Adrienne D. Mishkin, M.D., M.P.H.
Instructor of Psychiatry, Department of Psychiatry/Consultation-Liaison Psychiatry, Columbia University Medical Center, New York, New York

Philip R. Muskin, M.D., M.A.
Professor of Psychiatry, Columbia University Medical Center; Chief, Consultation-Liaison Psychiatry at New York-Presbyterian Hospital/Columbia Campus; Faculty, Columbia University Center for Psychoanalytic Training and Research, New York, New York

Sara Siris Nash, M.D.
Assistant Professor of Psychiatry and Assistant Attending, Department of Psychiatry/Consultation-Liaison Psychiatry, Columbia University Medical Center, New York, New York

Daniel P. Notzon, M.D.
Fellow in Substance Abuse Disorders, Columbia University Medical Center/New York State Psychiatric Institute, New York, New York

Divy Ravindranath, M.D., M.S.
Clinical Assistant Professor (Affiliated), Department of Psychiatry, Stanford University School of Medicine, Stanford, California; Staff Psychiatrist, VA Palo Alto Health Care System, Palo Alto, California

Michelle Riba, M.D., M.S.
Clinical Professor and Associate Chair for Integrated Medical and Psychiatric Services, Department of Psychiatry, University of Michigan, Ann Arbor, Michigan

Amy Rosinski, M.D.
Clinical Assistant Professor, Department of Psychiatry, University of Michigan Health System; Director, Consultation-Liaison Services, University Hospital, Ann Arbor, Michigan

Lisa S. Seyfried, M.D.
Assistant Professor, Department of Psychiatry, and Section Director, Psychiatry Hospital Services, University of Michigan, Ann Arbor, Michigan

Yvette Smolin, M.D.
Clinical Assistant Professor and Director, Consultation-Liaison Psychiatry/Psychosomatic Medicine Fellowship, New York Medical College at Westchester Medical Center, Valhalla, New York

Oliver M. Stroeh, M.D.
Clarice Kestenbaum, M.D. Assistant Professor of Education and Training in the Division of Child & Adolescent Psychiatry, Department of Psychiatry, Columbia University Medical Center; Associate Director, New York-Presbyterian Hospital Child and Adolescent Psychiatry Residency Training Program of Columbia and Cornell Universities, New York, New York

Wendy L. Thompson, M.D.
Clinical Professor, Department of Family and Community Medicine, New York Medical College, Valhalla, New York

Thomas E. Ungar, M.D., M.Ed., CCFP, FCFP, FRCPC, DABPN
Associate Professor, Department of Psychiatry, University of Toronto; Chief of Psychiatry and Chief of Staff, North York General Hospital, Toronto, Ontario, Canada

Disclosure of Competing Interests

The following contributors to this book have indicated a financial interest in or other affiliation with a commercial supporter, a manufacturer of a commercial product, a provider of a commercial service, a nongovernmental organization, and/or a government agency, as listed below:

John Luo, M.D.—*Consultant*: Otsuka Pharmaceuticals.

Thomas Ungar, M.D.—*Speaker honoraria/Advisory Board*: Lundbeck, Otsaka, and Actavis; *Innovation grant funding*: Movember Canada, Inc. (charity); *Owner*: Mental Health Minute, Inc.

The following contributors to this book have indicated no competing interests to disclose during the year preceding manuscript submission:

Iqbal "Ike" Ahmed, M.D., FRCPsych
Rachel Caravella, M.D.
Alanna Chait, M.D.
Stephanie Cheung, M.D.
Adam Critchfield, M.D.
Catherine Daniels-Brady, M.D.
Meena Dasari, Ph.D.
Anna L. Dickerman, M.D.
Elizabeth Evans, M.D.
Christina Kitt Garza, M.D.
Liliya Gershengoren, M.D.
Jennifer S. Harrington-Knopf, B.A.
Yael Holoshitz, M.D.
Sarah Richards Kim, M.D.
Daniel Knoepflmacher, M.D., M.F.A.
Adrienne D. Mishkin, M.D., M.P.H.
Philip R. Muskin, M.D., M.A.
Sara Siris Nash, M.D.
Daniel P. Notzon, M.D.
Divy Ravindranath, M.D., M.S.
Michelle Riba, M.D., M.S.
Amy Rosinski, M.D.
Lisa S. Seyfried, M.D.
Yvette Smolin, M.D.
Oliver M. Stroeh, M.D.
Wendy L. Thompson, M.D.

Preface

The creation of this study guide involved authors from the full career spectrum: medical students, fellows, junior faculty, and senior faculty. They considered themselves stakeholders, because taking the initial certification examination in psychiatry—or taking the 10-year recertification examinations—is something all would face. The allocation of questions per topic follows the Certification Examination in Psychiatry: 2015 Blueprint of the American Board of Psychiatry and Neurology (www.abpn.com/wp-content/uploads/2015/01/PsychCert2015_-Blueprint.pdf).

We used numerous textbooks and several journal articles to provide the subject matter for the study guide. All of the textbooks used are readily available. Each explanation contains a reference source for the content. Where it is appropriate, we provide an explanation for both the correct and incorrect options. This is a *study guide* for the psychiatry boards, both the initial examination for certification as well as the recertification examinations. The recommended use of the book is to ascertain your areas of strength and weakness, to test your knowledge, and to prepare yourself for the examination. We do not intend the study guide to be your only preparation for the examination. Using this book for self-guidance in your study for the examination is the recommended approach. As has been the case with all of our study guides, the honorarium will be donated to a mental health charitable foundation.

We are grateful for the opportunity to prepare this volume.

Philip R. Muskin, M.D.
Anna L. Dickerman, M.D.

Part I

Questions

Anthropology/Sociology/
Ethology/Psychology

Select the single best response for each question.

1.1   Which of the following statements is true regarding completed suicide among youth in the United States?

   A. The ratio of completed suicide is higher for females than males.
   B. Black youth have the highest suicide rate.
   C. American Indians/Alaska Natives have the highest suicide rate.
   D. Hispanic youth have the highest suicide rate.
   E. White youth have the highest rate of suicide attempts but the lowest rate of suicide.

1.2   Which of the following best defines *ethnicity*?

   A. Physical, biological, and genetic qualities of humans, particularly as these features lead to categorization of visible similarities or differences.
   B. Identity with a group of people sharing common origins, history, customs, and beliefs.
   C. A set of meaning, behavioral norms, and values used by members of a particular society as they construct their unique view of the world.
   D. An organized system of beliefs, principles, rituals, practices, and related symbols that brings individuals and groups to sacred or ultimate reality and truth.
   E. Religion and faith communities, not restricted to organized religion and group membership.

1.3   Which of the following is a true statement regarding culture-bound syndromes?

   A. Culture-bound syndromes are vague and diffuse.
   B. Culture-bound syndromes are not accepted as a specific disorder in the country of origin.
   C. Culture-bound syndromes occur less frequently in the "home" culture than in other cultures.

D. Culture-bound syndromes are a response to specific precipitants in that culture.

E. Culture-bound syndromes are common in childhood and adolescence.

1.4 Which of the following is true regarding dissociation in culturally diverse patients?

A. Some world religious traditions foster dissociation in rituals and practices.
B. Dissociation is rarely a part of isolated culture-bound syndromes.
C. Dissociation is an insignificant symptom in culturally diverse children.
D. Exposure to trauma is rarely associated with dissociation.
E. Dissociation occurs only as a single symptom and never as a disorder.

1.5 Which of the following is a true statement regarding culture and child/adolescent development?

A. There is a wealth of methodologically sound studies of development outside of Western Europe and North America.
B. Cross-cultural studies have consistently documented that there is little variation in temperament and mother-child interactions among different cultures.
C. There is little variation in the time and manner in which different cultures mark adulthood.
D. Public acknowledgment of maturation is not relevant for role development in most cultures.
E. Theory and practical study of child and adolescent development have been dominated by Western schemas.

1.6 Which of the following DSM-5 tools was created to operationalize a culturally sensitive psychiatric evaluation?

A. Outline for Cultural Formulation.
B. Glossary of Culture-Bound Syndromes.
C. Glossary of Cultural Concepts of Distress.
D. Cultural Formulation Interview.
E. Culture, Age, and Gender Features Profile.

1.7 When researchers at McGill University used the Outline for Cultural Formulation (OCF) to reassess the cases of 70 patients with a referral diagnosis of a psychotic disorder, what proportion were rediagnosed as having a nonpsychotic disorder?

A. 27%.
B. 35%.
C. 49%.
D. 63%.
E. 78%.

1.8   For which of the following clinician groups was the Cultural Formulation Interview (CFI) originally designed?

A. Psychiatrists trained in specific skills of cultural competence.
B. Clinicians working with racial/ethnic minorities.
C. Clinicians working with patients who speak a different language than their own.
D. Clinicians working with patients from a different cultural background than their own.
E. Any clinician working with any patient in any setting.

1.9   As of 2010, the rate of uninsurance was highest for which ethnic group in the United States?

A. African Americans.
B. Hispanics.
C. American Indians/Alaska Natives.
D. Native Hawaiians/Pacific Islanders.
E. Asian Americans.

1.10   In 2005, the lifetime prevalence of any psychiatric disorder among males in American Indian tribes exceeded that among the average U.S. male population by what percentage?

A. 1%–5%.
B. 6%–10%.
C. 11%–15%.
D. 16%–20%.
E. 21%–25%.

1.11   According to U.S. Census Bureau estimates for 2013, what proportion of people in the United States identify themselves as nonwhite (including Black or African American, American Indian and Alaska Native, Native Hawaiian and Other Pacific Islander, Asian, Hispanic or Latino) or of two or more races?

A. 37%.
B. 54%.
C. 11%.
D. 23%.
E. 6%.

1.12   Which of the following terms refers to cultural ways of expressing distress that provide shared ways of experiencing and talking about personal or social concerns?

A. Cultural syndromes.
B. Culture-bound syndromes.

C. Cultural explanations.
D. Cultural idioms.
E. Cultural perceived causes.

1.13   How does mental health service utilization among racial and ethnic minority groups differ from that among white populations?

A. Nonmajority groups are more likely to receive mental health care in emergency room settings.
B. Nonmajority groups are more likely to receive mental health care in outpatient community settings.
C. Nonmajority groups are less likely to receive mental health care in inpatient hospital settings.
D. Nonmajority groups are more likely to seek mental health care from specialty mental health sources.
E. Nonmajority groups are less likely to use traditional or spiritual healers.

1.14   Relying on knowledge without any insight into real emotional meaning is an example of extreme imbalance in which of the following?

A. Implicit mentalizing.
B. Affective mentalizing.
C. External mentalizing.
D. Cognitive mentalizing.
E. Internal mentalizing.

CHAPTER 2

Anxiety Disorders

Select the single best response for each question.

2.1 What is the minimum duration of symptom persistence required for a diagnosis of generalized anxiety disorder (GAD)?

A. 1 week.
B. 2 weeks.
C. 1 month.
D. 2 months.
E. 6 months.

2.2 According to twin studies, what is the estimated heritability of panic disorder?

A. 5%.
B. 10%.
C. 15%.
D. 20%.
E. 40%.

2.3 Which of the following anxiety disorders has the youngest median age at onset?

A. Separation anxiety disorder.
B. Panic disorder.
C. Agoraphobia.
D. Social anxiety disorder.
E. Generalized anxiety disorder.

2.4 Which of the following anxiety disorders has the oldest median age at onset?

A. Specific phobia.
B. Panic disorder.
C. Agoraphobia.
D. Social anxiety disorder.
E. Generalized anxiety disorder.

2.5   Which of the following disorders is included among the anxiety disorders in DSM-5?

    A. Obsessive-compulsive disorder.
    B. Posttraumatic stress disorder.
    C. Acute stress disorder.
    D. Panic disorder with agoraphobia.
    E. Separation anxiety disorder.

2.6   A 50-year-old man reports episodes in which he will suddenly and unexpectedly wake from his sleep feeling a surge of intense fear that peaks within minutes. During this time he experiences shortness of breath, heart palpitations, sweating, and nausea. His medical history is significant only for hypertension, which is well controlled with hydrochlorothiazide. As a result of these symptoms, he has begun to have anticipatory anxiety associated with going to sleep. Which of the following disorders is the most likely cause for the man's symptoms?

    A. Anxiety disorder due to a general medical condition (hypertension).
    B. Substance-induced anxiety disorder.
    C. Panic disorder.
    D. Sleep terrors.
    E. Panic attacks.

2.7   A 35-year-old man is in danger of losing his job; the job requires frequent long-range traveling, and for the past year he has avoided flying. Two years prior, he traveled on a particularly turbulent flight, and although he was not in any real danger, he was convinced that the pilot minimized the risk and that the plane almost crashed. He flew again a month later; although he experienced a smooth flight, the anticipation of turbulence was so distressing that he experienced a panic attack during the flight. He has not flown since. Which of the following disorders is the most likely cause of his anxiety?

    A. Agoraphobia.
    B. Acute stress disorder.
    C. Specific phobia—situational type.
    D. Social anxiety disorder.
    E. Panic disorder.

2.8   A 26-year-old man is brought to the emergency department complaining of the sudden onset of panic. He has no psychiatric history but reports that he took several doses of an over-the-counter cold medication for which he had to show his driver's license. Which of the following would be most suggestive that the man is suffering from a substance-induced anxiety disorder?

    A. The presence of mild symptoms that do not impair functioning.
    B. Symptoms that persist for a long time after the medication is stopped.

C. Somewhat similar symptoms that occurred once prior to taking the medication.
D. Presence of a delirium or gross confusion.
E. Lack of any history of an anxiety disorder or panic symptoms.

CHAPTER 3

Bipolar Disorders

Select the single best response for each question.

3.1 To receive a diagnosis of bipolar I disorder, a patient must have experienced which of the following?

    A. At least one manic episode and one major depressive episode (MDE).
    B. More than one manic episode.
    C. At least two manic episodes and one MDE.
    D. At least one manic episode.
    E. At least one manic or hypomanic episode.

3.2 To receive a diagnosis of bipolar II disorder, a patient must have experienced which of the following?

    A. At least one hypomanic episode and one MDE.
    B. At least one hypomanic episode.
    C. At least two hypomanic episodes and one MDE.
    D. More than one hypomanic episode.
    E. At least one manic or hypomanic episode.

3.3 A mood episode that meets full criteria for both mania and depression would be diagnosed as which of the following in DSM-5?

    A. A depressive episode, yielding a diagnosis of major depressive disorder.
    B. A manic episode, yielding a diagnosis of bipolar I disorder.
    C. A hypomanic episode, yielding a diagnosis of bipolar II disorder.
    D. A mixed episode, yielding a diagnosis of bipolar II disorder.
    E. A mixed episode, yielding a diagnosis of major depressive disorder with mixed features.

3.4 To receive a DSM-5 diagnosis of cyclothymic disorder, an adult patient must have experienced which of the following?

    A. Chronic subsyndromal symptoms of mood elevation and depression for at least 1 year.

B. Chronic subsyndromal symptoms of mood elevation and depression for at least 6 months.

C. Chronic subsyndromal symptoms of mood elevation and depression for at least 2 years.

D. At least one manic episode interposed with subsyndromal symptoms of mood elevation and depression.

E. At least one depressive episode and at least one manic episode interposed with subsyndromal symptoms of mood elevation and depression.

3.5   A patient with a history of bipolar disorder reports experiencing 1 week of elevated and expansive mood. Evidence of which of the following would suggest that the patient is experiencing a hypomanic, rather than manic, episode?

A. Irritability.

B. Decreased need for sleep.

C. Increased productivity at work.

D. Psychotic symptoms.

E. Good insight into the illness.

3.6   How do the depressive episodes associated with bipolar II disorder differ from those associated with bipolar I disorder?

A. They are less frequent than those associated with bipolar I disorder.

B. They are lengthier than those associated with bipolar I disorder.

C. They are less disabling than those associated with bipolar I disorder.

D. They are less severe than those associated with bipolar I disorder.

E. They are rarely a reason for the patient to seek treatment.

3.7   A 29-year-old woman with no prior psychiatric history is placed on prednisone for a flare of systemic lupus erythematosus. Several days later she develops pressured speech, sleeplessness, irritability, and paranoid ideation. Prednisone is stopped, and the patient's symptoms persist for 2 weeks before resolving. Neurological evaluation and imaging do not demonstrate any evidence of central nervous system lupus. Which of the following is the most likely DSM-5 diagnosis?

A. Substance-induced bipolar disorder.

B. Bipolar disorder due to another medical condition.

C. Other specified bipolar and related disorder.

D. Bipolar II disorder.

E. Cyclothymic disorder.

CHAPTER 4

Dangerousness

Select the single best response for each question.

4.1 How should a psychiatrist assess for homicidality during the psychiatric interview?

  A. By asking the patient about ideation, intent, and plan, as well as access to any weapons.
  B. Cautiously so as not to agitate the patient and cause him or her to act on these impulses.
  C. By threatening the patient with involuntary hospitalization.
  D. By relying on the patient's close friends and family rather than directly asking the patient.
  E. By asking the patient about perceptual disturbances.

4.2 A 32-year-old man presents with a history of frequent angry and impulsive outbursts. Which of the following instruments would be the most appropriate choice for assessing this patient's ability to control his anger?

  A. Overt Aggression Scale—Modified.
  B. Buss-Durkee Hostility Inventory.
  C. State-Trait Anger Expression Inventory—2.
  D. Anger, Irritability, and Assault Questionnaire.
  E. Overcontrolled Hostility Scale.

4.3 The landmark *Tarasoff* case (*Tarasoff v. Regents of the University of California* 1976) defined a therapist's duty to protect third parties. Which of the following is true of this ruling or the interpretation of the ruling?

  A. It is a federal ruling that sets a universal standard applicable in all states.
  B. There must be a threat of imminent danger.
  C. The only permissible action is to immediately warn the threatened individual.
  D. It may apply to failure to warn a patient about the risks of driving while psychotic.
  E. It can only be used if the patient is not psychotic.

4.4 Which of the following factors was a predictor of violence in schizophrenic patients in the Clinical Antipsychotic Trials of Intervention Effectiveness (CATIE)?

A. Living alone.
B. History of victimization.
C. History of substance abuse absent.
D. Preponderance of negative symptoms.
E. High socioeconomic status.

4.5 Patients with a history of violent behavior are more likely to have a lesion in which area of the brain?

A. Dorsal prefrontal cortex.
B. Prefrontal cortex.
C. Cingulate gyrus.
D. Left posterior middle temporal gyrus.
E. Superior temporal gyrus.

4.6 The diagnostic criteria of recurrent suicidal or self-injurious behaviors are included in which of the following DSM-5 diagnoses?

A. Paranoid personality disorder.
B. All personality disorders.
C. Antisocial personality disorder.
D. Borderline personality disorder.
E. Narcissistic personality disorder.

CHAPTER 5

Depressive Disorders

Select the single best response for each question.

5.1   What is the most likely DSM-5 (American Psychiatric Association 2013) diagnosis for a child presenting with persistent, chronic irritability and frequent episodes of extreme behavioral dyscontrol?

    A. Pediatric bipolar disorder.
    B. Disruptive mood dysregulation disorder.
    C. Oppositional defiant disorder.
    D. Attention-deficit/hyperactivity disorder.
    E. Major depressive disorder.

5.2   Which of the following agents is most likely to cause substance-induced depressive disorder in the context of withdrawal?

    A. Interferon.
    B. Reserpine.
    C. Propranolol.
    D. Dextroamphetamine.
    E. Prednisone.

5.3   Which of the following symptoms would suggest the presence of a major depressive episode *in addition to* a normal and expected response to a significant loss (e.g., bereavement, financial ruin, natural disaster)?

    A. Intense sadness.
    B. Ruminations about the loss.
    C. Insomnia.
    D. Poor appetite.
    E. Feelings of worthlessness.

5.4   Which of the following symptoms should alert the physician to the possible presence of depression in a patient with a serious medical condition?

A. Anhedonia.
B. Weight loss.
C. Fatigue.
D. Hypersomnia.
E. Insomnia.

5.5   A 30-year-old woman reports 2 years of persistently depressed mood, accompanied by loss of pleasure in all activities, ruminations that she would be better off
dead, feelings of guilt about "bad things" she has done, and thoughts about quitting work because of her inability to make decisions. Although she has never been
treated for depression, she feels so distressed at times that she wonders if she
should be hospitalized. She experiences an increased need for sleep but still feels
fatigued during the day. Her overeating has led to a 12-kg weight gain. She denies
drug or alcohol use, and her medical workup is completely normal, including laboratory tests of vitamins. The consultation was prompted by her worsened mood
for the past several weeks. What is the most appropriate DSM-5 diagnosis?

A. Major depressive disorder.
B. Persistent depressive disorder (dysthymia), with persistent major depressive
   episode.
C. Cyclothymia.
D. Bipolar II disorder.
E. Major depressive disorder, with melancholic features.

5.6   Which of the following is one of the core symptoms required to meet DSM-5 criteria for premenstrual dysphoric disorder?

A. Marked affective lability.
B. Decreased interest in usual activities.
C. Physical symptoms such as breast tenderness.
D. Marked change in appetite.
E. A sense of feeling overwhelmed or out of control.

CHAPTER 6

Development: Adulthood

Select the single best response for each question.

6.1 Socioemotional selectivity theory explains how older adults experience life events differently than younger adults, which may explain the lower frequency of major depression in the older adult community. Which of the following is a tenet of that theory?

   A. Younger adults are motivated by the pursuit of pleasure.
   B. Younger adults have much to learn and too little time to learn.
   C. Younger adults pursue knowledge augmented with emotional well-being.
   D. Older adults ruminate on their negative life experiences.
   E. Older adults prioritize emotionally meaningful goals.

6.2 Which of the following best describes the age at which individuals become aware of their sexual or gender identity?

   A. Childhood.
   B. Adolescence.
   C. Young adults.
   D. Midlife.
   E. It varies among different patients.

6.3 What is the name of the developmental stage when people transition from home to college, reflecting a shift in relationship to family and sense of autonomy and self-determination?

   A. Adolescence proper.
   B. Early adolescence.
   C. Middle adolescence.
   D. Late adolescence.
   E. Emerging adulthood.

6.4 James Arnett coined the term *emerging adulthood*, referring to a postponement of traditional adulthood markers such as marriage, starting a family, and independent living. Which of the following items is a criterion of this stage?

A. Financial explorations.
B. Stability.
C. Outward focus.
D. Feeling in-between.
E. Narrowing of possibilities.

6.5 According to James Arnett, which risky behavior peaks in emerging adulthood?

A. Alcohol abuse.
B. Amphetamine abuse.
C. Benzodiazepine abuse.
D. Cannabis abuse.
E. Cocaine abuse.

6.6 After a therapy session during which a patient expressed frustration at his job, the therapist relates to these feelings at her own workplace. This feeling of counter-transference, or emotional reaction of the therapist to the patient, may be affected by how the therapist hears the patient. Which of the following is the most likely to exert such an influence on the therapist?

A. The patient's transference to the therapist.
B. The therapist's conscious conflicts.
C. The increased clarity of the therapist's judgment.
D. The developmental period of the therapist's life.
E. The lack of intensity of the transference.

6.7 In some Asian cultures, women who graduate from college typically move back home while working in their first job after graduation. It is a cultural expectation that they live with their parents until they get married, and while living at home, they do not pay rent and remain somewhat dependent on their parents. This situation reflects which developmental phase?

A. Adolescence proper.
B. Early adolescence.
C. Middle adolescence.
D. Late adolescence.
E. Emerging adulthood.

6.8 Which of the following is a task of emerging adulthood?

A. Disregard the accepted path toward autonomous living.
B. Move back to the family to reassess the value of career achievements.
C. Complete identity exploration in the adult world.

D. Renegotiate family relationships toward inequality.

E. Postpone the capacity to love, commit to, and depend on a significant other.

6.9 Erik Erikson's stage theory of late-life development indicates that the major developmental task of older age is to look back and seek meaning across the lifespan, rather than looking forward. The task is to maintain more integrity than despair about one's life. Each earlier life stage conflict must be reconciled and integrated with the current stage, allowing resolution of earlier conflicts. Which of the following describes what might occur for persons with personality disorders in late life?

A. Have an easier time in accomplishing this resolution compared with others.

B. Have a similar path of accomplishing this resolution compared with others.

C. Have accomplished this resolution completely or not at all.

D. Have some conflict resolution and mellowing in their personality disorder.

E. Have no change since the factors that affect healthy adjustment do not change.

6.10 Adults acquire more wisdom as they age. Baltes and Staudinger (2000) consider wisdom to be an expert knowledge system concerning the fundamental pragmatics of life. Which of the following statements is most consistent with this definition of wisdom?

A. Factual knowledge is unrelated to wisdom.

B. Procedural knowledge is the only measure of wisdom.

C. Wise people have difficulty integrating life experiences.

D. Tolerance for differences in society is relatively unimportant.

E. Wise individuals can recognize and manage uncertainty.

C H A P T E R 7

Development: Infancy Through Adolescence

Select the single best response for each question.

7.1 Mary Ainsworth's "Strange Situation" research on patterns of attachment examined the quality of the mother-child relationship in children of what age?

   A. Age 2 months.
   B. Age 6 months.
   C. Age 12 months.
   D. Age 2 years.
   E. Age 3 years.

7.2 At what age do most children begin to develop a gendered sense of self?

   A. Age 14 months.
   B. Age 2 years.
   C. Age 3 years.
   D. Age 4 years.
   E. Age 5 years.

7.3 Using puppets, the following scenario is presented to a normally developing 5-year-old child: "Jane is playing with a doll in the bedroom she shares with her sister, Eliza. She places the doll on her bed, then leaves to go into the kitchen. While she is gone, her sister Eliza enters, plays with the doll, places it in the toy chest, and leaves the room. When Jane returns to the bedroom, where will she look first for the doll—on the bed or in the toy chest?" How would one expect this child to answer?

   A. "On the bed."
   B. "In the toy chest."
   C. "In the kitchen."
   D. A child would be unable to comprehend this question at 5 years of age.
   E. "Sister Eliza has the toy."

7.4 Which of the following is an innate behavior exhibited by newborns that elicits caregiver responsiveness and engagement?

A. Social referencing.
B. Separation anxiety.
C. Joint attention.
D. Stranger anxiety.
E. Sucking.

7.5 In the "still-face" experiment, the sudden loss of an affectively reciprocal interaction with the parent would likely cause a healthily attached infant to exhibit which of the following?

A. Acute distress, crying, and averting the gaze.
B. A mirrored impassive, unresponsive expression.
C. Social smiling with playful affect.
D. No change in affect or behavior.
E. Cooing and babbling.

7.6 At around what age do children begin to look at and attempt to "read" the facial expressions of others to obtain emotional clues to guide their own behavior?

A. Between 0 and 2 months.
B. Between 4 and 6 months.
C. Between 8 and 10 months.
D. Between 12 and 14 months.
E. Between 16 and 18 months.

7.7 In Mary Ainsworth's "Strange Situation," a child with secure attachment would be expected to behave in which of the following ways?

A. Exhibit minimal observable distress when the parent departs.
B. Show difficulty reuniting with the parent after the brief separation.
C. Display no distress when alone with the stranger.
D. Display difficult-to-control anger even before the mother has left the room.
E. Explore the environment comfortably while the mother is near.

7.8 At around what age do children become able to recognize themselves in a mirror?

A. Age 6 months.
B. Age 12 months.
C. Age 18 months.
D. Age 24 months.
E. Age 36 months.

7.9   Which of the following is a major developmental goal of late adolescence?

A. Exclusion of sexuality from the self-representation.
B. Dependence on parental values and morals.
C. Establishment of peer relationships and group activities.
D. Revision/reworking of the superego.
E. Use of sublimation to deal with feelings and impulses.

7.10   A 2-year-old mimics his mother vacuuming around the house. Which of the following describes this behavior?

A. Social fantasy play.
B. Basic early pretend play.
C. Parallel play.
D. Social referencing.
E. Joint attention.

7.11   What does the play of a 5-year-old boy with an imaginary companion suggest?

A. He is among a significant minority of children 5–12 years of age who report sharing such experiences.
B. He is likely psychotic and responding to hallucinations.
C. He may have exemplary communication skills.
D. He has never experienced any unwanted psychodynamic urges or impulses.
E. He inevitably will experience conflict with his parents regarding this companion.

7.12   As part of a school project, a 12-year-old girl designs a science experiment, beginning with the formulation of an initial hypothesis that she plans to test. This cognitive ability marks a transition to which of Piaget's stages?

A. Concrete operational stage.
B. Formal operational stage.
C. Preoperational stage.
D. Sensorimotor stage.
E. Presensorimotor stage.

7.13   What does a teenage girl's expression of disgust for her mother's professional career while idolizing a notorious drug abusing and sexually audacious celebrity suggest?

A. Second individuation.
B. Contingent response.
C. Decentering.
D. Sublimation.
E. Rapprochement crisis.

7.14 A child is first asked to make sure that the amounts of water in two identical beakers are the same. The water from one of the beakers is then transferred into a tall, narrow cylinder. The child is asked whether the remaining beaker contains the same amount of water as the tall, narrow cylinder. In which one of Piaget's stages of cognitive maturation would the child insist that because the tall, narrow cylinder is "higher," it must contain more liquid?

A. Preoperational stage.
B. Formal operational stage.
C. Concrete operational stage.
D. Sensorimotor stage.
E. Presensorimotor stage.

CHAPTER 8

Developmental Issues in Older Adults

Select the single best response for each question.

8.1 Which of the following is a characteristic sleep change occurring in later life?

A. Increased total sleep time.
B. Fewer nighttime arousals.
C. Increased Stage 1 and Stage 2 sleep.
D. Increased Stage 3 and Stage 4 sleep.
E. Increased rapid eye movement (REM) sleep latency.

8.2 When prescribing benzodiazepines for anxiety in geriatric patients, which of the following is an important consideration?

A. Benzodiazepine half-life is often decreased in older individuals; therefore, longer-acting agents are preferred.
B. Withdrawal symptoms are usually not a problem when older individuals are prescribed short-acting benzodiazepines.
C. Older individuals are more susceptible than younger adults to the side effects of fatigue, motor dysfunction, and memory impairment.
D. In some older patients, long-acting benzodiazepines may lead to withdrawal episodes and a rebound of anxiety.
E. Side-effect profiles of benzodiazepines tend to be relatively consistent across age groups.

8.3 Older adults have elevated levels of which of the following hormones?

A. Thyroid-stimulating hormone (TSH).
B. Corticotropin.
C. Epinephrine.
D. Dehydroepiandrosterone (DHEA).
E. Growth hormone.

8.4   Which of the following changes is seen in the elderly that could affect drug pharmacokinetics?

    A. Decreased hepatic conjugation.
    B. Increased protein binding.
    C. Decreased hepatic blood flow.
    D. Increased body water.
    E. Decreased gastric acid transit time.

8.5   Personality in older adults is characterized by higher levels of which of the following?

    A. Depression.
    B. Vulnerability to stress.
    C. Openness.
    D. Agreeableness.
    E. Sociability.

8.6   Personality development in healthy elderly is characterized by which of the following?

    A. Increase in neurotic defenses.
    B. Looking forward to meaning in life ahead.
    C. Denial of one's mortality.
    D. Tendency to remember more negative events.
    E. Expectation of death of loved ones.

8.7   Which of the following cognitive functions is the most likely to remain intact in
healthy older adults?

    A. Divergent thinking.
    B. Attentional capacity.
    C. Executive skills.
    D. Visual integration.
    E. Verbal abilities.

8.8   Which of the following memory abilities most likely remains intact in healthy older
adults?

    A. Working memory.
    B. Cued recall.
    C. Delayed free recall.
    D. Memory retrieval.

8.9   Which of the following best characterizes sexual activity in old age?

A. The frequency of sex decreases with age equally in both men and women.
B. Only a minority of women without partners masturbate.
C. Physical health is the most important factor in determining levels of sexual activity in women.
D. Past levels of sexual activity do not affect later levels of activity.
E. Single individuals are more sexually active than those with steady partners.

8.10   Normal age-related change in sexual functioning of women includes which of the following?

A. Libido may decrease due to decreased testosterone levels.
B. Vaginal size increases.
C. Blood supply to the pelvic region is increased.
D. Orgasm remains as intense.
E. Sexual arousal may occur faster due to increased vaginal congestion.

8.11   Which of the following differentiates bereavement in women compared with men after the death of their spouse?

A. Greater death rate in the next few years.
B. Greater risk of depression.
C. Greater life satisfaction.
D. Experience more personal growth.
E. Focus on restoration of their life pattern.

8.12   A recently retired 63-year-old woman with a history of depression, currently in remission, says that now that she has retired she is interested in an exercise routine. She has not exercised much before and is moderately overweight. She stresses that her primary motivation is preventing cognitive loss, which she greatly fears. She asks the psychiatrist's opinion regarding popular news items regarding preventing cognitive loss with exercise. Which of the following statements by the psychiatrist would be the most accurate reply?

A. Although unlikely to be helpful for preventing cognitive loss, exercise confers many other benefits, including preventing depression.
B. Positive studies show that only those who have been exercising for many years have benefited from exercise, and there is no evidence supporting later-life adoption.
C. Exercise has been shown to be primarily effective in men only, and studies in women have been more equivocal.
D. Evidence suggests that physical activity is associated with lower risk of cognitive decline compared with a sedentary lifestyle.
E. Early open trials showed positive effect of exercise on cognitive loss; however, more rigorous studies do not support any effect of exercise on any prevention of cognitive loss.

CHAPTER 9

Diagnostic Procedures

Select the single best response for each question.

Diagnostic Assessment and Rating Scales

9.1 Which of the following self-report assessment tools takes the least amount of time to administer?

   A. Symptom Checklist-90—Revised.
   B. Brief Symptom Inventory.
   C. Minnesota Multiphasic Personality Inventory—2.
   D. Personality Assessment Inventory.
   E. Positive and Negative Syndrome Scale.

9.2 Which of the following descriptions correctly matches the assessment tool with its targeted area of symptomatology?

   A. Alcohol Use Disorders and Associated Disabilities Interview Schedule, DSM-IV Version, assesses a patient's readiness to change in relation to the use of alcohol.
   B. Thematic Apperception Test assesses personality disorders.
   C. Reasons for Living Inventory assesses suicidal behavior.
   D. Eating Disorder Examination diagnoses binge-eating disorder.
   E. University of Rhode Island Change Assessment measures dependence-related symptoms.

9.3 Which of the following is the most widely used self-report inventory of depression?

   A. Positive and Negative Syndrome Scale.
   B. Schedule for Affective Disorders and Schizophrenia.
   C. Beck Depression Inventory—II.
   D. Beck Hopelessness Scale.
   E. Reasons for Living Inventory.

9.4   Which of the following instruments can be used to assess psychodynamic factors such as drives, unconscious wishes, conflicts, and defenses?

    A. Anger, Irritability, and Assault Questionnaire.
    B. Thematic Apperception Test.
    C. Wisconsin Card Sorting Test.
    D. Brief Psychiatric Rating Scale.
    E. Beck Depression Inventory—II.

9.5   The Global Assessment of Functioning Scale is useful for which of the following purposes?

    A. Rating patients on a hypothetical continuum from psychological sickness to mental health.
    B. Measuring the construct of quality of life.
    C. Assessing the patient's degree of social adjustment.
    D. Tracking the progress and impact of treatment.
    E. Assessing activity limitations and participation restrictions.

9.6   Which of the following instruments could provide information about the adequacy of the support system available to a 34-year-old schizophrenic man who lives alone?

    A. World Health Organization Disability Assessment Schedule 2.0.
    B. Independent Living Scale.
    C. Brief Psychiatric Rating Scale.
    D. Social Support Questionnaire.
    E. Positive and Negative Syndrome Scale.

Laboratory Monitoring

9.7   Which of the following screening tests is correctly matched to the clinical picture for recommended screening prior to initiating pharmacotherapy and at regular intervals during maintenance treatment?

    A. Potassium level in a 25-year-old man being started on carbamazepine.
    B. Complete blood count (CBC) for a 48-year-old woman being treated with fluoxetine.
    C. Electrocardiogram (ECG) for a 30-year-old man without any medical history being started on nortriptyline.
    D. Blood urea nitrogen (BUN) and creatinine for a 68-year-old man being treated with valproate.
    E. Follow-up CBC for a 13-year-old girl with bipolar disorder being treated with carbamazepine.

9.8 In which of the following options is the recommended laboratory test correctly matched to the medication scenario?

A. LFT for monitoring lithium therapy.
B. Renal function panel for monitoring valproate therapy.
C. Serum level for assessing clinical response to nortriptyline therapy.
D. Serum level for assessing clinical response to risperidone therapy.
E. ECG for monitoring carbamazepine therapy.

9.9 In which of the following options is the appropriate laboratory test matched to the medication scenario?

A. CBC monitoring during carbamazepine treatment.
B. Fasting serum glucose before initiating a tricyclic antidepressant.
C. Echocardiogram before initiating a tricyclic antidepressant.
D. LFT monitoring during lithium treatment.
E. Electroencephalogram before starting valproate.

9.10 Which of the following tests is routinely recommended as part of the initial diagnostic workup of a patient presenting with an altered mental status?

A. Ceruloplasmin.
B. Lead level.
C. Electromyogram.
D. Positron emission tomography scan.
E. HIV test.

9.11 A 48-year-old British man is admitted to the inpatient unit for progressive cognitive decline and abnormal jerky movements in his left leg over the last 2 months. The clinician suspects Creutzfeldt-Jakob disease. Which of the following laboratory studies could be helpful in confirming the diagnosis?

A. Lumbar puncture and cerebrospinal fluid biomarkers.
B. Serum iron level.
C. Liver function tests.
D. Lumbar puncture and culture.
E. Urinalysis.

Other Tests

9.12 Which of the following is a true statement about use of electroencephalography (EEG) in psychiatric diagnosis?

A. EEG is essential in evaluating a first episode of depression.
B. EEG is useful in the diagnosis of bipolar disorder.
C. EEG can always diagnose epilepsy.

D. EEG can be helpful in diagnosing sleep disorders.

E. EEG can help in differentiating types of dementias.

9.13 Which of the following statements correctly describes an advantage of computed tomography (CT) over magnetic resonance imaging (MRI)?

A. CT can acquire images in the axial, coronal, and sagittal planes, whereas MRI can acquire them only in the coronal and axial planes.

B. CT has superior visualization of brain tissue compared to MRI.

C. CT can be used in patients with pacemakers, whereas MRI is contraindicated in such patients.

D. There is less radiation exposure with CT than with MRI.

E. CT provides better visualization of the posterior fossa than does MRI.

9.14 In which of the following options is the appropriate imaging study matched to the clinical presentation?

A. MRI of the brain in a 60-year-old man with new-onset dementia.

B. A head CT scan in a 25-year-old man with new-onset depression.

C. Magnetic resonance spectroscopy in a 35-year-old woman with a first psychotic episode.

D. A head CT scan with contrast in a 45-year-old woman with a suspected infarct.

E. Diffusion tensor imaging in the evaluation of depression.

9.15 In which of the following options is the appropriate neuroimaging test ordered for the clinical presentation?

A. Single positron emission computed tomography (SPECT) scan for a 55-year-old man with hypertension and signs of a stroke.

B. MRI for a 30-year-old man with mild traumatic brain injury.

C. SPECT for a 23-year-old woman with mild traumatic brain injury.

D. Head CT scan with contrast for a 46-year-old woman with a history of chronic renal failure and a suspected brain hemorrhage after a hypertensive crisis.

E. PET scan for a 60-year-old man with a history of diabetes mellitus and suspected frontotemporal dementia.

9.16 In which of the following options is the screening test correctly matched to the clinical presentation?

A. Thyroid-stimulating hormone screening for a 27-year-old man with anhedonia, suicidal ideation, and newly diagnosed major depressive disorder.

B. Chest radiograph for a 55-year-old woman with first-episode delusions of jealousy.

C. Electrocardiogram for a 39-year-old woman starting on citalopram for anxiety.

D. Electroencephalogram for a 22-year-old woman with recurrent mania.

E. Head CT scan for a 70-year-old woman with a first episode of atypical depression.

CHAPTER 10

Disruptive Behavior Disorders

Select the single best response for each question.

10.1 Which of the following disorders is most commonly comorbid with oppositional defiant disorder (ODD)?

A. Attention-deficit/hyperactivity disorder (ADHD).
B. Major depressive disorder.
C. Conduct disorder (CD).
D. Bipolar disorder.
E. Specific learning disorder.

10.2 The presence of ODD with emotional symptoms predicts the future development of which of the following?

A. Anxiety disorders.
B. Personality disorders.
C. Psychotic disorders.
D. Eating disorders.
E. Substance abuse disorders.

10.3 A 21-year-old man with a history of oppositional defiant disorder presents with frequent impulsive behavioral outbursts that are grossly out of proportion to the stressor. He reports that he is unable to control himself and is worried that he might lose his job if his behavior continues. What is the most likely diagnosis?

A. Bipolar disorder.
B. Attention-deficit/hyperactivity disorder (ADHD).
C. Intermittent explosive disorder (IED).
D. Conduct disorder (CD).
E. Adjustment disorder.

10.4   Which of the following is true regarding the incidence and course of ODD?

   A. Symptoms of oppositional defiant disorder (ODD) usually emerge first in the
      school setting.
   B. The majority of patients with ODD will not develop conduct disorder (CD).
   C. The number of ODD symptoms is not positively correlated with the develop-
      ment of CD.
   D. Typical age at onset of ODD is between 10 and 12 years of age.
   E. Boys are twice as likely as girls to meet criteria for ODD at all ages.

10.5   Which of the following has been shown to be more effective for aggression in pa-
        tients with Cluster B personality disorders than in patients with IED?

   A. Fluoxetine.
   B. Divalproex.
   C. Risperidone.
   D. Lithium.
   E. Propranolol.

10.6   Which of the following is characteristic of pyromania?

   A. Fire setting for monetary gain.
   B. Fire setting for revenge.
   C. Fascination with fire.
   D. Fire setting due to impaired judgment.
   E. Delusional thinking.

CHAPTER 11

Dissociative Disorders

Select the single best response for each question.

11.1   Which of the following conditions is characterized by an inability to recall important personal information (including traumatic memories) that cannot be explained by ordinary forgetfulness, overt brain pathology, or substance use?

A. Dissociative amnesia.
B. Dissociative fugue.
C. Forgetfulness.
D. Derealization.
E. Posttraumatic stress disorder.

11.2   Which of the following conditions is characterized by persistent feelings of unreality, detachment, or estrangement from oneself?

A. Dissociative amnesia.
B. Dissociative fugue.
C. Depersonalization/derealization disorder.
D. Acute stress disorder.
E. Peritraumatic dissociation.

11.3   Recall of a personal experience identified with the self, such as attending a baseball game, involves which of the following types of memory?

A. Episodic memory.
B. Implicit memory.
C. Procedural memory.
D. Semantic memory.
E. Nondeclarative memory.

11.4   Which of the following statements best characterizes the nature of memory loss in dissociative amnesia?

A. The memory loss is procedural.
B. The memory loss is permanent.

C. The memory deficit typically involves an inability to lay down new episodic memories.
D. The amnesia is typically anterograde.
E. The memory loss is generally for traumatic or stressful events.

11.5 Experiencing of others as unreal, dreamlike, or foggy is an example of which of the following?

A. Delusional disorder.
B. Depersonalization.
C. Dissociative amnesia.
D. Impaired reality testing.
E. Derealization.

11.6 Which of the following statements regarding the treatment of dissociative identity disorder (DID) is most correct?

A. Hypnosis is the gold standard for diagnosis and treatment.
B. In psychotherapy, alters should be addressed by name rather than as identity states.
C. The goal of psychotherapeutic treatment is to facilitate integration of disparate elements.
D. It is unusual for a negative transference to develop between patients with DID and their therapists.
E. Short-acting barbiturates (e.g., sodium amobarbital) remain the pharmacological treatment of choice in treating DID.

CHAPTER 12

Elimination Disorders

Select the single best response for each question.

12.1 What is the earliest age at which a child can be diagnosed with enuresis according to DSM-5 criteria?

A. 3 years.
B. 4 years.
C. 5 years.
D. 6 years.
E. 7 years.

12.2 What is the most common cause of encopresis?

A. Intellectual disability.
B. Obsessive-compulsive disorder.
C. Sexual abuse.
D. Attention-deficit/hyperactivity disorder (ADHD).
E. Constipation.

12.3 What factors do enuresis and encopresis have in common?

A. Both enuresis and encopresis will not remit without treatment in most children.
B. Both enuresis and encopresis have a similar longitudinal trajectory.
C. Both enuresis and encopresis share the same treatment modality.
D. Both enuresis and encopresis are strongly associated with ADHD.
E. Both enuresis and encopresis have approximately the same incidence rate.

CHAPTER 13

Epidemiology and Public Policy: Health Care Economics/ Public Policy Issues

Select the single best response for each question.

13.1 The American Psychiatric Association principles of medical ethics prohibit serious boundary violations such as sexual contact with patients. Which of the following sets of physician risk factors are associated with sexual contact with patients?

A. Intense transference, isolation from colleagues, and narcissistic pathology.
B. Inadequate training, isolation from colleagues, and borderline personality.
C. Inadequate training, isolation from colleagues, and narcissistic pathology.
D. Intense transference, isolation from colleagues, and borderline personality.
E. Intense transference, inadequate training, and narcissistic pathology.

13.2 A cardiology resident is obtaining consent from a 65-year-old woman for cardiac catheterization and stent placement. The patient agrees to have the procedure because "whatever the doctor says is probably best." When asked about the procedure, the patient states, "I'm a homemaker and I can't really understand these things; it's something to do with the heart. I guess it will make me better. It'll probably be fine." Why would this patient's agreement *not* meet the standard for informed consent?

A. The patient's level of education does not provide for a thorough understanding of the procedure.
B. The important information necessary to make a decision was presented to the patient.
C. The patient cannot articulate an understanding of the procedure or of its risks, benefits, and alternatives.

D. The physician does not have an overall therapeutic relationship with the patient.

E. Informed consent is not important in this case, because the procedure is clearly in the patient's best interests.

13.3 Medical trainees often provide care beyond their current capabilities in order to learn skills that will ultimately benefit future patients. Which of the following safeguards is required to handle this ethical dilemma?

A. Safeguards to ensure that trainees practice only marginally beyond their current capabilities, with adequate supervision and informed consent of patients.

B. Safeguards to ensure that trainees practice only marginally beyond their current capabilities after a thorough orientation.

C. Safeguards to ensure that trainees practice only marginally beyond their current capabilities, with adequate supervision and thorough evaluations.

D. Safeguards to ensure that trainees practice well beyond their current capabilities, with adequate supervision and informed consent of patients.

E. Safeguards to ensure that trainees practice well beyond their current capabilities, with adequate supervision and thorough evaluations.

13.4 What is collaborative care?

A. Primary care physicians getting psychiatric consultations for depressed patients.

B. Psychiatrists getting medical consultations for patients.

C. An informal interaction between primary care physicians and psychiatrists.

D. An evidence-based, systematic approach in which primary care and behavioral health providers work closely together to deliver effective treatment.

E. Nonpsychiatrists providing mental health care to patients with serious mental illness.

13.5 Which of the following best describes the interaction between serious mental illness (SMI) and medical disorders?

A. People with SMI have lower rates of medical disorders than people in the general population.

B. Rates of disease in people with SMI are only increased for diabetes.

C. Cardiovascular disease is increased 2–3 times for people with schizophrenia.

D. Medical disorders are uncommon in adults with mental illness.

E. Cardiovascular disease occurs, but at an older age in persons with SMI.

13.6 Which of the following best describes a "health home"?

A. A living facility where persons with severe mental illness are housed.

B. A short-term service model of health care delivery.

C. Delivery of the full array of required services.

D. A cost-effective way to facilitate access to an interdisciplinary array of care.

E. Services that are only provided to adults.

13.7   What prompted Congress to enact the Nursing Home Reform Act as part of the Omnibus Budget Reconciliation Act of 1987?

A. Attempt to shift costs for patients' care to the federal government.

B. Attempt to put more elderly patients with mental health problems into nursing homes.

C. The misuse of physical and chemical restraints in nursing homes.

D. Patients with chronic psychiatric problems needing the type of care provided in nursing homes.

E. Overregulation of nursing facilities by the government.

13.8   What led Congress to the Mental Retardation Facilities and Community Mental Health Centers Construction Act in 1963?

A. Too many state-level child mental health systems.

B. The child guidance movement with a shift from a punishment model to a corrective model.

C. The underutilization of institutionalized care for children and adolescents.

D. Excessive reimbursement for school consultations.

E. Too many community mental health centers providing children's services.

13.9   Which of the following would fall into the "social" component of a biopsychosocial patient interview?

A. Asking about medications taken by the patient.

B. Asking about psychiatric symptoms.

C. Asking about family history.

D. Asking about spirituality.

E. Asking about other medical illness.

CHAPTER 14

Feeding and Eating Disorders

Select the single best response for each question.

14.1 Which of the following indicates a major change in the DSM-5 diagnostic criteria for anorexia nervosa in women compared with DSM-IV?

A. The criterion for menorrhagia has been eliminated.
B. The criterion for amenorrhea has been eliminated.
C. The criteria for both amenorrhea and menorrhagia have been eliminated.
D. Body weight is no longer a significant criterion.
E. Developmental stage is no longer a significant issue.

14.2 What is the change in the criteria for bulimia nervosa in DSM-5 compared with DSM-IV?

A. There is an increase in the required numbers of binge-eating episodes and inappropriate compensatory behaviors per week, from twice to three times weekly.
B. There is an increase in the numbers of episodes of using ipecac or vomiting per week, from three to four.
C. There is a reduction in the required minimum average frequency of binge eating and inappropriate compensatory behavior frequency, from twice to once weekly.
D. There is a requirement for an episode of pica, at least once in the last year.
E. There is a requirement for an electrolyte imbalance to be demonstrated, at least twice in the last 2 years.

14.3 The minimum average frequency of binge eating for a diagnosis of binge-eating disorder in DSM-5 requires which of the following time periods?

A. Once weekly over the last 3 months.
B. Once weekly over the last 4 months.
C. Every other week over the last 3 months.

D. Every other week over the last 4 months.

E. Once a month over the last 3 months.

14.4   What are the two subtypes of anorexia nervosa?

A. Restricting type and binge-eating/purging type.

B. Energy-sparing type and binge-eating/purging type.

C. Low-calorie/low-carb type and restricting type.

D. Low-carb/low-fat type and restricting type.

E. Restricting type and low-weight type.

14.5   Which are the three essential diagnostic features of anorexia nervosa in DSM-5?

A. Low self-confidence, low attention, and low motivation.

B. Low libido, disturbance in self-perceived weight or shape, and persistent energy restriction.

C. Low mood, low concentration, and low energy level.

D. Persistent energy restriction, behavior interfering with weight gain or fear of weight gain, and a disturbance in self-perceived weight or shape.

E. Persistent low attention, low motivation, and low mood.

14.6   What is the most effective treatment for osteopenia and osteoporosis in patients with anorexia nervosa?

A. Calcium.

B. Vitamin D.

C. Bisphosphonates.

D. Weight gain.

E. Hormone replacement therapy.

14.7   Which of the following is the most serious complication of weight restoration in patients with anorexia nervosa?

A. Refeeding syndrome.

B. High white blood cell count.

C. Hypocortisolism.

D. Hyperphosphatemia.

E. Hyperkalemia.

14.8   Which of the following medical problems is found in patients with anorexia nervosa but not in those with bulimia nervosa?

A. Enlarged parotid glands.

B. Malnutrition.

C. Dental enamel erosion.

D. Constipation.

E. Hematemesis.

14.9   Which of the following compensatory behaviors is most commonly used by patients with bulimia nervosa?

A. Self-induced vomiting.
B. Laxatives.
C. Diuretics.
D. Fasting.
E. Excessive exercise.

14.10 What is the only drug that currently has U.S. Food and Drug Administration (FDA) approval for bulimia nervosa?

A. Imipramine.
B. Sertraline.
C. Fluoxetine.
D. Citalopram.
E. Topiramate.

14.11 Which DSM-5 diagnostic criterion differentiates bulimia nervosa from binge-eating disorder?

A. Recurrent episodes of binge eating.
B. Recurrent inappropriate compensatory behavior aimed at preventing weight gain.
C. Binge-eating frequency of at least once a week for 3 months.
D. Eating, in a discrete period of time, an amount of food that is definitely larger than what most individuals would eat in a similar period of time.
E. A sense of loss of control over eating during binge episodes.

14.12 What is the most commonly abused substance among patients with binge-eating disorder?

A. Marijuana.
B. Cocaine.
C. Alcohol.
D. Tobacco.
E. Opiates.

14.13 Which of the following statements regarding pica is most accurate?

A. Ingestion of nonfood, nonnutritive substances must be sustained for at least 1 year.
B. Pica typically displays an onset in adolescence.
C. Common substances ingested include paper, soap, and soil.
D. Psychiatric comorbidities may include bipolar disorder and personality disorders.
E. Pica does not occur in adults.

14.14 Which of the following best describes the DSM-5 diagnosis of avoidant/restrictive food intake disorder (ARFID)?

A. ARFID replaces the diagnosis of feeding disorder of infancy or early childhood.
B. The main diagnostic feature of ARFID is disturbance of body image.
C. Somatic interventions are typically used to treat ARFID.
D. ARFID cannot be diagnosed in the presence of certain medical conditions.
E. ARFID tends to present similarly across different age groups.

CHAPTER 15

Law

Select the single best response for each question.

15.1 Who decides whether a patient is competent to stand trial?

    A. Any licensed physician.
    B. A jury.
    C. A psychiatrist.
    D. A judge.
    E. The patient.

15.2 In addition to communication of choice, understanding of relevant information provided, and appreciation of available options and consequences, what other standard is used to determine competency?

    A. Acting in one's own best interest.
    B. Deciding in a timely manner.
    C. Showing a stable choice over time.
    D. Rational decision making.
    E. Choosing what is medically indicated.

15.3 In the landmark case *Rennie v. Klein* (1978), the court recognized the right of psychiatric patients to refuse treatment but concluded that this right could be overridden in which of the following circumstances?

    A. The patient is psychotic.
    B. The patient denies having a mental illness.
    C. The patient is not acting in his or her best interest.
    D. The patient is charged with a crime.
    E. The patient is a danger to self or others.

15.4 What is the *most common* allegation when patients sue psychiatrists for inappropriate involuntary hospitalization?

    A. Abuse of authority.
    B. Assault and battery.

C. Malicious prosecution.
D. Intentional infliction of emotional distress.
E. Absence of "good faith" in the psychiatrists' behavior.

15.5   Which of the following is seclusion?

A. Informing the patient that he or she must remain in his or her room with the door open and a security guard sitting outside of the room.
B. Hospitalizing the patient involuntarily on a locked unit.
C. Instructing a patient, in the middle of the night, to return to his or her room.
D. Allowing a patient to remain in his or her room with the door closed.
E. Using physical force to limit freedom of movement.

15.6   According to federal law, which of the following is deemed a physical restraint?

A. Verbal commands.
B. Behavior contracts.
C. Medications.
D. Video surveillance cameras.
E. An aide assisting a patient who has difficulty walking.

CHAPTER 16

Mental Status

Select the single best response for each question.

16.1 A psychiatrist observes a sustained muscle contraction in the patient's right forearm, with a flexed wrist and extended fingers. In the write-up, this finding is documented as which of the following?

A. Dystonia.
B. Chorea.
C. Asterixis.
D. Myoclonus.
E. Akathisia.

16.2 A patient's speech is marked by lack of emotional expression. When documenting this type of speech in the mental status examination, which of the following is the correct term?

A. Stuttering.
B. Aprosodia.
C. Echolalia.
D. Palilalia.
E. Dysarthria.

16.3 "Misperceptions of actual sensory inputs" describes which of the following?

A. Hallucinations.
B. Derealization.
C. Illusions.
D. Depersonalization.
E. Delusions.

16.4 How is attention tested during the mental status examination?

A. By asking patients to name all the animals they can think of in 1 minute.
B. By asking patients where they were born.

C. By asking patients simple logic questions, such as "Does a stone float on water?"

D. By asking patients to subtract 7 from 100, and to keep subtracting 7 from the result for five responses.

E. By asking patients to state their name, the present location, and the date.

16.5   What is being measured when a clinician asks a patient to recall, after a few minutes, three unrelated objects, such as a penny, an apple, and a chair?

A. Short-term memory.
B. Orientation.
C. Long-term memory.
D. Judgment.
E. Immediate recall.

CHAPTER 17

Neurocognitive Disorders

Select the single best response for each question.

17.1   Which of the following laboratory results would be suggestive of Wilson's disease?

A. Low blood ceruloplasmin and low urinary copper.
B. Low blood ceruloplasmin and high urinary copper.
C. High blood ceruloplasmin and low urinary copper.
D. High blood ceruloplasmin and high urinary copper.
E. High blood ceruloplasmin and normal urinary copper.

17.2   Which of the following is a true statement about delirium?

A. Disorientation to person, place, or time must be present to meet DSM-5 criteria for delirium.
B. The hallmark of delirium is impaired attention.
C. Change in psychomotor activity is an uncommon clinical manifestation of delirium.
D. Delirium has a lower degree of personality disorganization and clouding of consciousness compared with mild or major neurocognitive disorder.
E. Delirium generally takes weeks to months to resolve.

17.3   What cerebrospinal fluid (CSF) findings would you expect in Alzheimer's disease?

A. Normal.
B. High β-amyloid 42 and low tau and phosphorylated tau.
C. Low β-amyloid 42 and high tau and phosphorylated tau.
D. High β-amyloid 42 and high tau and phosphorylated tau.
E. Low β-amyloid 42 and low tau and phosphorylated tau.

17.4 Which of the following neurocognitive disorders is associated with rapid eye movement (REM) sleep behavior disorder?

A. Alzheimer's disease.
B. Frontotemporal lobar degeneration.
C. Lewy body disease.
D. Cerebrovascular disease.
E. Neurocognitive disorder associated with traumatic brain injury.

17.5 Which of the following is a true statement about the diagnosis of language-variant frontotemporal lobar degeneration (FTLD)?

A. Language impairment is the principal cause of the impaired daily functioning.
B. Most often behavioral symptoms, such as disinhibition and hyperorality, are the most prominent clinical manifestations at symptom onset.
C. Language symptoms are directly related to the frequency of word use.
D. The prototypical language variant of FTLD is caused by Pick's disease.
E. FTLD has sudden onset and rapid progression.

17.6 Which of the following is a true statement about the categorization of aphasias in neurocognitive disorders?

A. In global aphasia, verbal fluency is impaired but repetition and naming are generally intact.
B. Anomic aphasia is uncommon in Alzheimer's disease.
C. Patients with Broca's aphasia can generally obey commands but have difficulty with repetition.
D. Unlike patients with Broca's aphasia, patients with Wernicke's aphasia have good comprehension.
E. In contrast to the naming difficulty in Wernicke's aphasia, the naming difficulty in Broca's aphasia is usually not helped by prompts.

17.7 What normal, age-related change in neurotransmitter input to the forebrain increases the likelihood of delirium from anticholinergic drugs?

A. Loss of pigmented cells in the substantia nigra, increasing the sensitivity of dopamine D_2 receptors.
B. Loss of neurons in the nucleus basalis of Meynert and septal nuclei, increasing the cholinergic input to the forebrain.
C. Loss of pigmented cells in the substantia nigra, reducing the sensitivity of D_2 receptors.
D. Loss of neurons in the nucleus basalis of Meynert and septal nuclei, reducing the cholinergic input to the forebrain.
E. Increase in pigmented cells in the substantia nigra, increasing the sensitivity of D_2 receptors.

17.8 Which of the following clinical features would support a diagnosis of neurocognitive disorder over a diagnosis of depression?

    A. Increased psychomotor activity.
    B. Mood-congruent auditory hallucinations.
    C. Frequent suicidal ideation.
    D. Marked change in appetite.
    E. Day/night confusion.

17.9 Which of the following is a true statement about management of delirium in an inpatient setting?

    A. Pharmacological intervention is indicated even in mild delirium that does not cause sleep disturbance or interfere with medical treatment.
    B. For delirium lasting longer than 7 days, providers should consider substance withdrawal as the likely cause.
    C. Rooms should be kept dimly lit to avoid overstimulating the patient.
    D. Mechanical restraints should be used in preference to sitters, because bedside companions often exacerbate confusion.
    E. Patients should be frequently reoriented to time, place, and staff members.

17.10 Which of the following cognitive abnormalities, if elicited on mental status examination of a patient with depression, would be most suggestive of an underlying comorbid neurocognitive disorder?

    A. Impaired episodic memory.
    B. Impaired attention.
    C. Impaired orientation.
    D. Reduced information-processing speed.
    E. Impaired working memory.

17.11 Which of the following statements correctly describes an advantage of the Montreal Cognitive Assessment (MoCA) over the Folstein Mini-Mental State Examination (MMSE)?

    A. The MoCA takes less time to administer than the MMSE.
    B. The MoCA has a larger scoring range than the MMSE.
    C. The MoCA takes into account differences in education level.
    D. The MoCA has greater sensitivity for detection of mild cognitive impairment.
    E. The MoCA is more widely used and therefore more acceptable to the public.

17.12 Which of the following is a true statement about cholinesterase inhibitors?

    A. They may improve cognitive performance in individuals with neurocognitive disorders, but they do not slow the rate of cognitive decline.
    B. Their use is absolutely contraindicated in individuals with bradycardia or bronchopulmonary disease.

C. They are effective only in major neurocognitive disorder due to probable Alzheimer's disease.

D. They are available only in oral formulations.

E. They are used as first-line monotherapy for patients with advanced major neurocognitive disorder.

17.13 An 88-year-old man with major neurocognitive disorder secondary to probable Parkinson's disease begins to develop paranoia and agitation over the course of several months. Behavioral interventions are ineffective, and there is concern about caregiver burnout. Which of the following is a true statement about pharmacological treatment of agitation with psychotic features during the course of a neurocognitive disorder?

A. Numerous antipsychotics have received U.S. Food and Drug Administration (FDA) approval for treatment of behavioral disturbances in persons with neurocognitive disorders.

B. High doses of antipsychotics should be employed initially in order to control the behavior, and then tapered as tolerated with close monitoring for symptom recurrence.

C. Psychotropic medications that are helpful should be continued indefinitely.

D. An antipsychotic would be the first choice for treatment of agitation with psychotic features.

E. FDA warnings have been issued about increased cerebrovascular adverse events and increased mortality with use of typical antipsychotics but not with atypical antipsychotics in older dementia patients.

17.14 Which of the following is a true statement about the treatment of depression in individuals with neurocognitive disorders?

A. Depression cannot be diagnosed in persons with a neurocognitive disorder, and therefore treatment is not indicated.

B. Serotonin reuptake agents have not been shown to have any benefit in persons with neurocognitive disorders.

C. Methylphenidate may be useful for reducing apathy and depression in Alzheimer's disease.

D. Stimulants are relatively safe agents with few side effects in persons with neurocognitive disorders.

E. Electroconvulsive therapy is the first-line treatment for depression in persons with neurocognitive disorders.

17.15 Which of the following is the most problematic limitation of high-dose vitamin E in the treatment of patients with neurocognitive disorders?

A. Association with increased cardiovascular adverse events.

B. Failure to significantly slow functional progression of the disease.

C. Potential to increase irritability, agitation, and psychosis in individuals with neurocognitive disorders.

D. Association with extrapyramidal side effects.

E. Association with postural hypotension and increased falls.

17.16 Which of the following is a true statement about the drug memantine?

A. Memantine is a reversible inhibitor of the enzyme acetylcholinesterase.

B. Memantine is typically dosed once daily.

C. Memantine is poorly absorbed and has a short half-life of 2.5 hours.

D. Memantine received FDA approval for early Alzheimer's disease.

E. Memantine may cause transient confusion or sedation during the titration phase but generally has few adverse effects.

17.17 Which of the following is a true statement about the use of antiandrogens in controlling inappropriate sexual behavior?

A. There is no report of successful pharmacotherapy for inappropriate sexual behavior in individuals with cognitive impairment.

B. The antiandrogen medroxyprogesterone is effective in reducing sexual drive and sexually aggressive acts both in men who are cognitively intact and in men with brain injury.

C. The drug medroxyprogesterone is available only in an oral formulation.

D. Women with brain injury who are hypersexual are effectively treated with estrogen patches.

E. Medroxyprogesterone carries the risk of deep vein thrombosis.

17.18 What is the most preventable cause of neurocognitive disorders in young adults?

A. Substance abuse.

B. Traumatic brain injury due to accidents.

C. HIV infection.

D. Depression.

E. Nutritional deficiency.

17.19 Which of the following is a true statement about the psychopharmacological treatment of insomnia or disturbed sleep in individuals with neurocognitive disorder?

A. Conventional hypnotics are not associated with ataxia.

B. Conventional hypnotics do not cause oversedation.

C. Mood stabilizers should be first-line treatment for insomnia in persons with neurocognitive disorder.

D. The most commonly employed hypnotics for these individuals are diazepam and chlordiazepoxide.

E. The REM sleep behavior disorder that is a frequent concomitant to Lewy body disease often responds to anticholinesterase treatment.

CHAPTER 18

Neurodevelopmental Disorders

Select the single best response for each question.

18.1 A 7-year-old boy in second grade displays significant delays in his ability to reason, problem solve, and learn from his experiences. He has been slow to develop reading, writing, and mathematics skills in school. Throughout his development, these skills have lagged behind those of his peers, although he is making slow progress. These deficits significantly impair his ability to play in an age-appropriate manner with peers and to begin to acquire independent skills at home. He requires ongoing assistance with basic skills (dressing, feeding, and bathing himself and doing any type of schoolwork) on a daily basis. Which DSM-5 diagnosis is most appropriate?

  A. Global developmental delay.
  B. Specific learning disorder.
  C. Intellectual disability (intellectual developmental disorder), moderate.
  D. Communication disorder.
  E. Autism spectrum disorder (ASD).

18.2 Which of the following is a characteristic feature of intellectual disability?

  A. Full-scale IQ less than 70.
  B. Inability to use money.
  C. Inability to make medical decisions.
  D. Inability to meet community standards of personal independence.
  E. In spite of other deficits, there are adequate communication skills for self-expression.

18.3 A 3½-year-old girl with a history of lead exposure and a seizure disorder demonstrates substantial delays across multiple domains of functioning, including communication, learning, attention, and motor development, which limit her ability to interact with same-age peers, and requires substantial support in all activities of daily living at home that are not typical for a child her age. Unfortunately, her mother is an extremely poor historian, and the child has received no formal psychological or learning evaluation to date. She is about to be evaluated by the Committee on Preschool Education. What is her most likely DSM-5 diagnosis?

A. Major neurocognitive disorder.
B. Developmental coordination disorder.
C. Autism spectrum disorder.
D. Global developmental delay.
E. Specific learning disorder.

18.4   A 7-year-old boy demonstrates deficits in social-emotional reciprocity, in nonverbal communication, and in developing and maintaining relationships. Symptoms were present in early childhood and caused significant impairment across domains. How many restricted, repetitive patterns of behavior, interests, or activities must he have from Criterion B of the new classification of ASD in DSM-5 to meet criteria for the diagnosis?

A. One symptom.
B. Two symptoms.
C. Three symptoms.
D. Four symptoms.
E. Five symptoms.

18.5   A 5-year-old boy has problems with initiating, sustaining, and having back-and-forth conversation; reading social cues; and sharing his feelings with others. He demonstrates a restricted interest in trains that seems abnormal in intensity and focus, has difficulty making friends, and demonstrates little imaginative or symbolic play. There are no clear deficits in his nonverbal communication; he makes good eye contact, has normal speech intonation, displays facial gestures, and has a range of affect that generally seems appropriate to the situation. His mother attends an autism conference and learns about the new diagnostic criteria for ASD in DSM-5. Which of these DSM-5 criteria does the boy seem to lack?

A. Deficits in social-emotional reciprocity.
B. Deficits in nonverbal communication behaviors used for social interaction.
C. Deficits in developing and maintaining friendships.
D. Two of the specified four categories of restricted, repetitive patterns of behavior, interests, or activities.
E. Symptoms dating to early childhood that cause clinically significant impairment.

18.6   A 7-year-old girl presents with a history of normal language skills (vocabulary and grammar intact) but is unable to use language in a socially pragmatic manner to share ideas and feelings. She has never made good eye contact and has difficulty reading social cues. Her difficulty making friends is, in part, due to her obsession with cartoon characters and her tendency to repetitively mimic conversations she hears in the cartoons. She tends to excessively smell objects and has difficulty getting dressed because she insists on wearing the same shirt and shorts every day, regardless of the season. These symptoms have dated from early childhood and cause significant impairment in her functioning. According to DSM-5, what diagnosis would she receive?

A. Asperger's disorder.
B. Autism spectrum disorder (ASD).
C. Pervasive developmental disorder not otherwise specified (PDD NOS).
D. Social (pragmatic) communication disorder.
E. Rett's disorder.

18.7 A 15-year-old boy has a long history of nonverbal communication deficits. As an infant he was unable to follow someone else directing his attention by pointing. As a toddler he was not interested in sharing events, feelings, or games with his parents. From school age into adolescence, his speech was odd in tonality and phrasing, and his body language was awkward. What do these behaviors represent?

A. Stereotypies.
B. Restricted range of interests.
C. Developmental regression.
D. Prodromal schizophreniform symptoms.
E. Deficits in nonverbal communication behaviors.

18.8 The parents of a 15-year-old female in tenth grade believe that she should be doing better in high school given that she seems bright and that she received mostly As through eighth grade. She hands in papers late and makes careless mistakes on examinations. Her handwriting has always been messy, and she procrastinates completing written assignments, although there has been some improvement since she started typing her responses. Neuropsychological testing is notable for verbal IQ of 125, Perceptual Reasoning Index of 122, Full Scale IQ of 123, Working Memory Index in the 55th percentile, and Processing Speed Index in the 50th percentile, as well as weaknesses in executive function. In a psychiatric evaluation, she reports a long history of failing to give close attention to details; difficulty sustaining attention while in class or doing homework; failing to finish chores and tasks; and significant difficulties with time management, planning, and organization. She says she is forgetful, often loses things, and is easily distracted. She has no history of restlessness or impulsivity and is well liked by her peers. What is her most likely DSM-5 diagnosis?

A. Adjustment disorder with anxiety.
B. Specific learning disorder.
C. Attention-deficit/hyperactivity disorder (ADHD), predominantly inattentive.
D. Developmental coordination disorder.
E. Major depressive disorder.

18.9 A 25-year-old man who was raised in the United States, but whose first language was Spanish, presents with avoidance of both leisure and work-related activities that involve reading, which is affecting his ability to function in both settings and is exacerbating feelings of inadequacy and anxiety. He was told that as a young child he was a late speaker of Spanish, and he recalls that he had difficulty learning to read in both languages. He received remediation that helped him, but in middle school he continued to have difficulties due to his slow rate of reading, which was complicated by his need to reread material to understand it. He also experienced difficulty with writing, which continued through high school and college. Currently, he is a poor speller and reads quite slowly. What likely conclusions can be drawn about the developmental course of his problems and treatment?

A. The young man has developed adult ADHD.
B. The source of the problem is that he is bilingual.
C. His anxiety symptoms and feelings of inadequacy are the primary issues.
D. This developmental course is somewhat typical for an individual with a specific learning disorder.
E. Treatment with a selective serotonin reuptake inhibitor (SSRI) will likely resolve his problems.

18.10 An 8-year-old boy comes to your office for his third office visit. He has a 6-month history of excessive eye blinking and intermittent chirping, but now the mother has noticed the development of grunting sounds since starting school this term. What is the most likely DSM-5 diagnosis?

A. Tourette's disorder.
B. Provisional tic disorder.
C. Temporary tic disorder.
D. Persistent vocal tic disorder.
E. Transient tic disorder, recurrent.

18.11 When considering the diagnosis of speech sound disorder, it is important to know that the speech of a young child should be fully intelligible by the age of ___, and full mastery of speech sounds of one's native language should occur by the age of ___.

A. 3 years; 10 years.
B. 4 years; 8 years.
C. 2 years; 6 years.
D. 2 years; 10 years.
E. 3 years; 7 years.

18.12 Which of the following dysfluencies involves changing around the order of words spoken?

A. Repetitions.
B. Dyslexia.
C. Circumlocutions.
D. Pauses.
E. Prolongations.

18.13 A 10-year-old girl with a seizure disorder has an IQ of 50, becomes agitated by bright light, and has limited interest in social interaction. What is the most likely diagnosis?

A. Intellectual disability.
B. Asperger's disorder.
C. Childhood disintegrative disorder.
D. Autism spectrum disorder.
E. Major depressive disorder.

18.14 A 6-year-old girl is noted to have poor motor coordination for her age. She often bumps into objects and is unable to catch a ball. Although her mother works with her to practice skills, the girl's play is significantly impacted. These symptoms seemed to have started before the girl was age 3 years. What is the most likely diagnosis?

A. Rett's disorder.
B. Childhood disintegrative disorder.
C. Autism spectrum disorder.
D. Developmental coordination disorder.
E. Cerebral palsy.

18.15 According to DSM-5, by what age must symptoms be present for a child to be diagnosed with ADHD?

A. 5 years.
B. 7 years.
C. 8 years.
D. 10 years.
E. 12 years.

18.16 Efficacy studies of clonidine in the treatment of pediatric ADHD have demonstrated which of the following?

A. Clonidine is more beneficial than methylphenidate for inattention symptoms.
B. Treatment with clonidine for 2–4 weeks may be necessary before its benefits can be adequately assessed.
C. Children with ADHD and comorbid tics have a more positive response to clonidine than children who have ADHD without tics.
D. Extended-release clonidine is similar to placebo in improvement of inattention and hyperactivity.
E. Clonidine and methylphenidate in combination is superior to either alone in the treatment of children with ADHD.

CHAPTER 19

Nonpharmacological Somatic Treatments

Select the single best response for each question.

19.1 How do the antidepressant effects and safety of daily left prefrontal transcranial magnetic stimulation (TMS) for 3 6 weeks compare with those of psychopharmacological treatments for depression?

A. TMS has a substantially greater risk of seizures.
B. Effect sizes are consistently smaller for TMS.
C. TMS results were not clinically meaningful.
D. TMS has been shown to be effective in "real-world" patients with treatment-resistant depression.
E. High rates of patient discontinuation of TMS limit its applicability in real-world populations.

19.2 A typical initial course of electroconvulsive therapy (ECT) involves administration ___ times per week for a total of ___ treatments?

A. Two times per week for a total of 9–12 treatments.
B. Three times per week for a total of 12–16 treatments.
C. Two to three times per week for a total of 8–12 treatments.
D. Two to three times per week for a total of 16–18 treatments.
E. Four to five times per week for a total of 16–18 treatments.

19.3 Approximately how strong a magnetic field is typically used in TMS?

A. 0.5 tesla.
B. 1.5 teslas.
C. 4 teslas.
D. 7 teslas.
E. 10 teslas.

19.4 Which of the following aspects of TMS has been useful for researchers studying the brain?

A. Repetitive TMS over a brain region can cause a temporary augmentation of a brain function controlled by that region.
B. Paired-pulse TMS can demonstrate the behavior of local interneurons in the motor cortex and indirectly measure serotonin activity.
C. Brain circuit excitation caused by TMS reverts to baseline when stimulation ends.
D. There is no evidence that TMS can induce neurogenesis, which can confound the collection of functional data.
E. TMS can be conducted in a magnetic resonance imaging (MRI) machine.

19.5 Which of the following statements best describes the relationship between TMS and seizures?

A. The site of stimulation is not significant in terms of the risk of a seizure.
B. Concurrent use of medications plays no role in seizure risk.
C. TMS intensity and frequency have no impact on the risk of a seizure.
D. The estimated risk of a seizure in ordinary clinical use is approximately 10%.
E. All TMS seizures have occurred during stimulation rather than later.

19.6 Which of the following brain stimulation treatments has been approved by the U.S. Food and Drug Administration (FDA) for the treatment of depression?

A. Focal electrically administered seizure therapy (FEAST).
B. Transcutaneous electrical nerve stimulation (TENS).
C. Magnetic seizure therapy (MST).
D. Repetitive transcranial magnetic stimulation (rTMS).
E. Deep brain stimulation (DBS).

19.7 How do functional brain changes seen in depressed patients after ECT compare with changes seen in depressed patients after TMS?

A. ECT increases global activity following the seizure.
B. TMS increases limbic activity.
C. Both TMS and ECT decrease limbic activity.
D. ECT increases prefrontal activity following the seizure.
E. No changes in brain activity are seen after TMS stimulation.

19.8 Which of the following is a true statement about transcranial direct current stimulation (tDCS)?

A. The costs and inconvenience of tDCS are major obstacles to its wider use.
B. The most promising effects of tDCS have been observed in depression studies.
C. tDCS affects neuronal excitability by causing neurons to fire at particular frequencies.

D. tDCS is a relatively safe treatment that can be administered in a patient's home.

E. tDCS dosing is based on motor threshold, similar to TMS.

19.9 How is vagus nerve stimulation (VNS) thought to impact neuropsychiatric disorders?

A. By blocking efferent motor and autonomic signals.
B. By modulating afferent fibers.
C. By directly increasing sympathetic tone.
D. By initiating seizures.
E. By modulating abdominal vagus tone.

19.10 Which of the following is a true statement about relapse after symptom remission in response to ECT?

A. Most patients who experience symptom remission in response to ECT will relapse after 6 months.
B. Remission is typically maintained for at least 12 months.
C. Medication does not affect the relapse rate after symptom remission with ECT.
D. A robust body of evidence shows that maintenance ECT prevents relapse.
E. ECT is the most effective treatment for both acute and chronic depression.

19.11 The FDA has approved VNS for treatment of which of the following conditions?

A. Treatment-resistant depression.
B. Obsessive-compulsive disorder.
C. Parkinson's disease.
D. Acute depression.
E. Chronic pain.

19.12 DBS has FDA approval for which of the following conditions?

A. Epilepsy.
B. Obsessive-compulsive disorder.
C. Parkinson's disease.
D. Depression.
E. Chronic pain.

19.13 What is the preferred electrical stimulation in current ECT treatment?

A. Long pulse widths.
B. Ultrabrief pulse widths.
C. Delivery through bilateral electrode placement.
D. Delivery through left electrode placement.
E. Application of the pulse after the neuron has depolarized.

19.14 Which of the following brain stimulation treatments targets the subcortical regions of the brain?

A. Electroconvulsive therapy (ECT).
B. Deep brain stimulation (DBS).
C. Transcranial magnetic stimulation (TMS).
D. Vagus nerve stimulation (VNS).
E. Transcutaneous electrical nerve stimulation (TENS).

19.15 Which of the following disorders has the *least* evidence supporting the use of ECT?

A. Catatonia associated with an underlying medical condition.
B. Depression in bipolar disorder.
C. Parkinson's disease.
D. Negative symptoms of schizophrenia.
E. Nonmelancholic symptoms of depression.

19.16 Which of the following is a true statement about the relationship between ECT and cognitive side effects?

A. Cumulative deterioration of cognitive functions should be expected.
B. Association between the magnitude of cognitive effects and ECT treatment parameters increases as time from ECT progresses.
C. During and shortly after a course of ECT, retrograde amnesia is greater for personal information than for impersonal or public events.
D. Cognitive side effects are the major factor limiting the use of ECT.
E. Patients' scores on intelligence tests will typically worsen shortly after ECT compared with scores obtained in the pretreatment depressed state.

19.17 Which of the following accurately describes the relationship between ECT treatment parameters and memory?

A. Unilateral placement of stimulus electrodes increases the risk of amnesia.
B. Lower stimulus intensity decreases the risk of amnesia.
C. Lower number of ECT treatments increases the risk of amnesia.
D. Higher doses of barbiturate anesthetic decrease the risk of amnesia.
E. More time between treatments increases the risk of amnesia.

19.18 What is the overall mortality rate for ECT?

A. 0.02 deaths per 100,000 treatments.
B. 0.2 deaths per 100,000 treatments.
C. 2 deaths per 100,000 treatments.
D. 20 deaths per 100,000 treatments.
E. 200 deaths per 100,000 treatments.

19.19 Which of the following is *not* considered to be a routine component of a pre-ECT evaluation?

A. Obtaining a thorough psychiatric history.
B. Obtaining a medical history and physical examination.
C. Obtaining a dental history and examination of teeth.
D. Eliciting a history of personal experiences with anesthesia.
E. Obtaining a neuropsychological assessment.

19.20 For which of the following patients would bright light therapy be a first-line treatment option?

A. Elderly moderately depressed patient.
B. Psychotically depressed patient.
C. Mildly depressed pregnant patient.
D. Bipolar I patient in a depressed phase.
E. Severely depressed pregnant patient.

19.21 A 55-year old woman with a history of major depressive disorder, gastroesophageal reflux disease (GERD), coronary artery disease, and asthma is admitted for ECT. Which of her currently prescribed medications should be discontinued prior to starting an index ECT course?

A. Metoprolol.
B. Lithium.
C. Ranitidine.
D. Albuterol.
E. Sertraline.

19.22 In a _____ patient receiving ECT, prolonged paralysis and associated apnea induced by _____ may occur.

A. Hyperkalemic; succinylcholine.
B. Hypokalemic; succinylcholine.
C. Hyperkalemic; rocuronium.
D. Hyponatremic; succinylcholine.
E. Hypercalcemic; rocuronium.

19.23 Biofeedback from electromyography (EMG) is used as a treatment for which of the following?

A. Migraine headaches.
B. Phantom limb pain.
C. Fibromyalgia.
D. Cancer pain.
E. Chronic regional pain syndrome.

19.24 Which of the following are the three key components of hypnosis?

    A. Distraction, dissociation, reattribution.
    B. Distraction, emotional processing, suggestibility.
    C. Absorption, emotional processing, reattribution.
    D. Absorption, dissociation, suggestibility.
    E. Distraction, dissociation, mentalization.

CHAPTER 20

Obsessive-Compulsive and Related Disorders

Select the single best response for each question.

20.1 Which of the following is a compulsion commonly seen in obsessive-compulsive disorder (OCD)?

A. Purging.
B. Fear of contamination.
C. Intrusive sexual thoughts.
D. Checking.
E. Skin picking.

20.2 Among individuals with OCD, what is the most common comorbid psychiatric diagnosis?

A. Obsessive-compulsive personality disorder.
B. Major depressive disorder.
C. Substance use disorder.
D. Generalized anxiety disorder.
E. Schizophrenia.

20.3 What are the concordance rates of OCD in monozygotic twins?

A. 5%–12%.
B. 10%–17%.
C. 24%–31%.
D. 80%–87%.
E. 93%–100%.

20.4 A patient presents with obsessive ruminations about a defect in the appearance of his genitalia that prevents him from sexual interaction with any partner. What is the most likely diagnosis?

A. Body dysmorphic disorder.
B. Major depressive disorder.
C. Anorexia nervosa.
D. Obsessive-compulsive disorder (OCD).
E. Schizophrenia presenting with somatic delusions.

20.5 Findings from studies examining psychiatric comorbidity in individuals with body dysmorphic disorder (BDD) show that approximately what percentage will experience OCD at some point in life?

A. 5%.
B. 10%.
C. 25%.
D. 33%.
E. 60%.

20.6 Which of the following is a true statement about treatment of hoarding disorder?

A. Patients with hoarding disorder are usually fairly agreeable to treatment.
B. Serotonin reuptake inhibitors (SRIs) are considered the first-line treatment for hoarding disorder.
C. Behavioral therapy is considered the first-line treatment for hoarding disorder.
D. Rates of response to behavioral therapy for hoarding disorder are similar to those for OCD.
E. There is no role for motivational interviewing in the treatment of hoarding disorder.

20.7 What is the DSM-5 definition of obsessions?

A. Chronic impulses that occur within a person's life but do not cause the patient internal distress.
B. Pursuits that give people pleasure, such as attending sporting events or shopping.
C. Recurrent delusions that are intrusive, causing a patient distress.
D. Behaviors meant to suppress thoughts through avoidance or suppression.
E. Recurrent thoughts that are experienced as intrusive and unwanted and that cause anxiety to the patient.

20.8   Which of the following is a true statement about hair-pulling disorder (trichotil-lomania)?

A. Trichotillomania occurs exclusively in times of elevated distress.
B. Trichotillomania is time limited in presentation and does not become chronic in the majority of patients.
C. Trichotillomania occurs more frequently in women than in men.
D. Trichotillomania does not respond to pharmacotherapy with antipsychotics.
E. Trichotillomania has a consistently high incidence of response to SRIs.

CHAPTER 21

Paraphilic Disorders

Select the single best response for each question.

21.1 Which of the following paraphilic disorders can be diagnosed only if a patient reports experiencing distress or psychosocial role impairment from the urges or behaviors?

   A. Exhibitionistic disorder.
   B. Fetishistic disorder.
   C. Frotteuristic disorder.
   D. Pedophilic disorder.
   E. Sexual sadism disorder.

21.2 To qualify for a diagnosis of pedophilia, an individual must have been at least how old at the onset of symptoms and be at least how many years older than the child?

   A. At least 16 years of age and at least 5 years older than the child.
   B. At least 16 years of age and at least 7 years older than the child.
   C. At least 18 years of age and at least 5 years older than the child.
   D. At least 18 years of age and at least 7 years older than the child.
   E. At least 18 years of age and at least 10 years older than the child.

21.3 Which of the following is a true statement about exhibitionistic disorder?

   A. It is generally thought to be a disorder of women.
   B. It is directed primarily at men.
   C. Its onset is almost invariably between ages 18 and 22 years.
   D. Seventy percent of the victims are adolescents.
   E. It is typically found in individuals who have high levels of sexual behavior in general.

21.4   What is the minimum time frame that symptoms must be present in order to meet diagnostic criteria for a paraphilic disorder?

A. 1 month.
B. 3 months.
C. 6 months.
D. 1 year.
E. 2 years.

21.5   A 25-year-old woman presents to your office and says that for the past year she has been into "rough sex," and has fantasies of being dominated or humiliated by a sexual partner. What other necessary piece of information do you need prior to diagnosing her with sexual masochism disorder?

A. Whether she has acted on these urges.
B. Whether she has these fantasies about men, women, or both.
C. What age these fantasies began.
D. Whether she is significantly distressed by these fantasies.
E. Whether she has a diagnosis of personality disorder.

CHAPTER 22

Personality Disorders

Select the single best response for each question.

22.1 What percentage of patients with borderline personality disorder (BPD) commit suicide?

A. 1%.
B. 10%.
C. 20%.
D. 30%.
E. 40%.

22.2 Which of the following personality disorders (PDs) is characterized by an excessive need to be cared for by others, leading to submissive and clinging behavior and excessive fears of separation?

A. Narcissistic PD.
B. Antisocial PD.
C. Borderline PD.
D. Dependent PD.
E. Schizotypal PD.

22.3 Which of the following is a key element in Linehan's concept of BPD?

A. In contrast to psychodynamic theories, it is silent on the importance of the development of a stable sense of self.
B. It downplays the importance of physiological responses to emotional arousal.
C. It defines a major problem in BPD as a difficulty in inhibiting inappropriate behavior related to intense affect.
D. It considers refocusing of attention as a maladaptive defense mechanism.
E. It downplays the importance of developing interpersonal strategies when setting interpersonal goals.

22.4 In a randomized controlled trial of transference-focused psychotherapy, dialectical behavior therapy, and supportive therapy, which treatment modality achieved an increased number of patients classified as secure after treatment?

A. Treatment results were inconclusive.
B. Transference-focused psychotherapy.
C. Dialectical behavior therapy.
D. Supportive therapy.
E. Treatment has no effect on attachment

22.5 Criterion A of the general criteria for the diagnosis of PD in the alternative DSM-5 model of PD requires moderate or greater impairment in which of the following personality functioning?

A. Conscientiousness.
B. Emotional stability.
C. Extraversion.
D. Lucidity.
E. Self/interpersonal relatedness.

22.6 Why were PDs initially placed on a separate axis (Axis II) of the multiaxial system in DSM-III?

A. Assessment for presence of additional disorders is often overlooked in the presence of an Axis I disorder.
B. The diagnostic construct of PD did not evolve over time.
C. To enhance recognition of the instability of both Axis I and Axis II PDs.
D. To encourage clinicians to focus on a specific disorder.
E. To enhance recognition of the pattern of instability of personality traits.

22.7 A patient describes excessive anxiety in social situations and in intimate relationships. Although she would like to have more friends, she avoids others because of fears of being ridiculed, criticized, rejected, or humiliated. What is the most likely PD diagnosis for this patient?

A. Paranoid PD.
B. Avoidant PD.
C. Schizoid PD.
D. Schizotypal PD.
E. Dependent PD.

CHAPTER 23

Principles of Psychopharmacology

Select the single best response for each question.

23.1   Which second-generation antipsychotic is most likely to cause hyperprolactinemia?

    A. Quetiapine.
    B. Ziprasidone.
    C. Risperidone.
    D. Aripiprazole.
    E. Olanzapine.

23.2   Which of the following describes a *pharmacodynamic* interaction?

    A. Two medications with similar or opposing effects are combined.
    B. One medication blocks the absorption of another medication.
    C. One medication enhances the distribution of another medication.
    D. One medication induces the metabolism of another medication.
    E. One medication inhibits the excretion of another medication.

23.3   What is the proposed mechanism for the parkinsonian side effects seen with antipsychotic medications?

    A. Nigrostriatal dopamine receptor blockade.
    B. Muscarinic cholinergic receptor blockade.
    C. Tuberoinfundibular dopamine receptor blockade.
    D. Hypothalamic histaminergic H_1 receptor blockade.
    E. α_1-Adrenergic receptor antagonism.

23.4   A 34-year-old woman with comorbid attention-deficit/hyperactivity disorder and depression is treated with selegiline 45 mg/day for 6 months. Although her depressive symptoms resolve, she continues to experience difficulty with attention. Her psychiatrist suggests treatment with dextroamphetamine. How long should the psychiatrist wait after discontinuing selegiline before starting the stimulant?

A. 0 days.
B. At least 3 days.
C. At least 7 days.
D. At least 14 days.
E. At least 28 days.

23.5 Concomitant use of which of the following medications might be responsible for an increase in plasma clozapine levels in an adherent patient?

A. Carbamazepine.
B. Clonazepam.
C. Fluvoxamine.
D. Propranolol.
E. Temazepam.

23.6 Which of the following is a common side effect of MAOIs?

A. Anxiety.
B. Leukopenia.
C. Hypertensive crisis.
D. Orthostatic hypotension.
E. Urinary retention.

23.7 Discontinuation of which of the following selective serotonin reuptake inhibitor (SSRI) medications would be most likely to result in withdrawal symptoms?

A. Citalopram.
B. Escitalopram.
C. Fluoxetine.
D. Sertraline.
E. Paroxetine.

23.8 Which of the following is *not* considered a common side effect of SSRIs?

A. Acne.
B. Dry mouth.
C. Sexual dysfunction.
D. Impaired sleep.
E. Sweating.

23.9 A 47-year-old man presents to the emergency department after being found wandering aimlessly in the street. Upon examination, he is disoriented, his skin is hot and dry, he has dilated pupils, and he has absent bowel sounds. An electrocardiogram reveals a supraventricular arrhythmia. The patient most likely overdosed on which of the following medications?

A. Amitriptyline.
B. Bupropion.
C. Fluoxetine.
D. Sertraline.
E. Venlafaxine.

23.10 What are the main mechanisms of action of mirtazapine?

A. Inhibition of serotonin and norepinephrine reuptake transporters.
B. Increases norepinephrine and serotonin via blockade of inhibitory receptors.
C. Antagonism of norepinephrine type $\alpha 1$, muscarinic, and histamine receptors.
D. Partial agonism at serotonin type 1A (5-HT_{1A}) receptors.
E. Norepinephrine and dopamine modulation.

23.11 A 30-year-old woman with no medical problems and a history of two major depressive episodes is evaluated for medication consultation. She has a history of involuntary inpatient hospitalization for suicidal ideation 1 year ago. Six months ago her maintenance dose of fluoxetine 40 mg/day was reduced to 10 mg/day under psychiatric supervision. She subsequently suffered a severe depression relapse. Fluoxetine was then increased to 40 mg/day, and the patient has been euthymic since then. She just discovered that she is pregnant. How should she be advised about the risks of fluoxetine during her pregnancy?

A. Recommend continuing fluoxetine because exposure to fluoxetine has no significant adverse fetal effects.
B. Recommend discontinuing fluoxetine because the risks of fluoxetine are greater than the risks of maternal depression.
C. Recommend continuing fluoxetine because maternal depression carries a significant risk of adverse fetal effects.
D. Recommend discontinuing fluoxetine because the risk of depression relapse is decreased during pregnancy.
E. Recommend continuing fluoxetine because fluoxetine has independently been found to improve neonatal outcomes.

23.12 What are the adverse effects frequently observed with clozapine?

A. Dry mouth and impaired thermoregulation.
B. Activation and hyperprolactinemia.
C. Akathisia and diabetic ketoacidosis.
D. Tardive dyskinesia and sedation.
E. Seizures and hypotension.

23.13 What is the initial standard of treatment for neuroleptic malignant syndrome (NMS)?

A. Dantrolene started immediately for all cases of suspected NMS.
B. Expectant management on the psychiatric unit because this is a self-limited illness.
C. Rapid cessation of antipsychotics, lithium, and antiemetics.
D. Initiation of benzodiazepines until vital signs stabilized then taper.
E. Switch to a less potent dopamine D_2 blocking agent until symptoms resolve.

23.14 Which benzodiazepine would be an appropriate choice for the inpatient treatment of mild to moderate acute alcohol withdrawal in an elderly man with known liver cirrhosis?

A. Midazolam.
B. Diazepam.
C. Triazolam.
D. Oxazepam.
E. Alprazolam.

23.15 A 37-year-old woman with schizophrenia is brought to the clinic by her mother. She has a history of five hospitalizations in the last 7 years for severe psychotic symptoms in the setting of nonadherence to oral medications. You consider using risperidone long-acting injectable (LAI) and propose a treatment plan to the team. The patient has not used risperidone in the past. What is your plan for initiation of this medication?

A. Initial injection of risperidone LAI 25 mg intramuscularly today without oral medication.
B. Initial treatment with risperidone oral for 2 weeks and then switch to LAI.
C. Initial treatment with risperidone oral until tolerability is established and continued for 3 weeks after LAI is administered.
D. Initial treatment with risperidone oral and LAI today for 2 weeks, then LAI monotherapy.
E. Initial treatment with risperidone LAI today with plan to titrate LAI dose weekly to desired efficacy.

23.16 You are evaluating a patient who has developed acute symptoms suggestive of either serotonin syndrome or NMS. The patient was recently started on fluoxetine, olanzapine, trazodone, and as-needed intramuscular haloperidol. Which of the following signs or symptoms is more indicative of serotonin syndrome than of NMS?

A. Spontaneous or inducible clonus.
B. Tachycardia.
C. Elevated body temperature.
D. Elevated creatine phosphokinase.
E. Diaphoresis.

23.17 A 46-year-old man with bipolar I disorder and a co-occurring seizure disorder is maintained on valproate extended release for mood stabilization and seizure prophylaxis. His neurologist has suggested adding lamotrigine for adjunctive seizure prophylaxis given a recent increase in number of partial seizures. What is the appropriate recommendation?

A. Decrease the maintenance dose of valproate.
B. Increase the maintenance dose of valproate.
C. Start the patient on a lower than usual dose of lamotrigine.
D. Start the patient on a higher than usual dose of lamotrigine.
E. No change in doses of either medication.

23.18 A 28-year-old man with schizophrenia with poor medication adherence presents to the emergency department with severe agitation. He receives haloperidol 20 mg and lorazepam 4 mg intramuscularly over the next 12 hours. On examination, his neck is flexed to the left and he is unable to turn it to the right. He is able to breathe, and his vital signs are normal. Which medication is first-line treatment for this patient's motor condition?

A. Amantadine.
B. Benztropine.
C. Clozapine.
D. Dantrolene.
E. Propranolol.

23.19 A 45-year-old man has a history of diabetes, hyperlipidemia, chronic low back pain, and recurrent major depressive disorder. He has a history of medication nonadherence with paroxetine and fluoxetine, due to complaints of sedation and sexual side effects. He is requesting treatment for symptoms consistent with a recurrent episode of major depression. What regimen will you recommend considering his prior medication nonadherence?

A. Restart paroxetine daily in the morning.
B. Start duloxetine in twice-daily dosing.
C. Start fluvoxamine daily.
D. Restart fluoxetine daily at night.
E. Start bupropion daily in the morning.

23.20 A 72-year-old woman living with her daughter has a history of depression. She was fully independent in activities of daily living at her last follow-up appointment 1 month ago but needed assistance with shopping and bill paying. She has been maintained on a stable dose of amitriptyline for the last 25 years without symptoms of depression. She also takes cyclobenzaprine as needed for muscle relaxation in the evening. At the evaluation today, her daughter tells you that the patient has experienced mild confusion during the day and difficulty urinating in the last 2 weeks. On examination, she is oriented to place and season only, and demonstrates mild impairment in attention and memory. On review of her medication list, you learn that her primary care physician started meclizine daily for dizziness. What is your treatment recommendation?

A. Discontinue meclizine and call the primary care physician.
B. Direct hospital admission for stroke evaluation.
C. Increase amitriptyline for depression leading to pseudodementia.
D. Initiate donepezil treatment for dementia.
E. Refer patient to memory disorders clinic for likely Alzheimer's dementia.

23.21 What is the function of the CYP450 enzymes?

A. Phase I oxidative metabolism.
B. Phase II glucuronidation.
C. P-glycoprotein efflux transportation.
D. Renal elimination.
E. Regulation of protein binding.

23.22 What is an anticipated protein-binding interaction?

A. Drugs competing to bind at a receptor, leading to an additive effect at that receptor.
B. Drugs competing to bind with a plasma protein, leading to an increase in the level of circulating free drug of the first medication.
C. Drugs competing to bind with a plasma protein, leading to a decrease in the level of circulating free drug of the first medication.
D. Drugs competing to bind with a plasma protein, leading to negligible changes in the level of circulating free drug of the first medication.
E. Drugs competing to be metabolized by a CYP450 enzyme, leading to increased enzyme inhibition.

23.23 What is a critical substrate drug?

A. A drug with a wide therapeutic window and a single CYP enzyme mediating its metabolism.
B. A drug with a wide therapeutic window and multiple CYP enzymes mediating its metabolism.
C. A drug with a narrow therapeutic window and a single CYP enzyme mediating its metabolism.
D. A drug with a narrow therapeutic window and multiple CYP enzymes mediating its metabolism.
E. A drug with a narrow therapeutic window metabolized outside the CYP450 system.

23.24 A 25-year-old woman presents to you for treatment of her first episode of moderate depression. She has never taken antidepressants. After deciding that she can be treated as an outpatient, you prescribe fluoxetine 20 mg/day. Six weeks later, she reports no side effects but still has significant symptoms of depression without notable improvement. What do you recommend next?

A. Wait an additional 4 weeks before considering a dose change.
B. Discontinue fluoxetine and initiate sertraline.
C. Augment fluoxetine by initiating bupropion.
D. Increase fluoxetine dose to 80 mg/day and reassess in 4 weeks.
E. Increase fluoxetine dose to 40 mg/day and reassess in 4 weeks.

23.25 How do generic medications compare with brand-name medications?

A. Generic and brand-name medications are equivalent biochemically and therapeutically.
B. Generic and brand-name medications are bioequivalent but may have different clinical effects.
C. Generic medications often have 20%–30% differences in potency.
D. Generic and brand-name medications have identical active ingredients, but the bioavailability can vary.
E. Generic and brand-name medications may have different chemical structure but must be similar therapeutically.

CHAPTER 24

Professionalism

Select the single best response for each question.

24.1 Intrinsic consequences of boundary violations may include which of the following?

   A. Ethics complaint to the professional society.
   B. Civil lawsuit.
   C. Board of registration complaint.
   D. Criminal lawsuit.
   E. Patient suicide.

24.2 When a boundary crossing occurs in therapy, it is essential to first do which of the following?

   A. Discuss with the patient at the next available occasion.
   B. Apologize to the patient at the next session.
   C. Only discuss it if the patient brings it up at the next session.
   D. Transfer the patient to another therapist.
   E. Emphasize to the patient that this is considered a normal part of therapy.

24.3 Which of the following is defined as the "red flag" that should alert a therapist of an impending boundary violation with a patient who has borderline personality disorder (BPD)?

   A. The therapist's realization that an exception to his or her usual practice is about to be made.
   B. The patient's sense of entitlement and of being "special."
   C. A history of early sexual trauma in the patient.
   D. The therapist's recognition of the patient's unconscious manipulation.
   E. Recognition of "borderline rage" in a patient.

24.4   Which of the following is the definition of *integrity*?

A. The virtue of truthfulness.
B. The virtue of fully regarding and according intrinsic value to someone or something.
C. The virtue of promise keeping.
D. The virtue of acting for the good of another person rather than for oneself.
E. The virtue of coherence and adherence to professionalism in intention and action.

24.5   Posting a photograph of someone identified as a patient on Facebook is acceptable under which of these circumstances?

A. If it is a former patient.
B. Under no circumstances.
C. If the patient is not identified.
D. If the patient is a Facebook "friend."
E. If appropriate privacy settings are used.

24.6   Which of the following scenarios exemplifies a "dual agency" conflict?

A. While moonlighting in an emergency room, a psychiatrist evaluates a patient she has treated in another mental health facility.
B. A military psychiatrist lives on a military base near his patients who are currently enlisted for active duty.
C. A psychiatrist works in a correctional facility treating prisoners for mental health issues.
D. A psychiatrist is asked to complete disability forms for someone who is his patient.
E. A psychiatrist is asked to evaluate a police officer's fitness for duty after the officer completed a drug rehabilitation program.

CHAPTER 25

Psychiatric Consultation

Select the single best response for each question.

25.1 A surgeon requests a capacity consultation for a patient with colon cancer. The patient is refusing surgery that has a high probability of a cure. In assessing this patient's capacity, you elect to follow the four-pronged approach developed by P. S. Appelbaum and T. Grisso. Which of the following is *not* one of the four factors requiring consideration in this model?

   A. Rational manipulation of information.
   B. Absence of a serious mental disorder.
   C. Preference.
   D. Appreciation of the facts presented.
   E. Factual understanding of the procedure.

25.2 In recent years, the clinical and ethical appropriateness of the use of physical restraints in the medical setting has come under increasing scrutiny, leading to an evolution in medical and nursing practice regarding the use of restraints. In regard to the ethics of restraint use for an acutely agitated and confused medical patient, which of the following statements is true?

   A. Agitated and confused patients should never be restrained.
   B. Agitated and confused patients may be restrained only after a formal determination of decision-making capacity.
   C. Immediate safety concerns transcend ethics discussions and allow for restraint as the unequivocal standard of care in acute agitation and confusion.
   D. Restraints may be legally permissible but are always unethical.
   E. Refusal of care by an agitated and confused patient should be treated no differently from refusal of care by a competent and informed patient.

25.3 Which of the following clinical scenarios would *not* routinely prompt early use of neuroimaging for evaluation?

   A. Acute onset of psychotic illness, without delirium, in a previously healthy patient.
   B. First presentation of apparent dementia.

C. Pretreatment workup for electroconvulsive therapy (ECT) in a patient with psychotic depression.

D. Mental status changes associated with lateralizing neurological signs.

E. Delirium following documented overdose with anticholinergic medication with normal motor examination.

25.4 Treatment of anxiety disorders in terminally ill patients may require modification of usual psychopharmacological practices. For example, many terminally ill patients can no longer reliably take oral medications. Which of the following benzodiazepines can be administered rectally?

A. Oxazepam.

B. Clonazepam.

C. Lorazepam.

D. Diazepam.

E. Temazepam.

25.5 Suicide accounts for a very low number of deaths in cancer patients. Which of the following risk factors has been reported?

A. The risk of suicide in cancer patients was five times that in the general population.

B. Female cancer patients had a higher suicide rate than male patients.

C. Caucasians had a lower rate of suicide than other racial groups.

D. Young age at cancer diagnosis predicted suicide risk.

E. Head and neck cancers were associated with a notably high suicide risk.

25.6 A patient you treat in the HIV/AIDS clinic exhibits a change in his level of alertness, confusion, headache, fever, and focal neurological signs. The brain computed tomography (CT) scan shows multiple bilateral, ring-enhancing lesions in the basal ganglia. What is the *most likely* medical diagnosis for this patient?

A. Cytomegalovirus.

B. Cryptococcal meningitis.

C. Progressive multifocal leukoencephalopathy.

D. Toxoplasmosis.

E. Central nervous system (CNS) lymphoma.

25.7 The personality type of a hospitalized patient may elicit various countertransference responses from the treating physician. A physician notices that she feels little connection with a patient and finds the patient difficult to engage. Which of the following personality types might elicit this countertransference response?

A. Masochistic.

B. Histrionic.

C. Paranoid.

D. Narcissistic.

E. Schizoid.

25.8 Which of the following statements is true about the use of electroencephalograms (EEGs) in psychiatric diagnosis?

A. There are clear guidelines for use of EEGs in routine screening of psychiatric patients.

B. An EEG is considered an invasive recording of electrical activity of the brain.

C. An EEG can always diagnose epilepsy.

D. An EEG can be helpful in diagnosing sleep disorders.

E. Patients without epilepsy have a normal EEG.

CHAPTER 26

Psychiatric Interview

Select the single best response for each question.

26.1   Which of the following is true regarding the use of outside information when gathering data on a patient?

A. It is safe to assume that medications previously taken by the patient were of therapeutic dose and duration and were prescribed for U.S. Food and Drug Administration–indicated psychiatric conditions.
B. If a patient has a diagnostic code written in his or her electronic health record, it is not necessary to verify the symptoms and chronology of that disorder before recommending treatment for it.
C. Psychiatrists may not contact a patient's relatives against his or her wishes, even in the setting of acute risk.
D. It would be rare for a patient's situation to evolve between a previous psychiatric evaluation and the current one.
E. In the event that a psychiatrist must obtain information from a patient's family member in an emergency situation, the psychiatrist must make every effort to not unnecessarily disclose confidential information.

26.2.   Which of the following describes the most appropriate approach to interviewing a patient with distinguishing sociological, religious, racial, or ethnic characteristics?

A. The examiner should draw on prior reading or experience with the subgroup of interest to appear as an expert.
B. It is best to ignore socioeconomic status, race, ethnicity, and sexual orientation, because these factors have little bearing on patients' experiences and symptoms.
C. To understand the relevance of the sociological characteristic to the patient's presenting complaint, the examiner should ask the patient for his or her perspective.
D. If the examiner shares a trait with the patient (such as race, religion, or sexual orientation), the examiner should proceed as if his or her experiences are the same as the patient's.
E. The "social" aspects of a patient's background are not clinically relevant.

26.3. A psychiatrist is interviewing a new patient in the emergency room. No previous health records are available on the patient, and no collateral informants are available. The patient exhibits psychomotor agitation, threatening behavior, and rapid/tangential speech. Which of the following would be a recommended early interview question?

A. "Have you ever used drugs or been admitted to a psychiatric unit?"
B. "You are too excited right now to be safe. Would you like to remain quietly in the room to get calm or would you prefer medication to help you?"
C. "How long have you been off your medications for bipolar disorder?"
D. "Is there a history of mental illness in your blood relatives?"
E. "Have you ever been in psychoanalytic treatment?"

26.4. Which of the following terms refers to anything that prevents a patient from talking openly to an interviewer?

A. Resistance.
B. Countertransference.
C. Catatonia.
D. Affect.
E. Mood.

26.5. A psychiatrist is interviewing a patient to determine suitability for psychotherapy in an outpatient office setting. Which of the following is consistent with usual interviewing technique?

A. The examiner starts the interview with directive questioning.
B. The examiner in this situation should avoid the interview technique of confrontation, because it is likely to be experienced as an attack by a patient.
C. The examiner may reflect content and feelings to help the patient feel heard and to encourage the patient to continue speaking.
D. It is important to offer solutions early in the interview to develop positive transference; full understanding of the situation is not necessary before offering solutions.
E. The interviewer's eye contact and tone of voice are unlikely to be important in the building of the therapeutic alliance.

CHAPTER 27

Psychoanalysis

Select the single best response for each question.

27.1 What is a concordant countertransference reaction?

A. The therapist experiences the patient's feelings or emotional position.
B. The therapist empathizes with the feelings of someone in the patient's life.
C. The therapist feels frustrated with the patient due to the therapist's own conflict.
D. The therapist enacts a similar transference reaction with his or her own therapist.
E. The therapist feels that his or her emotions about the patient obscure his or her judgment.

27.2 What defense mechanism is represented when children who have been abused become abusers themselves in adulthood?

A. Denial.
B. Displacement.
C. Reaction formation.
D. Identification with the aggressor.
E. Sublimation.

27.3 A patient receives a bill that overcharges him for the most recent month of therapy. Which essential concept in psychodynamic psychotherapy is illustrated at the next appointment when this patient worries that his therapist is angry with him?

A. Countertransference.
B. Identification with the aggressor.
C. Transference.
D. Resistance.
E. Projection.

27.4 What is the focus of the drive theory perspective of psychodynamic psycho-therapy?

A. Wishes and feelings.
B. Defense mechanisms, cognitive style.
C. Regulation of self-esteem.
D. Internalized memories of interpersonal relationships.
E. Infant-caregiver attachment.

27.5 Which of these defense mechanisms is considered to be "primitive"?

A. Repression.
B. Reaction formation.
C. Splitting.
D. Sublimation.
E. Intellectualization.

CHAPTER 28

Psychological Testing

Select the single best response for each question.

28.1 Which of the following terms refers to the ability of a test to produce stable scores when readministered at different times?

A. Content validity.
B. Criterion related validity.
C. Alternate-form reliability.
D. Split-half reliability.
E. Test-retest reliability.

28.2 In order for a test to demonstrate construct validity, which of the following conditions must apply?

A. The test score correlates with other measurements of the same area of activity.
B. The test measures a theoretical construct of interest, and scores on the test reflect this construct.
C. The test yields comparable scores at two proximate points in time.
D. Two forms of the same test yield comparable scores.
E. Subgroups of items yield scores comparable to those of other subgroups of items.

28.3 For what assessment is the Minnesota Multiphasic Personality Inventory (MMPI) most useful?

A. Assessing affective disorders and personality symptoms and disorders.
B. Assessing thought disorders and personality symptoms and disorders.
C. Assessing personality symptoms and disorders only.
D. Assessing a variety of symptom patterns, including thought disorders, affective disorders, and personality symptoms.
E. Assessing a variety of symptom patterns but not personality disorders.

28.4   The Beck Anxiety Inventory is a self-report questionnaire that is best used for which of the following?

   A. Assessing whether a patient meets criteria for any mood disorder.
   B. Assessing whether a patient meets criteria for panic disorder.
   C. Differentiating between panic disorder and generalized anxiety disorder.
   D. Distinguishing between somatic and nonsomatic symptoms of generalized anxiety disorder.
   E. Discriminating between anxiety and depression.

28.5   A 22-year-old woman comes to you for treatment and reports a history of thinking about hurting herself. Which of the following is a general psychiatric assessment tool that also includes a specific measure for suicidal ideation?

   A. Beck Hopelessness Scale.
   B. University of Rhode Island Change Assessment.
   C. Minnesota Multiphasic Personality Inventory—2.
   D. Suicide Intent Scale.
   E. Positive and Negative Syndrome Scale.

28.6   A 72-year-old man is brought in by his family for evaluation because he has been having problems functioning at work and frequently misplaces objects around the house. After the patient receives neuroimaging, you also send him for neuropsychological testing. Which of the following neuropsychological instruments would yield the most useful information about this patient's executive functioning?

   A. WAIS-IV Digit Span Test.
   B. California Learning Test II.
   C. Token Test.
   D. Wisconsin Card Sorting Test.
   E. Judgment of Line Orientation Test.

CHAPTER 29

Psychopharmacology

Select the single best response for each question.

29.1 A 65-year-old woman with diabetes mellitus type 2, neuropathic pain, and normal renal function reports depressive symptoms that adversely affect her functioning. Which of the following antidepressants would be the best choice for this patient?

A. Bupropion.
B. Citalopram.
C. Duloxetine.
D. Fluoxetine.
E. Mirtazapine.

29.2 A 42-year-old woman in good physical health with mild depressive symptoms is eager to quit smoking. Which of the following antidepressants has been demonstrated to increase rates of smoking cessation?

A. Bupropion.
B. Fluoxetine.
C. Fluvoxamine.
D. Sertraline.
E. Venlafaxine.

29.3 A 35-year-old man with generalized anxiety disorder treated with sertraline develops lethargy, confusion, restlessness, flushing, tremors, diaphoresis, and myoclonic jerks when he is started on an antibiotic. Which of the following antibiotic medications could have been responsible for these symptoms?

A. Erythromycin.
B. Ceftriaxone.
C. Ciprofloxacin.
D. Linezolid.
E. Trimethoprim/sulfamethoxazole.

29.4 Following administration of a medication to treat agitation, a patient develops confusion, autonomic instability, and rigidity. Which of the following agents is most likely to have caused the patient's symptoms?

A. Diphenhydramine.
B. Clozapine.
C. Haloperidol.
D. Lorazepam.
E. Valproate.

29.5 What is the primary mechanism of action of buspirone?

A. Direct binding to γ-aminobutyric acid (GABA) subtype A.
B. Serotonin reuptake inhibition.
C. Partial agonism of serotonin type 1A (5-HT$_{1A}$) receptor.
D. α_2 Agonism.
E. β-Blockade.

29.6 Which of the following benzodiazepines would be the best choice for treating acute anxiety in a patient with liver failure?

A. Alprazolam.
B. Lorazepam.
C. Clonazepam.
D. Diazepam.
E. Chlordiazepoxide.

29.7 An unconscious 34-year-old man with newly diagnosed schizoaffective disorder is brought to the emergency department. He is stuporous, has dysarthric speech, walks with an ataxic gait, and exhibits nystagmus and myoclonus on examination. An electrocardiogram (ECG) reveals inverted T waves, and his blood work is remarkable for preserved renal function and a lithium level of 5.2 mEq/L. Which of the following is the most appropriate treatment?

A. Dantrolene.
B. Forced diuresis.
C. Activated charcoal.
D. Potassium supplementation.
E. Hemodialysis.

29.8 Which of the following antidepressants has been associated with dose-dependent QTc interval prolongation, resulting in a U.S. Food and Drug Administration (FDA) warning about its use?

A. Bupropion.
B. Citalopram.
C. Duloxetine.

D. Fluoxetine.

E. Venlafaxine.

29.9 Which of the following antipsychotics is approved by the FDA for vocal and motor tics in children and adults with Tourette's syndrome?

A. Olanzapine.

B. Risperidone.

C. Haloperidol.

D. Ziprasidone.

E. Quetiapine.

29.10 Which of the following antipsychotic medications is *least* likely to prolong the QTc interval?

A. Haloperidol.

B. Aripiprazole.

C. Thioridazine.

D. Ziprasidone.

E. Droperidol.

29.11 Weight gain is a common and problematic side effect of mood stabilizers. Which of the following mood stabilizers is associated with the greatest degree of weight gain?

A. Gabapentin.

B. Carbamazepine.

C. Topiramate.

D. Lamotrigine.

E. Valproate.

29.12 Which of the following atypical antipsychotics is associated with the lowest risk of extrapyramidal symptoms (EPS)?

A. Ziprasidone.

B. Quetiapine.

C. Aripiprazole.

D. Risperidone.

E. Asenapine.

29.13 Which of the following nonbenzodiazepine sedatives is a melatonin agonist?

A. Eszopiclone.

B. Zopiclone.

C. Ramelteon.

D. Zolpidem.

E. Zaleplon.

29.14 A 36-year-old man with chronic schizophrenia has had minimal relief of symptoms with three antipsychotic trials. At best, he has experienced partial relief from positive symptoms of schizophrenia but no relief from negative symptoms of schizophrenia. You are considering recommending clozapine for him. What is the correct regimen of blood count monitoring for patients taking clozapine?

A. Weekly red blood cell counts during the first 3 months of treatment, followed by bimonthly counts.
B. Weekly red blood cell and white blood cell counts during the first 3 months of treatment, followed by bimonthly counts.
C. Weekly white blood cell counts during the first 6 months of treatment, followed by biweekly counts.
D. Weekly platelet counts during the first year of treatment and then monthly counts.
E. Bimonthly plasma cell counts.

29.15 A 29-year-old woman with chronic generalized anxiety disorder has achieved partial remission with fluoxetine 60 mg/day. You are reluctant to increase the dose and are considering adding another medication for adjunctive treatment of her anxiety disorder. Which of the following medications would be appropriate in this case?

A. Aripiprazole.
B. Gabapentin.
C. Quetiapine.
D. Olanzapine.
E. Risperidone.

29.16 A 56-year-old woman with chronic alcohol dependence has achieved periods of sobriety following residential treatment for up to a few months at a time. She attended 12-step groups regularly; however, these interventions have not been sufficient in keeping her from craving alcohol or from relapsing to alcohol when things get more stressful. You are considering a pharmacological option to help her manage her alcohol use disorder. With consideration for efficacy and tolerability, which of the following medications has the most evidence to support its use?

A. Acamprosate.
B. Bupropion.
C. Fluoxetine.
D. Naltrexone.
E. Oxcarbazepine.

29.17 A 73-year-old nursing home resident with moderate to severe dementia experiences intermittent episodes of agitation, most commonly at times when staff encourage and assist him with bathing and grooming. As a result of the agitation, the patient is not receiving optimal care, although the agitation is not so severe as to seriously compromise patient or staff safety. The patient is receiving sertraline

100 mg/day and donepezil 10 mg/day. You are considering prescribing risperidone 0.25 mg for use as needed to address periods of agitation. This is an off-label use of this medication. In this case, which of the following side effects is particularly important to discuss with the patient's next of kin prior to obtaining consent and prescribing the medication?

A. Constipation.
B. Death.
C. Headache.
D. Dizziness.
E. Xerostomia.

29.18 You are taking care of a 28-year-old man with schizophrenia who has had paranoid thoughts and feelings. You have been seeing him once a month for about 3 years and feel that he is starting to trust you; however, he has intermittently stopped taking the prescribed oral antipsychotic medication that you have prescribed. You have tried two different antipsychotics as well as clozapine. You have a discussion about long-acting injectable (LAI) neuroleptic medication. What is the major and significant issue to discuss with him about the LAI?

A. Whether he trusts that the LAI will be helpful.
B. Whether he wants to see another psychiatrist.
C. How his cultural background may affect his decision.
D. How his childhood might have led to the diagnosis of schizophrenia.
E. Why he could not tolerate clozapine.

29.19 An 8-year-old girl with difficulty attending at school and at home also has trouble remembering instructions. She gets into trouble for fidgeting in her seat and for talking with her peers when she is supposed to be paying attention in class. She exhibits involuntary movements of her eyebrows and hands that she is able to suppress for a short time. These movements are distressing and embarrassing for her. Which of the following treatment options for attention-deficit/hyperactivity disorder (ADHD) is most appropriate for this patient?

A. Amphetamine salts.
B. Fluoxetine.
C. Clonidine.
D. Gabapentin.
E. Methylphenidate.

29.20 A 67-year-old man with chronic paranoid schizophrenia had been stable on oral medications. He is hospitalized with an ileus and is placed on bowel rest with nothing through the mouth. The surgical team is worried that he will become psychotic when not taking medication. Which of the following medications would be appropriate in this case?

A. Olanzapine.
B. Aripiprazole.

C. Risperidone.

D. Asenapine.

E. Perphenazine.

29.21 A 46-year-old man with bipolar II disorder has chronic migraines. His neurologist recently added an antiepileptic medication to his regimen. During his most recent clinic visit, he complained of feeling that his memory was worse On examination, he seemed to be experiencing more psychomotor retardation and difficulty with sequencing. You suspect that the new antiepileptic medication is to blame for these mental status findings. Which of the following is the medication that was most likely added by the neurologist?

A. Gabapentin.

B. Lamotrigine.

C. Valproate.

D. Topiramate.

E. Pregabalin.

CHAPTER 30

Psychosocial Interventions

Select the single best response for each question.

30.1 Which of the following psychosocial interventions has been shown to reduce relapse rates in patients with schizophrenia?

    A. Personal therapy.
    B. Compliance therapy.
    C. Supported employment.
    D. Family psychoeducation.
    E. Social skills training.

30.2 Which of the following is an example of a psychosocial intervention for a patient with schizophrenia?

    A. Long-acting injectable antipsychotic.
    B. Combination of antidepressant and antipsychotic medications.
    C. Assertive community treatment.
    D. Long-term hospitalization.
    E. Psychological testing.

30.3 What is the core principle of supported employment for patients with schizophrenia?

    A. All patients should work whether they want to or not.
    B. What the person does in terms of employment does not matter.
    C. Taking a long period of time to find a job is essential.
    D. Any person who wants to work should be offered assistance.
    E. Once the person has the job, he or she no longer needs assistance.

30.4 Which of the following statements regarding 12-step mutual-help organizations (MHOs) is true?

    A. There is extensive randomized-control trial evidence to support their efficacy.
    B. They extend the benefits of professionally delivered treatment for substance use disorders (SUDs).

C. The magnitude of benefit is significantly lower than that achieved with professional intervention efforts.

D. People with dual diagnoses are unlikely to benefit from attendance.

E. They are most beneficial as a short-term adjunct to outpatient professional intervention efforts.

30.5 Twelve-step facilitation (TSF) is a professionally delivered intervention designed to support engagement with MHOs such as Alcoholics Anonymous (AA). Which of the following patient characteristics is most important to consider when deciding whether to provide a standard or intensive referral to a 12-step group?

A. Age.

B. Gender.

C. Spiritual beliefs.

D. Prior experience with 12-step programs.

E. Comorbid psychiatric diagnosis.

30.6 Which cognitive MHO mechanism of change is most strongly associated with recovery in adolescents?

A. Enhanced self-efficacy.

B. Identifying coping strategies.

C. Motivation for abstinence.

D. Increased religiosity.

E. Reduction in anger.

30.7 MHO participation has been associated with which of the following?

A. Increased health care costs.

B. Increased patient reliance on professional services.

C. Abstinence rate one-third lower than that achieved by patients treated in cognitive-behavioral therapy (CBT) programs.

D. Improved outcomes in adults but not in adolescents.

E. Helping individuals change their social networks in support of recovery.

30.8 What was the clinical significance of the CASA Substance Abuse Research Demonstration (CASASARD) study?

A. Intensive Case Management (ICM) clients were significantly more likely to have completed treatment, be abstinent from substances, and be employed than those who received the usual screening and referral to treatment.

B. Drug courts showed significant reduction in drug and alcohol use and improved family relationships.

C. Brief motivational interviewing techniques increased tobacco quit rates 2%–8% compared to brief advice.

D. In substance-abusing individuals, approaches using therapeutic communities, psychosocial rehabilitation, 12-step programs, and enhancement of supportive relationships were all successful.

E. Adding a family-based treatment component to a family treatment drug court (FTDC) program was shown to improve the chances that an at-risk child would remain in the family.

30.9 Which of the following is true about group therapy for patients with SUDs?

A. Group therapy is used primarily in inpatient and residential settings.

B. Group therapy is only indicated for patients without co-occurring psychiatric disorders.

C. Group therapy may be problematic for use in managed care settings because of cost.

D. Group therapy is not helpful for the symptoms and adverse effects that are the consequences of substance abuse.

E. Group psychotherapy is the psychosocial treatment of choice for most patients with SUDs.

30.10 A 36-year-old woman with a severe alcohol use disorder and bipolar I disorder (three past hospitalizations for mania) has started attending AA meetings. She is trying to identify a sponsor. Which of the following traits in a sponsor might be most beneficial for this patient?

A. A sponsor with a similar co-occurring psychiatric disorder.

B. A sponsor with many years of sobriety and experience in AA.

C. A sponsor willing to regularly speak with the patient's psychiatrist about the patient by phone.

D. A sponsor with similar sociodemographic characteristics to the patient.

E. A sponsor who continues to attend meetings at a high frequency.

30.11 What is an effective target of contingency management (CM) treatment for substance abuse disorders as demonstrated by research studies?

A. Doing homework assignments in CBT.

B. Looking for a job.

C. Finding a sober friend.

D. Entering treatment.

E. Going to an AA meeting.

30.12 A company decides to adopt a CM strategy to curb alcohol use among its employees. Most employees who drink alcohol also smoke cigarettes. What is the recommended action for the company to take?

A. To target only alcohol, because there is no clinically significant relationship between alcohol use and smoking cigarettes.

B. To target abstinence from all substances to avoid "substitution," namely, increased smoking to compensate for stopping drinking.
C. To target abstinence from all substances, which is the usual recommendation despite lack of clear research evidence.
D. To target only smoking, because smoking and drinking are related, smoking cessation is the easier goal to achieve, and dual-substance interventions are not supported by the evidence base.
E. To seek a non-CM intervention because CM interventions for SUDs are ineffective in company settings because of conflicting interests, including patient confidentiality and employees' fear of repercussion due to treatment failure.

CHAPTER 31

Psychotherapies

Select the single best response for each question.

31.1 In research on the treatment of personality disorders (PDs), which of the following is the most robust predictor of treatment outcome?

A. Therapeutic alliance.
B. Duration of therapy.
C. Therapeutic modality.
D. Socioeconomic factors.
E. Self-harm history.

31.2 When providing therapy to a person with borderline PD (BPD), which of the following approaches carries the greatest risk of rupturing the therapeutic alliance?

A. Supportive psychotherapy.
B. Cognitive-behavioral therapy (CBT).
C. Psychoeducation.
D. Medication management.
E. Transference interpretations.

31.3 During an inpatient hospitalization of a patient with BPD, the treatment team encounters escalating conflict with each other about the treatment. Which of the following is the recommended action?

A. Transfer the patient to a different unit.
B. Change the attending psychiatrist.
C. Have team members independently assess the patient and contribute opinions.
D. Request a second opinion to decide on treatment.
E. Hold a team meeting to communicate and have a common united approach.

31.4 What is a typical way that patients with PDs reveal their pathology that can facilitate group treatment?

A. Describing in words.
B. Demonstrating in interpersonal actions.

C. Dealing with internally.
D. Defending against subconsciously.
E. Deliberating carefully.

31.5 What is the role of the therapist when a patient is identified as a difficult group member?

A. Ask the patient to leave the group.
B. Discern whether the individual's behavior may be serving a defensive function for the group.
C. Ask the patient during the group why he or she is being difficult so that the group can contribute to the discussion.
D. Avoid bringing attention to the problem so that the patient's feelings are not hurt.
E. Invite the patient to join an alternative group to see if the problems continue.

31.6 Which of the following is a typical characteristic focus of dialectical behavior therapy (DBT)?

A. Suicidal and self-injurious behaviors.
B. Countertransference.
C. Defense mechanisms.
D. Insecure attachment.
E. Socioeconomic status.

31.7 Which core component is least consistently found in psychoeducational programs?

A. Education.
B. Problem solving.
C. Social support.
D. Skills training.
E. Bibliotherapy.

31.8 In which psychoeducation program does the patient assume the role of coteacher to inform and educate those people important to him or her?

A. Gunderson's Multifamily Groups.
B. Systems Training for Emotional Predictability and Problem Solving (STEPPS).
C. Family Connections.
D. DBT–Family Skills Training (DBT-FST).
E. Certified Peer Specialist Program.

31.9 "Attentiveness to thinking and feeling in self and others" defines which of the following terms?

A. Transference.
B. Countertransference.

C. Mentalizing.
D. Psychological mindedness.
E. Mindfulness.

31.10 The concept of therapeutic alliance is attributed to which of the following people?

A. Gerald Adler.
B. Heinz Kohut.
C. Otto Kernberg.
D. Sigmund Freud.
E. Donald Winnicott.

31.11 Which of the following psychological mechanisms is/are most central to a psychoanalytic understanding of severe PDs?

A. Repression and reaction formation.
B. Splitting and projective identification.
C. Humor and sublimation.
D. A neurotic level of personality organization.
E. A significant absence of reality testing.

31.12 Which of the following describes the current American Psychiatric Association (APA) treatment guideline for patients with BPD?

A. Pharmacotherapy only.
B. Primary treatment of pharmacotherapy with adjunctive psychotherapy.
C. Primary treatment of CBT.
D. Primary treatment of psychotherapy with adjunctive, symptom-targeted pharmacotherapy.
E. Pharmacotherapy with psychotherapy for anxiety, depressive, or substance abuse disorders as indicated.

31.13 Which of the following is a newer form of CBT that is currently being explored and adapted to treatment of PDs?

A. Dialectical behavior therapy.
B. Psychodynamic therapy.
C. Acceptance and commitment therapy.
D. Interpersonal therapy.
E. Schema-focused therapy.

31.14 Which of the following therapeutic strategies is likely to be employed during a brief psychodynamic therapy session?

A. The therapist emphasizes that change cannot occur until the patient develops full insight into his or her drives.

B. The therapist focuses on historical patterns within the therapeutic relationship.

C. The therapist takes a passive role in the therapeutic process.

D. The therapist involves himself or herself in the core conflictual relationship patterns.

E. The therapist uses interpretation as the chief therapeutic tool.

31.15 A patient in psychodynamic psychotherapy describes being angry with his boss, upon whom he is dependent for employment and financial stability. However, instead of expressing the anger to his boss, he screamed at one of his children over a minor offense later in the day. What defense mechanism is illustrated?

A. Denial.

B. Displacement.

C. Reaction formation.

D. Repression.

E. Sublimation.

31.16 What is the focus of the object relations perspective of psychodynamic psychotherapy?

A. Wishes and feelings.

B. Maladaptive cognitive defense mechanisms.

C. Regulation of self-esteem.

D. Internalized memories of interpersonal relationships.

E. Infant-caregiver attachment.

31.17 During a session in a couple's treatment, the husband voices concerns about rejection from his wife and his tendency to avoid intimate interactions with her. He reports that his overall functioning at work and with interpersonal relationships is positive. Which of the following would be a reason for the therapist to use solution-focused brief therapy?

A. The problem is clearly a result of only one party.

B. The couple is invested in exploring childhood and formative experiences.

C. The husband is interested in a formulation of his personality.

D. The husband can identify problem-free areas of his life where the symptom does not occur.

E. The couple has multiple presenting concerns.

31.18 Which of the following is a true statement about brief psychotherapies?

A. The brief therapies are similar in both duration and focus on the present.

B. All of the brief therapies stress in-session experience as central to change.

C. All of the brief therapies are manualized.

D. All of the brief therapies set limits on the number of sessions at the outset of treatment.

E. In all brief therapies, it is the therapist who maintains the treatment focus from session to session.

31.19 Which of the following terms refers to a therapist's emotional reaction to a patient that emanates from the therapist's own past?

A. Countertransference.
B. Identification with the aggressor.
C. Transference.
D. Resistance.
E. Projection.

31.20 Mentalization-based therapy (MBT) was originally developed for the treatment of which of the following conditions?

A. Borderline PD.
B. Major depressive disorder.
C. Anxiety disorders.
D. Substance use disorders.
E. Psychotic disorders.

31.21 What is the "negative cognitive triad" of depression proposed by Beck and colleagues in the cognitive model?

A. Self, world/environment, and future.
B. Stimulus, response, reward versus punishment.
C. Misperception, error in logic, misattribution.
D. Cognition distortion, depression, reinforcing behavior.
E. Dysphoric mood, maladaptive behavior, negative cognition.

31.22 Exposure and response prevention (ERP), a specialized CBT technique, has been shown to be most effective and widely used for which disorder?

A. Posttraumatic stress disorder.
B. Acute stress disorder.
C. Panic disorder.
D. Social phobia.
E. Obsessive-compulsive disorder.

31.23 Which of the following is a component of a CBT case conceptualization?

A. Selecting a manual to allow the therapist to use a standard approach to treatment.
B. Choosing CBT interventions based on a unique working hypothesis of the patient.

C. Adhering to and maintaining the same formulation throughout the duration of treatment.

D. Identifying fantasies and linking them to developmental history.

E. Describing the connections between thoughts, emotions, and early relationships.

31.24 Under which of the following circumstances might transference be discussed in supportive psychotherapy?

A. A negative transference interferes with treatment.

B. A positive transference becomes apparent.

C. The therapist experiences countertransference.

D. The patient's attitudes toward his mother are displaced onto the therapist.

E. The patient mistakes the therapeutic relationship for a real relationship.

31.25 Which of the following has been shown to predict a positive outcome in both brief supportive psychotherapy and supportive-expressive psychotherapy?

A. An absence of countertransference.

B. A positive transference.

C. Frequent discussions about the therapeutic relationship.

D. A strong therapeutic alliance.

E. A relaxed patient-therapist relationship in which both participants feel free to express negative emotions.

31.26 How might supportive psychotherapy be beneficial to patients with substance use disorders?

A. Helping patients admit to being powerless over their substance use.

B. Helping patients discover their spiritual side.

C. Helping patients make amends to those they have harmed.

D. Helping patients rediscover old hobbies.

E. Helping patients develop coping strategies to control their substance use.

31.27 Which two specific psychotherapies have been shown to be very effective in treatment of depressive disorders?

A. Dialectical behavior therapy (DBT) and cognitive-behavioral therapy (CBT).

B. Mentalization-based therapy (MBT) and interpersonal psychotherapy (IPT).

C. MBT and CBT.

D. MBT and DBT.

E. IPT and CBT.

31.28 Which treatment component is considered most effective and linked to greatest symptom reduction for patients with an anxiety disorder?

A. Transference interpretations.
B. Exposure to anxiety-provoking situations.
C. Avoidance of anxiety-provoking situations.
D. Focus on therapeutic boundaries.
E. Supportive reassurance.

CHAPTER 32

Research/Biostatistics

Select the single best response for each question.

32.1 Which of the following is a true statement regarding case-control studies?

A. Results of a case-control study are considered as definitive as those of a randomized controlled trial (RCT).
B. Control groups should include subjects with the disease of interest.
C. A comparison is made prospectively between two identical populations, one exposed to the factor of interest and the other not.
D. Case-control studies generally cost less than a prospective RCT.
E. Case-control studies are not very valuable sources of data.

32.2 Which of the following best describes Phase II of a human clinical trial?

A. Testing of multiple doses of a drug for bioavailability, pharmacokinetics, and side effects.
B. Dose-finding studies in patients with a given disorder.
C. Pivotal double-blind trials for demonstrating efficacy and safety/tolerability.
D. Trials to help clarify potential uses of a drug.
E. Assessment of drug bioavailability, metabolism, and toxicity.

32.3 Which of the following statements is true regarding use of placebo controls in pharmacology research?

A. Placebo controls are not necessary if treatment is randomized.
B. Placebo response is consistent across patient groups.
C. For most psychiatric disorders, no treatment can be considered effective without a placebo control.
D. A placebo group is not needed to accurately assess a new drug's value if it is equivalent to the standard treatment.
E. Demonstrating statistical superiority to placebo is sufficient to convey a drug's clinical relevance.

32.4 Which of the following is the mode in this list of test scores: 3, 4, 5, 5, 5, 6, 6, 7, 9, 10?

A. 2.049.
B. 6.
C. 5.
D. 5.5.
E. 7.

32.5 The investigation by which of the following individuals led to the creation of institutional review boards?

A. Walter Mondale.
B. Andrew Ivy.
C. Henry Beecher.
D. Benjamin Rush.
E. Samuel Woodward.

32.6 A psychiatrist wants to learn more about the patients treated in her practice by performing structured diagnostic interviews at intake on all patients over the course of 1 year. These data are recorded, along with results from measures of depression and anxiety, at intake and at all subsequent visits. At the end of the year, she has a database of 150 patients. In the statistical analysis, which of the following is a *descriptive* statistical analysis?

A. Testing hypotheses regarding treatment decisions.
B. Testing hypotheses regarding outcomes for patients with different diagnoses.
C. Calculating whether men have more diagnoses of schizophrenia than women.
D. Deciding whether male patients have different anxiety disorders than female patients.
E. Calculating the percentage of patients in her practice who have mood disorders.

CHAPTER 33

Schizophrenia Spectrum and Other Psychotic Disorders

Select the single best response for each question.

33.1   Which of the following symptoms is associated with a worse prognosis in schizophrenia?

    A. Hallucinations.
    B. Disorganization.
    C. Delusions.
    D. Paranoia.
    E. Mood lability.

33.2   Which of the following is a risk factor for suicide among patients with schizophrenia?

    A. Older age at symptom onset.
    B. Low premorbid functioning.
    C. Reduced awareness of symptoms.
    D. Female sex.
    E. High personal expectations.

33.3   Which of the following symptoms would be most likely to fluctuate when a patient has reached the chronic-residual stage of schizophrenia?

    A. Anhedonia.
    B. Social withdrawal.
    C. Cognitive symptoms.
    D. Stereotyped thinking.
    E. Hallucinations.

33.4 Antipsychotic medication is most likely to improve which of the following schizophrenia symptoms?

A. Social withdrawal.
B. Stereotyped thinking.
C. Muscle rigidity.
D. Disorganization.
E. Autonomic instability.

33.5 Which of the following has been found in neuroimaging studies of patients with schizophrenia?

A. Decreased size of lateral and third ventricles.
B. Increased prefrontal cortex.
C. Increased superior temporal lobe.
D. Increased thalamic volume.
E. Decreased volume in the hippocampus.

33.6 Which of the following distinguishes between brief psychotic disorder and schizophreniform disorder?

A. Delusions are present in brief psychotic disorder but not in schizophreniform disorder.
B. Duration of the disturbance is less than 1 month in brief psychotic disorder and less than 6 months in schizophreniform disorder.
C. Brief psychotic disorder cannot occur with catatonia.
D. Schizophreniform disorder symptoms last less than 1 month.
E. Presence of stressors rules out a diagnosis of brief psychotic disorder.

33.7 Which of the following is a true statement regarding delusional disorder?

A. Symptoms are present for less than 1 month.
B. Hallucinations are prominent.
C. Individuals tend to behave and appear appropriately when their delusions are not being discussed or acted upon.
D. Functioning is markedly impaired.
E. Hallucinations are not typically related to delusional content.

33.8 Which of the following is a DSM-5 diagnostic criterion for schizoaffective disorder?

A. Delusions or hallucinations must occur for 2 or more weeks in the absence of a major mood episode during the lifetime duration of the illness.
B. Delusions or other psychotic symptoms occur exclusively during manic or depressive episodes.

C. Major mood episodes must be present for one quarter of the total duration of illness.
D. Social and occupational functioning must be impaired.
E. Major mood symptoms must occur for 2 or more weeks in the absence of delusions or hallucinations.

Sexual Dysfunction/ Gender Dysphoria

Select the single best response for each question.

Sexual Dysfunction

34.1   A 22-year-old man is diagnosed with schizophrenia and treated with risperidone titrated up to 3 mg twice a day. After 2 weeks, he reports clear thinking and cessation of auditory hallucinations; however, he is bothered by the fact that his ejaculation is delayed. What is the best first course of action in this case?

A. Lower the dose of risperidone.
B. Add aripiprazole.
C. Switch to perphenazine.
D. Switch to haloperidol.
E. Add sildenafil.

34.2   In a 50-year-old obese man who smokes and presents with erectile dysfunction, which of the following clinical tests would you prioritize?

A. Nocturnal tumescence.
B. Nerve conduction studies.
C. A lipid panel.
D. Testosterone level.
E. A complete blood count.

34.3   How is the diagnosis of substance/medication-induced sexual dysfunction usually made?

A. By noting that sexual dysfunction occurs with 25%–50% of occasions of sexual activity.
B. By noting that the sexual difficulties increase when the medication is withdrawn and disappear upon reintroduction of the medication.

C. By noting that sexual dysfunction occurs with 50%–75% of occasions of sexual activity.

D. By noting a close temporal relationship between the initiation of a medication or dose increase and the occurrence of the sexual problem.

E. By noting that sexual function is unchanged from baseline prior to initiating pharmacotherapy.

34.4   A 30-year-old woman comes to your office and reports that she is there only because her mother pleaded with her to see you. She tells you that although she has a good social network with friends of both sexes, she has never had any feelings of sexual arousal in response to men or women, does not have any erotic fantasies, and has little interest in sexual activity. She has found other like-minded individuals, and she and her friends accept themselves as asexual. Which of the following best describes her diagnosis?

A. Female sexual interest/arousal disorder, early onset, mild.

B. Female sexual interest/arousal disorder, early onset, severe.

C. Sexual aversion disorder.

D. No diagnosis, because she does not have the minimum number of symptoms required (Criterion A) for female sexual interest/arousal disorder.

E. No diagnosis, because she does not have clinically significant distress or impairment.

34.5   Which of these statements is most correct about sexual dysfunctions that occur in the context of other social, medical, or psychiatric factors?

A. If the sexual symptoms are fully explainable by another psychiatric diagnosis, you should *not* give a sexual dysfunction diagnosis.

B. If the person has a concurrent medical condition that contributes to his or her sexual symptoms, you should give a psychiatric diagnosis.

C. If the sexual symptoms are fully explainable by the use of or discontinuation from a drug or other substance, you should *not* give a psychiatric diagnosis.

D. If the sexual symptoms are fully explainable by relationship distress or partner violence, you should diagnose a sexual dysfunction with a specifier for relationship factors.

E. Only the three most significant contributing factors/specifiers should be included.

34.6   Which of the following statements is most correct with regard to the diagnosis of male hypoactive sexual desire disorder?

A. The individual must have a low or absent desire for sex, as well as deficient or absent sexual thoughts and fantasies.

B. The prevalence rates of low desire across cultures are remarkably consistent.

C. A severity of "mild" is given if the presence of the symptoms is "rare to occasional."

D. The symptoms must be present for a minimum of 3 months.

E. A pattern of noninitiation of sexual activity is always a valid indicator of low or absent desire for sex.

Gender Dysphoria

34.7 Which of the following refers to the "watchful waiting" approach to gender dysphoria in children?

A. Deferring treatment until the child declares his or her sexual orientation.

B. Deferring treatment until the child undergoes puberty.

C. Treatment whose primary goal is for the child and family to function optimally while waiting to see if the child's gender dysphoria continues into adolescence.

D. Treatment whose primary goal is to contain symptoms until they make it difficult for the child to function at home or at school.

E. Deferring treatment until the child asks to be treated.

34.8 What is the beginning phase of the treatment of adult gender dysphoria?

A. Hormone therapy.

B. Bilateral orchiectomy in men and bilateral mastectomy and optional hysterectomy in women.

C. Encouraging the patient to live in the world in the cross-gender role.

D. Cognitive therapy designed to minimize the patient's dissatisfaction with his or her birth gender.

E. Referral to an endocrinologist and a surgeon.

34.9 Which of the following is a true statement about adolescents with gender dysphoria?

A. Childhood gender dysphoria usually persists into adolescence.

B. Adolescent patients generally do not require endocrinological screening unless there is suspicion of a hormonal disorder.

C. Early surgical intervention is recommended because of better outcomes in terms of healing and scarring.

D. If the behavior has persisted from childhood into adolescence, it is likely to persist into adulthood.

E. Adolescent patients do not require a psychiatric examination unless a specific psychiatric problem is suspected.

34.10 In DSM-5, which of the following statements is true about the words gender and transgender?

A. Gender refers to the biological indicators of male or female seen in an individual.

B. Gender refers to the individual's initial assignment of male or female, usually given at birth.

C. Gender refers to the individual's lived role in society or identification as male or female.

D. A transgender individual is someone who has undergone a social transition from male to female or female to male.

E. A transgender individual is someone who has sought sex reassignment treatment of some kind.

34.11 Which of the following is true for adults suffering from gender dysphoria?

A. There can be a specifier added for a posttransition phase of the disorder.

B. For this diagnosis to be made, the individual must seek some kind of sex reassignment treatment.

C. For this diagnosis to be made, the individual must have a strong desire to be the other gender or must insist that he or she is the other gender.

D. For this diagnosis to be made, there must be an associated disorder of sex development.

E. For this diagnosis to be made, the individual must engage in cross-dressing behavior.

34.12 Which of the following *must* be present to make a diagnosis of gender dysphoria in children?

A. There must be a co-occurring disorder of sex development.

B. There must be a strong desire to be the other gender or an insistence that the person is the other gender.

C. There must be a strong dislike of one's sexual anatomy.

D. The child must have stated a wish to change gender.

E. There must be a strong desire for the primary and/or secondary sex characteristics that match the experienced gender.

CHAPTER 35

Sleep-Wake Disorders

Select the single best response for each question.

35.1 Which of the following best characterizes the electroencephalogram (EEG) tracing of rapid eye movement (REM) sleep?

A. Low-voltage fast activity.
B. Delta waves.
C. Theta waves.
D. High-voltage slow activity.
E. Nonspecific changes.

35.2 Rapid eye movement (REM) sleep behavior disorder is characterized by which of the following?

A. Episode occurrence during the first part of the sleep period.
B. Muscle atonia during REM sleep.
C. Open eyes during REM sleep.
D. Shortened episodes of REM sleep.
E. Loss of muscle atonia during REM sleep.

35.3 Which of the following symptoms is characteristic of patients with NREM sleep arousal disorder?

A. Cataplexy.
B. Chronic insomnia.
C. Sleepwalking with eyes closed.
D. Total or partial amnesia for nighttime events.
E. Passive behavior.

35.4 Which of the following commonly prescribed hypnotic medications is a melatonin agonist?

A. Zaleplon.
B. Temazepam.
C. Ramelteon.

D. Eszopiclone.

E. Doxepin.

35.5 A 48-year-old woman with uterine fibroids and mild hypertension reports symptoms of waking discomfort, occasional pain, and the urge to move her legs that occur almost every night. The discomfort is somewhat relieved by leg movement. Which of the following would be an appropriate initial treatment for this patient?

A. Pramipexole.

B. Oxycodone.

C. Gabapentin.

D. Iron replacement if necessary.

E. Zolpidem.

35.6 Which of the following brain structures controls circadian rhythms?

A. Locus coeruleus.

B. Pineal gland.

C. Mesopontine junction.

D. Pedunculopontine nucleus.

E. Suprachiasmatic nucleus.

CHAPTER 36

Somatic Symptom and Related Disorders

Select the single best response for each question.

36.1   Which of the following statements about illness anxiety disorder is true?

   A. Patients with this diagnosis bear no relationship to patients diagnosed with hypochondriasis.
   B. A person with this disorder has no significant somatic symptoms.
   C. A negative medical workup usually alleviates the anxiety of patients with this disorder.
   D. A history of parental overprotection has not been associated with the development of this disorder.
   E. Given the delusional basis for the disorder, it can be expected that pharmacotherapy with antipsychotic medication may have some utility.

36.2   A patient with illness anxiety disorder would most likely benefit from which of the following?

   A. Medical hospitalization.
   B. Pharmacotherapy with antipsychotics.
   C. Pharmacotherapy with selective serotonin reuptake inhibitors (SSRIs).
   D. Additional medical tests.
   E. Psychiatric hospitalization.

36.3   After a medical illness is ruled out, how should treatment of factitious disorder be approached?

   A. The physician should aggressively confront the patient with the fact that no legitimate medical illness is present.
   B. The treatment team should confront the patient with the diagnosis of factitious disorder.
   C. The treatment team should confront the patient with his or her deception after conferring with hospital administration.

D. The physician should inform the patient of a treatment plan and attempt to enlist him or her in that plan, with minimal expectation that the patient will "confess" to the deception.

E. The physician should inform the patient of a treatment plan and attempt to enlist him or her in that plan, resorting to psychiatric admission only if the patient refuses to acknowledge the deception.

36.4 What percentage of neurology outpatients has been found to have a history of conversion symptoms?

A. 4%–15%.
B. 25%–40%.
C. 50%.
D. 1%–3%.
E. 75%–90%.

36.5 Which of the following is the most active symptomatic phase for somatization disorder?

A. Childhood.
B. Adolescence.
C. Early adulthood.
D. Middle age.
E. Old age.

36.6 Which of the following complications of somatization disorder (DSM-5 somatic symptom disorder) are likely to be preventable if the disorder is recognized and symptoms managed appropriately?

A. Surgical procedures and drug dependence.
B. Marital discord and occupational dysfunction.
C. Separations and divorces.
D. Suicide attempts and completions.
E. Drug addiction and mortality.

36.7 Which of the following is a true statement about the DSM-5 diagnostic criteria for somatic symptom disorder?

A. A minimum number of symptoms must be present to qualify for the diagnosis.
B. The requirement that the symptoms be medically unexplained has been eliminated.
C. The criteria no longer stipulate that the patient's somatic symptoms be accompanied by abnormal thoughts, feelings, or behaviors.

D. Somatic symptom disorder is no longer defined by the presence of somatic symptoms.

E. The DSM-5 diagnosis of somatic symptom disorder replaces and incorporates the previous DSM-IV/DSM-IV-TR diagnoses of hypochondriasis and pain disorder.

36.8 In patients with somatization disorder (DSM-5 somatic symptom disorder), which of the following, when combined with a psychiatric consultation, was found to be more effective in improving symptoms and functioning than a psychiatric consultation alone?

A. Cognitive-behavioral therapy (CBT).

B. Hospitalization for a more in-depth medical evaluation.

C. Supportive psychotherapy.

D. Psychoanalytic psychotherapy.

E. Dynamic psychotherapy.

36.9 Which of the following is the *least* likely condition to be included in the differential diagnosis of illness anxiety disorder?

A. Adjustment disorder.

B. Generalized anxiety disorder.

C. Obsessive-compulsive disorder.

D. Major depressive disorder.

E. Schizophrenia.

36.10 Research and clinical experience with illness anxiety disorder (DSM-IV/DSM-IV-TR hypochondriasis) suggest better outcomes for patients treated with which of the following approaches?

A. Reassurance by the treatment provider that the symptoms are not serious.

B. Medical evaluation and treatment only.

C. Psychiatric evaluation as a replacement for continued medical care.

D. Direct referral for psychiatric evaluation and treatment.

E. Early confrontation about the irrational fears of illness.

36.11 Which of the following is a recommended treatment approach for illness anxiety disorder?

A. Gradual redirection of focus from interpersonal difficulties to symptoms during office visits.

B. Regular office visits focused on evaluation of symptoms.

C. Consistent treatment by the same primary care physician, with supportive, regularly scheduled office visits.

D. Extensive medical tests to clarify the clinical picture of the patient.

E. Supportive therapy to help the patient adjust to a state of chronic illness and disability.

36.12 How does DSM-5 differ from DSM-IV/DSM-IV-TR in its conceptualization of conversion disorder?

    A. In DSM-5, a patient's symptoms must be fully explainable by culturally sanctioned behavior.
    B. In DSM-5, the requirement that symptoms be produced unintentionally has been eliminated.
    C. In DSM-5, the symptoms must be temporally associated with an identifiable stressor.
    D. In DSM-5, the requirement that symptoms be incompatible with any recognized neurological or medical condition has been removed.
    E. In DSM-5, the symptoms may involve pain or sexual dysfunction in addition to motor or sensory dysfunction.

36.13 Which of the following is a core feature of the DSM-5 diagnosis of psychological factors affecting other medical conditions?

    A. Presence of both a medical condition and a mental disorder.
    B. Preoccupation with having or acquiring a serious illness.
    C. Clinical evidence of incompatibility between patients' symptoms and recognized medical conditions.
    D. Documented falsification or self-induction of medical symptoms.
    E. Presence of a psychological or behavioral factor that adversely affects a medical condition.

36.14 Which of the following is a true statement about conversion disorder?

    A. The onset of conversion disorder is generally acute, but it may be characterized by gradually increasing symptomatology.
    B. The typical course of individual conversion symptoms is generally lengthy.
    C. Among patients whose symptoms disappear, 5%–10% will relapse within 1 year.
    D. A factor traditionally associated with good prognosis is late onset.
    E. There are no clear precipitants to an episode of conversion disorder.

CHAPTER 37

Special Topics: Seclusion/ Risk Management/ Abuse and Neglect

Select the single best response for each question.

37.1 Testimonial privilege statutes protect a patient from having his or her treating clinician testify about protected health information in court. There are several common exceptions to testimonial privilege statutes. Which of the following patient behaviors would constitute such an exception?

A. Perpetrating child abuse.
B. Engaging in an extramarital affair.
C. Driving while intoxicated.
D. Engaging in tax fraud.
E. Using illicit drugs.

37.2 If a patient commits suicide, which of the following circumstances renders the psychiatrist most vulnerable to a wrongful death claim?

A. The psychiatrist is never vulnerable to a wrongful death claim when a patient commits suicide.
B. The suicide was not foreseeable, and the psychiatrist did not implement precautions.
C. The suicide was not foreseeable, and the psychiatrist implemented reasonable precautions.
D. The suicide was foreseeable, and the psychiatrist implemented reasonable precautions.
E. A suicide contract between the clinician and patient was in place.

37.3 A managed care company refuses to authorize payment for an extended hospital stay for a patient who is deemed violent by the hospital's doctors. Which of the following entities is most likely to carry the burden of liability if this patient commits a violent act soon after discharge?

A. The managed care company.
B. The psychiatric hospital.
C. The outpatient psychiatrist.
D. The inpatient psychiatrist.
E. The patient.

37.4 A 33-year-old woman has been treated with psychodynamic psychotherapy for major depressive disorder and borderline personality disorder since age 20. She has been stable for many years. When her treating psychiatrist decides to retire from practice, he informs the patient and begins to help her prepare for his departure. As they discuss the issue in sessions over the ensuing several months, the patient becomes regressed and angry with him. He ultimately retires, transfers his patient's care to another psychiatrist (with whom she resumes treatment), and moves out of state. A month later, he learns that the patient is suing him for abandonment and receives a subpoena to appear in court. Why would this case *not* be considered patient abandonment?

A. The psychiatrist informed the patient with adequate notice that he was closing his practice.
B. The psychiatrist transferred his patient's care to another physician, and the situation was not an emergency.
C. Physicians can choose whom they serve.
D. The patient was clinically stable.
E. Retirement is a legitimate reason to stop treating patients.

37.5 Which of the following describes the importance of the psychiatrist's maintaining therapeutic boundaries?

A. Because boundaries are only important in treatment of psychiatric illness.
B. Because the psychiatrist can terminate treatment at any time.
C. Because sexual relationships with patients are acceptable in some circumstances.
D. Because of the intimacy of the psychotherapeutic relationship.
E. Because there are no time constraints or financial requirements imposed on the therapeutic encounter.

37.6 There are many strategies for helping psychiatrists to ensure that role conflicts do not distort their professional judgments. Which of the following is *not* an appropriate safeguard against role conflicts?

A. Disclosure and documentation.
B. Focused supervision.

C. Oversight committees.
D. Medical education seminars sponsored by pharmaceutical companies.
E. Retrospective review.

37.7 Which of the following is a true statement regarding the use of seclusion?

A. Seclusion is the direct application of physical force to an individual to restrict his or her freedom of movement.
B. Federal law permits the use of seclusion and restraint only as a last resort to protect the patient's safety and dignity.
C. Seclusion orders do not typically require specific time periods.
D. Once a patient has been placed in seclusion, no further review of the seclusion order is required.
E. Any mental health staff member can write orders to place a patient in seclusion if the patient is considered imminently dangerous to self or others.

37.8 There are certain instances when a nonconsenting patient may have the privilege of confidentiality suspended based on the physician's overriding duties to others. In which of the following situations would suspension of confidentiality be most appropriate?

A. A patient admits to shoplifting numerous times.
B. A patient admits to use of intravenous heroin using a dirty needle.
C. A patient admits to frequent episodes of unprotected sex.
D. A patient admits to child abuse.
E. A patient admits to suicidal thoughts.

37.9 Which of the following statements is most accurate regarding seclusion and restraint?

A. Legal regulation of seclusion and restraint has become less stringent over time.
B. Legal challenges to the use of seclusion and restraint are uncommon.
C. Most states have developed requirements designed to minimize and avoid the use of seclusion and restraint.
D. Federal requirements regarding seclusion and restraint may never be superseded.
E. Federal law does not include the use of drugs in the definition of restraint.

37.10 Under which of the following circumstances is it permissible to treat an adult patient without obtaining informed consent?

A. The patient lacks decision-making capacity and has a surrogate decision maker.
B. The patient has been legally declared incompetent and has a guardian.
C. There is a medical emergency.
D. The treatment is in the patient's best interests.
E. It is never permissible to treat without informed consent.

37.11 Under what circumstances can a physician bypass informed consent because of "therapeutic privilege"?

A. The physician has more clinical knowledge than the patient, making the informed consent process unnecessary.
B. The physician knows confidential information about the patient, making the informed consent process unnecessary.
C. Complete disclosure of risks and alternatives might harm the patient's health and welfare.
D. The physician is the surrogate decision maker.
E. There is a medical emergency.

37.12 According to the Health Insurance Portability and Accountability Act (HIPAA), under which of the following circumstances is it permissible for a provider to disclose a patient's health care information without prior patient authorization?

A. It is never permissible to disclose a patient's health care information without prior consent.
B. The patient's spouse asks for an update.
C. The patient's friend asks for an update.
D. A researcher is recruiting subjects for a clinical trial.
E. The requesting party is another clinician on the patient's treatment team.

37.13 When state law regarding patient confidentiality disagrees with federal law, which regulation should the physician follow?

A. The more protective rule.
B. The less restrictive rule.
C. The state law.
D. The federal law.
E. Whatever a "reasonable physician" would do.

37.14 A patient who is deemed not competent to enter into a marriage contract refuses to take his prescribed psychotropic medications. What would be the most appropriate course of action for the treating clinician?

A. Medicate over objection because the patient is incompetent.
B. Identify a surrogate decision maker.
C. Transfer the patient to a higher level of care.
D. Ask the court to conduct another competency assessment.
E. Wait and see if the patient's decision changes.

CHAPTER 38

Spirituality

Select the single best response for each question.

38.1 Which of the following is not true of the research regarding Alcoholics Anonymous (AA) and spirituality?

A. Outpatient clients who attend AA meetings may report having had a spiritual awakening as a result of their AA attendance.
B. Spirituality is uniformly discussed in mainstream AA meetings regardless of differences in perceived AA group social dynamics.
C. Spirituality is measured by asking only about the extent that God is discussed in meetings.
D. Exposure to AA is associated with increased spirituality.
E. Gains in spiritual practices among AA members is a significant predictor of later abstinence.

38.2 Which of the following is a true statement regarding the relationship between religion/spirituality and late-life depression?

A. Religious involvement is not a common coping behavior used by older adults.
B. Religious involvement has been shown to predict faster recovery from depression in older adults.
C. Religious coping has been found to have a positive association with depressive symptoms in older adults with or without medical illness.
D. Older men are more likely than older women to use religious involvement to cope with stress.
E. Older adults with medical illness who use religion to cope experience no improvement in depressive symptoms over time.

38.3 Which of the following statements is true regarding the relationship between religious coping and bereavement course?

A. Personal religiosity has been shown in some cultures to decrease the negative psychological effects of losing a spouse.

B. There is no association between religious coping and resilience for individuals in the postloss period.
C. Patients with chronic grief are the most likely to use religious coping.
D. Resilient patients are less likely than other groups of bereaved patients to use religious coping.
E. Patients with chronic grief, resilience, and relief, are equally likely to use religious coping.

38.4 Which of the following statements is true regarding the role of religion and spirituality in therapist selection among older adults?

A. Older adults care more about therapist gender than religion.
B. Older adults feel more comfortable receiving care from practitioners who share the same race but not necessarily the same religion.
C. Spiritual concerns and values are not important factors in therapist selection among older adults.
D. Older adults feel more comfortable receiving care from practitioners who share the same religion.

38.5 Which of the following is a true statement regarding the FICA religion/spirituality screening tool?

A. It was primarily developed for use with children and adolescents.
B. It was developed for evaluating families in the medical setting.
C. It involves assessment of ethics and value systems.
D. It is a self-assessment tool that the patient completes independently.
E. It is a tool for obtaining basic information about a patient's religious and spiritual experiences.

CHAPTER 39

Substance-Related and Addictive Disorders

Select the single best response for each question.

39.1 What is thought to be the mechanism of action of hallucinogens such as lysergic acid diethylamide (LSD)?

A. Antagonism of the adenosine A_{2A} receptor.
B. Agonism of the nicotinic acetylcholine (nAChR) receptor.
C. Agonism of the serotonin 5-HT_{2A} receptor.
D. Agonism of the μ receptor.
E. Agonism of the cannabinoid CB_1 receptor.

39.2 What percentage of individuals with alcohol use disorder undergoing severe withdrawal exhibit seizures that require emergent hospital care?

A. Less than 5%.
B. 10%.
C. 15%.
D. 25%.
E. 50%.

39.3 You admit a 40-year-old patient with alcohol use disorder to your service. To manage his withdrawal, you would like to use a symptom-triggered approach (rather than fixed multiple daily dosing). Which one of the following should you use to assess the severity of alcohol withdrawal symptoms?

A. CAGE questions.
B. Clinical Institute Withdrawal Assessment for Alcohol Scale—Revised.
C. Alcohol Use Disorders Identification Test.
D. Michigan Alcoholism Screening Test.
E. TWEAK questionnaire.

39.4 Which of the following medications has as its mechanism of action the inhibition of aldehyde dehydrogenase?

    A. Acamprosate.
    B. Diazepam.
    C. Disulfiram.
    D. Buprenorphine.
    E. Naltrexone.

39.5 Which of the following is a true statement about the epidemiology of alcohol use disorders?

    A. Females have higher rates of drinking than males.
    B. The association of heavy alcohol use with death from hepatocellular carcinoma is greater for females than for males.
    C. Individuals with preexisting schizophrenia or bipolar disorder, blunted response to alcohol, and impulsivity are at low risk for developing alcohol use disorders.
    D. Family history of alcohol use disorder poses no significant risk for development of the condition.
    E. The prevalence of binge drinking is highest in Asian populations.

39.6 Which of the following is a true statement about opioid intoxication?

    A. Respiratory depression leading to overdose is due to opiate receptors located in the locus coeruleus.
    B. The "high" from opioids occurs only when the rate of change in brain dopamine is slow.
    C. Route of administration is not associated with the clinical aspects of opioid abuse.
    D. The burst of locus coeruleus activity is associated with the "high" of all abused drugs.
    E. Large, rapidly administered doses of opiates block GABA release.

39.7 Which of the following antidepressants has approval from the U.S. Food and Drug Administration (FDA) as pharmacotherapy for smoking cessation?

    A. Fluoxetine.
    B. Venlafaxine.
    C. Nortriptyline.
    D. Bupropion.
    E. Phenelzine.

39.8   Which of the following statements about the epidemiology of cannabis use is true?

A. The number of daily users in the 12- to 17-year-old age group rose sharply from 2009 to 2011.
B. Less than half of new users of cannabis in 2010 were younger than 18 years.
C. Use of cannabis among adolescents plateaued over the decade 2001–2011.
D. In the decade prior to 2009, the number of youths who were daily users dramatically increased.
E. The numbers of treatment admissions for cannabis use disorders in the United States have stayed the same over the past decade.

39.9   Which of the following is an FDA-approved pharmacotherapy for stimulant dependence?

A. Modafinil.
B. Acamprosate.
C. Disulfiram.
D. Buprenorphine.
E. There are no FDA-approved pharmacotherapies for stimulant dependence.

39.10   Which of the following is a symptom of acute benzodiazepine toxicity?

A. Agitation.
B. Sweating.
C. Seizures.
D. Tachycardia.
E. Anterograde amnesia.

C H A P T E R   4 0

Suicidality

Select the single best response for each question.

40.1   A patient at risk for suicide signs a safety contract, promising to call for help rather than act on suicidal impulses. This contract is most likely to accomplish which of the following?

A. Reduce the need for hospitalization.
B. Reduce the patient's suicide risk.
C. Protect the psychiatrist from a malpractice lawsuit.
D. Substitute for a detailed risk assessment.
E. Help foster a therapeutic alliance.

40.2   Which of the following is true regarding passive suicidal ideation?

A. It is relatively uncommon.
B. It frequently leads to involuntary hospitalization.
C. Discussion of such thoughts often damages the therapeutic alliance.
D. It requires no further evaluation on the Beck Scale for Suicide Ideation.
E. It is integral to the evaluation of thought content.

40.3   Which of the following is the most consistently described risk factor for a completed suicide?

A. Past history of suicide attempts.
B. Female sex.
C. Increased age.
D. Living in a group home.
E. Being married.

40.4 Beck and coworkers have proposed that people with depression are prone to cognitive distortions in three major areas—self, world, and future (i.e., the "negative cognitive triad"). Which of the following dysphoric perspectives deriving from cognitive distortions about the *future* has been found to be highly associated with suicide risk?

A. Pessimism.
B. Suspiciousness.
C. Hopelessness.
D. Fear of harm.
E. Self-criticism.

40.5 What is the topic of the U.S. Food and Drug Administration (FDA) black box warning carried by all antidepressants?

A. Increased risk of suicidality in pediatric patients.
B. Increased risk of violence in pediatric patients.
C. Increased risk of cerebrovascular accidents in pediatric patients.
D. Increased risk of sudden death in pediatric patients.
E. Increased risk of hepatic disease in pediatric patients.

40.6 Therapist effects were found to be significant in the Borderline Personality Disorder Study of Cognitive Therapy, a well-designed randomized clinical trial to test efficacy of CBT (Davidson et al. 2006). With which of the following provided by the therapists did patients have two to three times greater improvement in suicide-related outcomes?

A. Emergency services and medication management.
B. Cognitive techniques to modify core beliefs and schemas.
C. Behavioral strategies to promote adaptive functioning.
D. Higher quantity and more competent delivery of CBT.
E. Exposure to situations that triggered emotional distress.

40.7 What are the findings of studies defining the structural, metabolic, and functional biology of brain circuits mediating personality traits in subjects at high risk for suicidal behavior?

A. Hippocampal volume gain in structural magnetic resonance imaging (MRI) studies of patients with BPD.
B. Increase of gray matter concentrations in insular cortex of those who attempt suicide compared with those who do not attempt it.
C. Improved executive cognitive functioning in subjects with BPD under stress leading to suicidal behavior.
D. Excessive cortical inhibition in functional MRI (fMRI) studies of subjects with BPD.
E. Hyperarousal of the amygdala and other limbic structures in fMRI studies of subjects with BPD.

40.8   In the acute-on-chronic risk model for suicidality in patients with personality disorders (PDs), which of the following is considered an acute risk?

A. Childhood sexual abuse.
B. Poor employment history.
C. Multiple prior treaters.
D. Discharge from the hospital.
E. Low socioeconomic status.

40.9   Suicide mortality is lowest for which of the following groups?

A. Women ages 15–24.
B. Men ages 15–24.
C. Women ages 65 and older.
D. Men ages 65 and older.
E. Women ages 60–64.

40.10   Research on suicidality in patients with BPD has indicated the possibility of two patient groups with distinct patterns over time: a group with repeated high-lethality attempts and a group with repeated low-lethality attempts. The group with repeated low-lethality attempts is notable for which of the following?

A. Older age.
B. More psychiatric hospitalizations.
C. Comorbid histrionic or narcissistic PDs.
D. Poor baseline psychosocial functioning.
E. Recruitment for studies from inpatient populations.

40.11   Which of the following is the best description of the stress-diathesis causal model of suicidal behavior?

A. A model suggesting an underlying neurobiological vulnerability to suicidal behavior in times of stress.
B. Another way to assess and communicate risk of suicide in clinical situations in the acute-on-chronic model.
C. A theory specifically discounting a patient's core personality traits.
D. A model for suicidal behavior developed exclusively for patients with PDs.
E. A model for suicide to be assessed only in retrospective studies.

CHAPTER 41

Trauma- and Stressor-
Related Disorders

Select the single best response for each question.

41.1 Which class of medication has been shown to be effective in reducing the full range of symptoms in adults with posttraumatic stress disorder (PTSD)?

A. Benzodiazepines.
B. Second-generation antipsychotic medications.
C. Selective serotonin reuptake inhibitors (SSRIs).
D. Anticonvulsants.
E. α_1-Adrenergic receptor antagonists.

41.2 What is the most prominent focus of prolonged exposure therapy (PE) for the treatment of PTSD?

A. Targeted homework assignments designed to reshape dysfunctional cognitive beliefs that interfere with recovery.
B. Mindfulness exercises to enhance coping strategies.
C. Conjoint sessions to reduce the impact of the patient's PTSD symptoms on his or her intimate partner.
D. Repeated imaginal and in vivo exposures to enhance extinction of traumatic memories and decrease cue reactivity.
E. Intensive debriefing to prevent consolidation of traumatic memories.

41.3 In studies examining biological responses to trauma-related stimuli in subjects with PTSD, which of the following findings has been repeatedly confirmed?

A. Increased heart rate.
B. Decreased skin conductance.
C. Decreased facial electromyographic reactivity.
D. Decreased startle response.
E. Increased cortisol levels.

41.4 Which of the following statements regarding the DSM-5 criteria for acute stress disorder (ASD) is correct?

 A. The diagnosis requires the presence of symptoms including marked avoidance, marked anxiety or increased arousal, at least one of six reexperiencing symptoms, and at least three of five dissociative symptoms.
 B. The diagnosis requires at least two symptoms in each of the following five categories: intrusion symptoms, negative mood, dissociative symptoms, avoidance symptoms, and arousal symptoms.
 C. The time course for ASD requires symptoms beginning and worsening after the traumatic event and persisting for 2 days until 1 month after the trauma.
 D. The diagnosis includes but does not require dissociative symptoms.
 E. The reexperiencing symptoms apply not only to directly experienced exposures but also to exposure through electronic media, television, movies, or pictures, regardless of whether the exposure was work related.

41.5 Which of the following best describes the prevalence rates of suicidality in patients with adjustment disorders?

 A. 0%.
 B. 0–25%.
 C. 25%–50%.
 D. 50%–75%.
 E. 75%–100%.

41.6 An 85-year-old woman who lost her husband to cancer more than a year ago is sent to you for consultation. Since her husband's death, she has experienced intense sorrow and longing for him. In addition, on most days she has difficulty accepting that he is dead and often blames herself for his death. She feels alone and desires "to be with him"; however, she has been eating and sleeping acceptably. She recently was able to enjoy attending the college graduation of one of her adult grandchildren. What is the most appropriate diagnosis?

 A. Reactive attachment disorder.
 B. Major depressive disorder.
 C. Normal bereavement.
 D. Adjustment disorder with depressed mood.
 E. Other specified trauma- and stressor-related disorder.

Part II

Answer Guide

CHAPTER 1

Anthropology/Sociology/ Ethology/Psychology

1.1   Which of the following statements is true regarding completed suicide among youth in the United States?

   A. The ratio of completed suicide is higher for females than males.
   B. Black youth have the highest suicide rate.
   C. American Indians/Alaska Natives have the highest suicide rate.
   D. Hispanic youth have the highest suicide rate.
   E. White youth have the highest rate of suicide attempts but the lowest rate of suicide.

The correct response is option C: American Indians/Alaska Natives have the highest suicide rate.

The rate of completed suicide among youth is significantly higher for males than females, with a ratio of nearly 5 to 1 in 2010 (Centers for Disease Control and Prevention 2010) (option A). In general, the suicide rate in the United States is higher among white than nonwhite youth (option B). However, American Indians/ Alaska Natives (not Hispanic youth [option D]) exhibit the highest suicide rate of all ethnic groups in the United States (Centers for Disease Control and Prevention 2010) (option C). With regard to suicide attempt, 1-year incidence rates are greater among black (8.3%) and Hispanic (10.2%) youth than among white youth (6.2%), whereas white (15.5%) and Hispanic (16.7%) youth endorse greater rates of suicidal ideation compared with black youth (13.2%; Eaton et al. 2012) (option E). **(Dulcan M [ed]: Dulcan's Textbook of Child and Adolescent Psychiatry, 2nd Edition, Chapter 27, p. 572)**

1.2   Which of the following best defines *ethnicity*?

   A. Physical, biological, and genetic qualities of humans, particularly as these features lead to categorization of visible similarities or differences.

B. Identity with a group of people sharing common origins, history, customs, and beliefs.

C. A set of meaning, behavioral norms, and values used by members of a particular society as they construct their unique view of the world.

D. An organized system of beliefs, principles, rituals, practices, and related symbols that brings individuals and groups to sacred or ultimate reality and truth.

E. Religion and faith communities, not restricted to organized religion and group membership.

The correct response is option B: Identity with a group of people sharing common origins, history, customs and beliefs.

The Committee on Cultural Psychiatry for the Group for the Advancement of Psychiatry (2002) defines *culture* (option C) as "a set of meaning, behavioral norms, and values used by members of a particular society as they construct their unique view of the world." *Ethnicity* (option B) encompasses one's identity with a group of people sharing common origins, history, customs, and beliefs. Race (option A) refers to physical, biological, and genetic qualities of humans, particularly as these features lead to categorization of visible similarities or differences. *Religion* (option D) is an organized system of beliefs, principles, rituals, practices, and related symbols that brings individuals and groups to sacred or ultimate reality and truth. *Spirituality* (option E) includes religion and faith communities but is not restricted to organized religion and group membership. **(Dulcan M [ed]: Dulcan's Textbook of Child and Adolescent Psychiatry, 2nd Edition, Chapter 26, pp. 560, 562–563)**

1.3   Which of the following is a true statement regarding culture-bound syndromes?

A. Culture-bound syndromes are vague and diffuse.

B. Culture-bound syndromes are not accepted as a specific disorder in the country of origin.

C. Culture-bound syndromes occur less frequently in the "home" culture than in other cultures.

D. Culture-bound syndromes are a response to specific precipitants in that culture.

E. Culture-bound syndromes are common in childhood and adolescence.

The correct response is option D: Culture-bound syndromes are a response to specific precipitants in that culture.

The term *culture-bound syndromes* was introduced in 1967 to describe disorders that are 1) discrete and well defined (option A), 2) accepted as a specific disorder in the country of origin (option B), 3) a response to specific precipitants in that culture (option D), and 4) found to occur much more in the "home" culture than in other cultures (option C) (Guarnaccia and Rogler 1999; Levine and Gaw 1995). While important to adult cultural psychiatry, little evidence exists that the symptoms and behaviors of specific culture-bound syndromes are common in childhood or adolescence (option E). **(Dulcan M [ed]: Dulcan's Textbook of Child and Adolescent Psychiatry, Chapter 34, p. 519)**

1.4   Which of the following is true regarding dissociation in culturally diverse patients?

A. Some world religious traditions foster dissociation in rituals and practices.
B. Dissociation is rarely a part of isolated culture-bound syndromes.
C. Dissociation is an insignificant symptom in culturally diverse children.
D. Exposure to trauma is rarely associated with dissociation.
E. Dissociation occurs only as a single symptom and never as a disorder.

The correct response is option A: Some world religious traditions foster dissociation in rituals and practices.

Clinicians should be alert to dissociation in culturally diverse children (option C), both as a single symptom and as a disorder (option E). Exposure to trauma, as either witnesses or victims, may result in children distancing themselves from real or perceived experiences as a defense mechanism (option D). The clinician should always inquire about and be alert to indications of rape, torture, or abuse. On the other hand, some world religious traditions foster dissociation in rituals and practices (option A), or dissociation may be a part of isolated culture-bound syndromes (option B) (American Psychiatric Association 2000; Tseng 2003). **(Dulcan M [ed]: Dulcan's Textbook of Child and Adolescent Psychiatry, Chapter 34, p. 520)**

1.5   Which of the following is a true statement regarding culture and child/adolescent development?

A. There is a wealth of methodologically sound studies of development outside of Western Europe and North America.
B. Cross-cultural studies have consistently documented that there is little variation in temperament and mother-child interactions among different cultures.
C. There is little variation in the time and manner in which different cultures mark adulthood.
D. Public acknowledgment of maturation is not relevant for role development in most cultures.
E. Theory and practical study of child and adolescent development have been dominated by Western schemas.

The correct response is option E: Theory and practical study of child and adolescent development have been dominated by Western schemas.

Theory and practical study of child and adolescent development have been dominated by Western schemas, especially Freud's psychosexual, Piaget's cognitive, and Erikson's psychosocial frameworks (option E). Methodologically sound studies of development outside of Western Europe and North America are few (option A), although scholarship on cross-cultural child development generally spans a continuum. Cross-cultural studies have consistently documented that certain qualities of temperament and mother-child interactions are found more often in certain cultures than in others (option B). Later in development, different cultures mark adulthood at varying times, some with unique rites or rituals of passage often tied temporally to puberty (option C). Young people tend to take on adult roles and responsibilities after such a public acknowledgment of their maturation, especially in non-Western cultures (option D) (Tseng 2001). **(Dulcan M [ed]: Dulcan's Textbook of Child and Adolescent Psychiatry, 2nd Edition, Chapter 26, p. 561)**

1.6   Which of the following DSM-5 tools was created to operationalize a culturally sensitive psychiatric evaluation?

A. Outline for Cultural Formulation.
B. Glossary of Culture-Bound Syndromes.
C. Glossary of Cultural Concepts of Distress.
D. Cultural Formulation Interview.
E. Culture, Age, and Gender Features Profile.

The correct response is option D: Cultural Formulation Interview.

The DSM-5 Cultural Formulation Interview (CFI) is a standardized 16-item questionnaire that operationalizes the Outline for Cultural Formulation (OCF) (option D). The CFI questions are intended for use at the very beginning of the initial assessment of patients and cover the same topical areas as the OCF.

The OCF (option A), which first appeared in DSM-IV/DSM-IV-TR (American Psychiatric Association 1994, 2000) and was updated in DSM-5 (American Psychiatric Association 2013), provides a useful framework for culturally competent assessment that is both sensitive and responsive to the person's cultural background. The main goal of the OCF is to help clinicians identify cultural contextual factors affecting the patient that are relevant to diagnosis and treatment (Mezzich et al. 2009).

The DSM-IV/DSM-IV-TR Glossary of Culture-Bound Syndromes (option B) was replaced in DSM-5 with the Glossary of Cultural Concepts of Distress (option C). Finally, the subsection "Specific Culture, Age, and Gender Features" (option E) that appeared in the description of each DSM-IV/DSM-IV-TR disorder was disaggregated in DSM-5 into two separate subsections: "Culture-Related Diagnostic Issues" and "Gender-Related Diagnostic Issues." **(Hales RE, Yudofsky SC, Roberts LW [eds]: APP Textbook of Psychiatry, 6th Edition, Chapter 36, pp. 1272–1273, 1280–1284)**

1.7   When researchers at McGill University used the Outline for Cultural Formulation (OCF) to reassess the cases of 70 patients with a referral diagnosis of a psychotic disorder, what proportion were rediagnosed as having a nonpsychotic disorder?

A. 27%.
B. 35%.
C. 49%.
D. 63%.
E. 78%.

The correct response is option C: 49%.

Researchers at McGill University in Montreal, Quebec, demonstrated the utility of the OCF in identifying misdiagnosis of psychotic disorders among ethnic minority and immigrant patients referred to a cultural consultation service (Adeponle et al. 2012). In this study, use of the DSM-IV/DSM-IV-TR OCF for case reassessment of 323 patients referred over a 10-year period resulted in 34 (49%) of 70 cases with a referral diagnosis of a psychotic disorder being rediagnosed as having a nonpsychotic disorder, and 12 (5%) of 253 cases with a referral diagnosis of a nonpsychotic disorder being rediagnosed as having a psychotic disorder. The cultural consultation service utilized 60 cultural and linguistic brokers, 1.5-hour clinical assessments, and a 2-hour case conference in addition to the OCF (Kirmayer et al. 2003). **(Hales RE, Yudofsky SC, Roberts LW [eds]: APP Textbook of Psychiatry, 6th Edition, Chapter 36, p. 1280)**

1.8   For which of the following clinician groups was the Cultural Formulation Interview (CFI) originally designed?

A. Psychiatrists trained in specific skills of cultural competence.
B. Clinicians working with racial/ethnic minorities.
C. Clinicians working with patients who speak a different language than their own.
D. Clinicians working with patients from a different cultural background than their own.
E. Any clinician working with any patient in any setting.

The correct response is option E: Any clinician working with any patient in any setting.

An aspect of the CFI that bears noting is that it is not intended exclusively for the evaluation of members of nondominant cultural groups, such as racial/ethnic minorities (option B). Instead, it is intended for use by any clinician (option A) with any patient, regardless of cultural background (option E). Even patients and clinicians who appear to share the same cultural background (option D) and speak the same language (option C) may differ in ways that are relevant to care. **(Hales RE, Yudofsky SC, Roberts LW [eds]: APP Textbook of Psychiatry, 6th Edition, Chapter 36, p. 1284)**

1.9   As of 2010, the rate of uninsurance was highest for which ethnic group in the United States?

A. African Americans.
B. Hispanics.
C. American Indians/Alaska Natives.
D. Native Hawaiians/Pacific Islanders.
E. Asian Americans.

The correct response is option B: Hispanics.

The lack of medical insurance is a major barrier to receipt of psychiatric care. In 2010–2011, the rate of uninsurance was 20% for African Americans, 30% for Hispanics, 27% for American Indians/Alaska Natives, 19% for Native Hawaiians/Pacific Islanders, and 18% for Asian Americans, compared with 11% for whites (non-Hispanic) (DeNavas-Walt et al. 2012). **(Hales RE, Yudofsky SC, Roberts LW [eds]: APP Textbook of Psychiatry, 6th Edition, Chapter 36, p. 1269)**

1.10   In 2005, the lifetime prevalence of any psychiatric disorder among males in American Indian tribes exceeded that among the average U.S. male population by what percentage?

A. 1%–5%.
B. 6%–10%.
C. 11%–15%.
D. 16%–20%.
E. 21%–25%.

The correct response is option B: 6%–10%.

It is important to understand the epidemiological differences that exist in diverse racial and ethnic groups compared with whites. In American Indian tribes, the lifetime prevalence of any psychiatric disorder (50%–54% in men) has been found to exceed that of the U.S. population (44% in men; option B) (Beals et al. 2005). **(Hales RE, Yudofsky SC, Roberts LW [eds]: APP Textbook of Psychiatry, 6th Edition, Chapter 36, p. 1269)**

1.11   According to U.S. Census Bureau estimates for 2013, what proportion of people in the United States identify themselves as nonwhite (including Black or African American, American Indian and Alaska Native, Native Hawaiian and Other Pacific Islander, Asian, Hispanic or Latino) or of two or more races?

A. 37%.
B. 54%.
C. 11%.
D. 23%.
E. 6%.

The correct response is option A: 37%.

According to U.S. Census Bureau estimates released on June 27, 2013 (http://quickfacts.census.gov/qfd/states/00000.html), 37% of Americans self-identify as nonwhite (including Black or African American, American Indian and Alaska Native, Native Hawaiian and Other Pacific Islander, Asian, Hispanic or Latino) or of two or more races. Taken together, these groups represent an emerging majority—by 2050, nonwhites are expected to account for more than half of the U.S. population (Passel et al. 2012). **(Hales RE, Yudofsky SC, Roberts LW [eds]: APP Textbook of Psychiatry, 6th Edition, Chapter 36, p. 1266)**

1.12   Which of the following terms refers to cultural ways of expressing distress that provide shared ways of experiencing and talking about personal or social concerns?

A. Cultural syndromes.
B. Culture-bound syndromes.
C. Cultural explanations.
D. Cultural idioms.
E. Cultural perceived causes.

The correct response is option D: Cultural idioms.

DSM-5 (American Psychiatric Association 2013) replaced the older conceptual description of *culture-bound syndromes* (option B) with three concepts having greater clinical utility: *Cultural syndromes* (option A) are clusters of symptoms and attributions that tend to co-occur among individuals in specific cultural groups, communities, or contexts and that are recognized locally as coherent patterns of experience. *Cultural idioms of distress* (option D) are ways of expressing distress that may not involve specific symptoms or syndromes but that provide shared ways of experiencing and talking about personal or social concerns (e.g., everyday talk about "nerves" or "depression"). *Cultural explanations* (option C) or *perceived causes* (option E) are labels, attributions, or features of an explanatory model that indicate culturally recognized meanings or etiologies for symptoms, illness, or distress (Groleau et al. 2006; Hinton and Lewis-Fernández 2010; Nichter 1981). **(Hales RE, Yudofsky SC, Roberts LW [eds]: APP Textbook of Psychiatry, 6th Edition, Chapter 36, p. 1285)**

1.13   How does mental health service utilization among racial and ethnic minority groups differ from that among white populations?

A. Nonmajority groups are more likely to receive mental health care in emergency room settings.
B. Nonmajority groups are more likely to receive mental health care in outpatient community settings.
C. Nonmajority groups are less likely to receive mental health care in inpatient hospital settings.

D. Nonmajority groups are more likely to seek mental health care from specialty mental health sources.

E. Nonmajority groups are less likely to use traditional or spiritual healers.

The correct response is option A: Nonmajority groups are more likely to receive mental health care in emergency room settings.

Mental health service utilization varies greatly among racial and ethnic minority groups. In a study of Medicaid beneficiaries with mental illness, nonmajority patients were more likely than whites to receive mental health care in inpatient (option C) and emergency room hospital settings (option A) and less likely to receive such care in outpatient community settings (option B) (Samnaliev et al. 2009). Among people with past-year depression, 69% of Asians, 64% of Latinos, and 59% of African Americans sought no mental health care, compared with 40% of non-Latino whites (Alegría et al. 2008). There are also disparities in help seeking that revolve around the use of alternative sources of care outside conventional Western medicine. For example, American Indian adults with a diagnosis of depression, anxiety, or substance use disorder are significantly less likely to seek help from specialty mental or behavioral health or other medical sources (option D) than from a traditional or spiritual healer (option E) (Beals et al. 2005; Walls et al. 2006). **(Hales RE, Yudofsky SC, Roberts LW [eds]: APP Textbook of Psychiatry, 6th Edition, Chapter 36, pp. 1269–1270)**

1.14   Relying on knowledge without any insight into real emotional meaning is an example of extreme imbalance in which of the following?

A. Implicit mentalizing.
B. Affective mentalizing.
C. External mentalizing.
D. Cognitive mentalizing.
E. Internal mentalizing.

The correct response is option D: Cognitive mentalizing.

The focus in *cognitive* mentalizing is thoughts and beliefs (option D), whereas the focus in *affective* mentalizing (option B) is emotions and feelings. Extreme imbalance in either direction poses challenges for psychotherapy. For example, patients with an overreliance on cognition might be adept at generating explicit reasons for their own or others' behavior, but such insight—devoid of any real emotional meaning—does not promote change. Conversely, patients who are more prone to being flooded with affect are employing implicit processes conducive to emotional contagion and impaired self-other differentiation. For patients at both ends of this spectrum, mentalizing emotion—thinking and feeling about thinking and feeling—is a crucial therapeutic goal. *External* mentalizing (option C) entails responsiveness to external, observable aspects of behavior—most prominently facial expressions but also voice tone and posture. In contrast, *internal* mentalizing (option E) requires inference and imagination in the service of understanding the mental states conjoined with external behavior (i.e., desires, feelings, beliefs, and relationship proclivities). *Implicit* mentalizing (option A) is relatively automatic, procedural, and nonconscious. In general, people rely on implicit mentalizing when all goes smoothly in interactions. **(Hales RE, Yudofsky SC, Roberts LW [eds]: APP Textbook of Psychiatry, 6th Edition, pp. 1096–1098 and Table 31–1, p. 1097)**

References

Adeponle AB, Thombs BD, Groleau D, et al: Using the cultural formulation to resolve uncertainty in diagnoses of psychosis among ethnoculturally diverse patients. Psychiatr Serv 63(2):147–153, 2012 22302332

Alegría M, Chatterji P, Wells K, et al: Disparity in depression treatment among racial and ethnic minority populations in the United States. Psychiatr Serv 59(11):1264–1272, 2008 18971402

American Psychiatric Association: Diagnostic and Statistical Manual of Mental Disorders, 4th Edition. Washington, DC, American Psychiatric Association, 1994

American Psychiatric Association: Diagnostic and Statistical Manual of Mental Disorders, 4th Edition, Text Revision. Washington, DC, American Psychiatric Association, 2000

American Psychiatric Association: Diagnostic and Statistical Manual of Mental Disorders, 5th Edition. Arlington, VA, American Psychiatric Association, 2013

Beals J, Novins DK, Whitesell NR, et al: Prevalence of mental disorders and utilization of mental health services in two American Indian reservation populations: mental health disparities in a national context. Am J Psychiatry 162(9):1723–1732, 2005 16135633

Centers for Disease Control and Prevention: WISQARS (Web-based Injury Statistics Query and Reporting System). Atlanta, GA, Centers for Disease Control and Prevention, 2010. Available at: http://www.cdc.gov/injury/wisquars/.

DeNavas-Walt C, Proctor BD, Smith JC: Income, Poverty, and Health Insurance Coverage in the United States: 2011. Current Population Reports. Washington, DC, U.S. Census Bureau, U.S. Department of Commerce, September 2012. Available at: http://www.census.gov/prod/2012pubs/p60–243.pdf. Accessed October 15, 2012.

Eaton DK, Kann L, Kinchen S , et al: Youth risk behavior surveillance—United States, 2011. MMWR Surveill Summ 61(4):1–162, 2012 22673000

Groleau D, Young A, Kirmayer LJ: The McGill Illness Narrative Interview (MINI): an interview schedule to elicit meanings and modes of reasoning related to illness experience. Transcult Psychiatry 43(4):671–691, 2006 17166953

Group for the Advancement of Psychiatry: Committee on Cultural Psychiatry: Cultural Assessment in Clinical Psychiatry. Washington, DC, American Psychiatric Publishing, 2002

Guarnaccia PJ, Rogler LH: Research on culture-bound syndromes: new directions. Am J Psychiatry 156(9):1322–1327, 1999 10484940

Hinton DE, Lewis-Fernández R: Idioms of distress among trauma survivors: subtypes and clinical utility. Cult Med Psychiatry 34(2):209–218, 2010 20407812

Kirmayer LJ, Groleau D, Guzder J, et al: Cultural consultation: a model of mental health service for multicultural societies. Can J Psychiatry 48(3):145–153, 2003 12728738

Levine RE, Gaw AC: Culture-bound syndromes. Psychiatr Clin North Am 18(3):523–536, 1995 8545265

Mezzich JE, Caracci G, Fabrega H Jr, Kirmayer LJ: Cultural formulation guidelines. Transcult Psychiatry 46(3):383–405, 2009 19837778

Nichter M: Idioms of distress: alternatives in the expression of psychosocial distress: a case study from South India. Cult Med Psychiatry 5(4):379–408, 1981 7326955

Passel J, Livingston G, Cohn D: Explaining why minority births now outnumber white births. Pew Social and Demographic Trends. Pew Research Center. Released May 17, 2012. Available at: http://www.pewsocialtrends.org/2012/05/17/explaining-why-minority-births-now-outnumber-white-births. Accessed October 22, 2012.

Samnaliev M, McGovern MP, Clark RE: Racial/ethnic disparities in mental health treatment in six Medicaid programs. J Health Care Poor Underserved 20(1):165–176, 2009 19202255

Tseng W-S: Handbook of Cultural Psychiatry. San Diego, CA, Academic Press, 2001

Tseng W-S: Clinician's Guide to Cultural Psychiatry. San Diego, CA, Academic Press, 2003

Walls ML, Johnson KD, Whitbeck LB, Hoyt DR: Mental health and substance abuse services preferences among American Indian people of the northern Midwest. Community Ment Health J 42(6):521–535, 2006 17143732

CHAPTER 2

Anxiety Disorders

2.1 What is the minimum duration of symptom persistence required for a diagnosis of generalized anxiety disorder (GAD)?

A. 1 week.
B. 2 weeks.
C. 1 month.
D. 2 months.
E. 6 months.

The correct response is option E: 6 months.

The diagnosis of GAD requires characteristic *chronic* symptoms of nervousness, somatic symptoms, and excessive anxiety or worry. Although several studies had suggested that persistence of symptoms for 1–3 months was associated with a similar course, comorbidity, and functional impairment as persistence for 6 or more months (Andrews et al. 2010), DSM-5 (American Psychiatric Association 2013) retained the 6-month minimum duration for diagnosis. **(Hales RE, Yudofsky SC, Roberts LW [eds]: APP Textbook of Psychiatry, 6th Edition, Chapter 12, p. 416; DSM-5, Anxiety Disorders, p. 222)**

2.2 According to twin studies, what is the estimated heritability of panic disorder?

A. 5%.
B. 10%.
C. 15%.
D. 20%.
E. 40%.

The correct response is option E: 40%.

Twin studies suggest that panic disorder is moderately heritable (~40%) (Gelernter and Stein 2009). From a genetic perspective, it is believed that panic disorder, like other psychiatric disorders, is a complex disorder with multiple genes confer-ring vulnerability through as-yet largely undetermined pathways (Manolio et al. 2009; Smoller et al. 2009). **(Hales RE, Yudofsky SC, Roberts LW [eds]: APP Text-book of Psychiatry, 6th Edition, Chapter 12, p. 408)**

2.3   Which of the following anxiety disorders has the youngest median age at onset?

   A. Separation anxiety disorder.
   B. Panic disorder.
   C. Agoraphobia.
   D. Social anxiety disorder.
   E. Generalized anxiety disorder.

The correct response is option D: Social anxiety disorder.

Among the anxiety disorders, social anxiety disorder (social phobia) has the youngest median age at onset, at 15 years (option D). Median onset age is 16 years for separation anxiety disorder (option A), 23 years for panic disorder (option B), 18 years for agoraphobia (option C), and 30 years for GAD (option E) (Kessler et al. 2012). **(Hales RE, Yudofsky SC, Roberts LW [eds]: APP Textbook of Psychia-try, 6th Edition, Chapter 12, pp. 391–392 and Table 12–1, p. 393)**

2.4   Which of the following anxiety disorders has the oldest median age at onset?

   A. Specific phobia.
   B. Panic disorder.
   C. Agoraphobia.
   D. Social anxiety disorder.
   E. Generalized anxiety disorder.

The correct response is option E: Generalized anxiety disorder.

Among the anxiety disorders, GAD has the oldest median age at onset, at 30 years (option E). Median onset age is 15 years for specific phobia (option A), 23 years for panic disorder (option B), 18 years for agoraphobia (option C), and 15 years for so-cial anxiety disorder (option D) (Kessler et al. 2012). **(Hales RE, Yudofsky SC, Rob-erts LW [eds]: APP Textbook of Psychiatry, 6th Edition, Chapter 12, pp. 391–392 and Table 12–1, p. 393)**

2.5   Which of the following disorders is included among the anxiety disorders in DSM-5?

   A. Obsessive-compulsive disorder.
   B. Posttraumatic stress disorder.
   C. Acute stress disorder.
   D. Panic disorder with agoraphobia.
   E. Separation anxiety disorder.

The correct response is option E: Separation anxiety disorder.

The DSM-5 Anxiety Disorders section contains a number of additions and deletions when compared with DSM-IV (American Psychiatric Association 1994). A number of anxiety disorders formerly classified in DSM-IV as disorders usually first diagnosed in infancy and childhood or adolescence are now included among the anxiety disorders; these include separation anxiety disorder and selective mutism (option E). DSM-5 removed several disorders from the anxiety disorders, including obsessive-compulsive disorder, posttraumatic stress disorder, and acute stress disorder (options A–C). This reorganization was the result of a scientific review that concluded that these were distinct disorders that were not sufficiently described by the presence of anxiety symptoms. Agoraphobia has been separated from panic disorder as a distinct disorder, which includes a panic attack specifier when they co-occur (option D). **(DSM-5, Anxiety Disorders, pp. 189–191, 214)**

2.6   A 50-year-old man reports episodes in which he will suddenly and unexpectedly wake from his sleep feeling a surge of intense fear that peaks within minutes. During this time he experiences shortness of breath, heart palpitations, sweating, and nausea. His medical history is significant only for hypertension, which is well controlled with hydrochlorothiazide. As a result of these symptoms, he has begun to have anticipatory anxiety associated with going to sleep. Which of the following disorders is the most likely cause for the man's symptoms?

A. Anxiety disorder due to a general medical condition (hypertension).
B. Substance-induced anxiety disorder.
C. Panic disorder.
D. Sleep terrors.
E. Panic attacks.

The correct response is option C: Panic disorder.

Panic disorder refers to recurrent unexpected panic attacks. Panic attacks (option E) are a syndrome, not a disorder, and can occur with a variety of disorders. General medical conditions, substance-related disorders, and other psychiatric disorders must be ruled out; in this case the patient's well-controlled hypertension (option A) or use of a diuretic (option B) is unlikely to be a cause of his attacks. Nocturnal panic attacks associated with sleep are an example of an unexpected panic attack, not of sleep terrors, in which situation awareness is usually not present (option D). Although sleep-related disorders should be ruled out, this man's classic presentation makes panic disorder the most likely explanation (option C). **(DSM-5, Anxiety Disorders, pp. 208–214)**

2.7   A 35-year-old man is in danger of losing his job; the job requires frequent long-range traveling, and for the past year he has avoided flying. Two years prior, he traveled on a particularly turbulent flight, and although he was not in any real danger, he was convinced that the pilot minimized the risk and that the plane almost crashed. He flew again a month later; although he experienced a smooth flight, the anticipation of turbulence was so distressing that he experienced a panic attack during the flight. He has not flown since. Which of the following disorders is the most likely cause of his anxiety?

A. Agoraphobia.
B. Acute stress disorder.
C. Specific phobia—situational type.
D. Social anxiety disorder.
E. Panic disorder.

The correct response is option C: Specific phobia—situational type.

Specific phobia is characterized by the marked fear or anxiety of a specific object or situation, which is perceived as being dangerous (option C). This differs from agoraphobia (option A), in which the focus of the anxiety is on the possibility of having panic or other incapacitating symptoms, and from social anxiety disorder (option D), in which the focus is on being scrutinized by others. Trauma-related disorders should be considered in the differential; however, the lack of any real danger makes such diagnoses unlikely, and the time course is not compatible with the criteria for acute stress disorder (option B). Although the man did experience a panic attack, patients with many disorders, including specific phobia, can experience such attacks. Panic disorder should only be diagnosed when the attacks are unexpected and not otherwise explained by other disorders (option E). **(DSM-5, Anxiety Disorders, pp. 197–202)**

2.8   A 26-year-old man is brought to the emergency department complaining of the sudden onset of panic. He has no psychiatric history but reports that he took several doses of an over-the-counter cold medication for which he had to show his driver's license. Which of the following would be most suggestive that the man is suffering from a substance-induced anxiety disorder?

A. The presence of mild symptoms that do not impair functioning.
B. Symptoms that persist for a long time after the medication is stopped.
C. Somewhat similar symptoms that occurred once prior to taking the medication.
D. Presence of a delirium or gross confusion.
E. Lack of any history of an anxiety disorder or panic symptoms.

The correct response is option E: Lack of any history of an anxiety disorder or panic symptoms.

Many substances can potentially cause anxiety symptoms and it can, at times, be difficult to determine whether medication use is etiologically related to the onset of anxiety symptoms. Evidence to support the presence of a substance-induced anxiety disorder includes temporal associations and symptoms that are consistent with the medication and dose (option E). In this case, the patient is likely taking a medication containing pseudoephedrine, which requires the purchaser to show a driver's license. By definition, a substance-induced anxiety disorder must cause significant distress or impairment in functioning (option A), and it cannot occur exclusively during the course of a delirium (option D). According to criterion C of the diagnostic criteria, the disturbance cannot be better explained by evidence of an independent anxiety disorder such as symptoms preceding the onset of substance/medication use or persisting following the discontinuation of the substance (options B, C). **(DSM-5, Anxiety Disorders, pp. 226–230)**

References

American Psychiatric Association: Diagnostic and Statistical Manual of Mental Disorders, 4th Edition. Washington, DC, American Psychiatric Association, 1994

American Psychiatric Association: Diagnostic and Statistical Manual of Mental Disorders, 5th Edition. Arlington, VA, American Psychiatric Association, 2013

Andrews G, Hobbs MJ, Borkovec TD, et al: Generalized worry disorder: a review of DSM-IV generalized anxiety disorder and options for DSM-V. Depress Anxiety 27(2):134–147, 2010 20058241

Gelernter J, Stein MB: Heritability and genetics of anxiety disorders, in Handbook of Anxiety Disorders. Edited by Antony MM, Stein MB. New York, Oxford University Press, 2009, pp 87–96

Kessler RC, Petukhova M, Sampson NA, et al: Twelve-month and lifetime prevalence and lifetime morbid risk of anxiety and mood disorders in the United States. Int J Methods Psychiatr Res 21(3):169–184, 2012 22865617

Manolio TA, Collins FS, Cox NJ, et al: Finding the missing heritability of complex diseases. Nature 461(7265):747–753, 2009 19812666

Smoller JW, Block SR, Young MM: Genetics of anxiety disorders: the complex road from DSM to DNA. Depress Anxiety 26(11):965–975, 2009 19885930

CHAPTER 3

Bipolar Disorders

3.1 To receive a diagnosis of bipolar I disorder, a patient must have experienced which of the following?

A. At least one manic episode and one major depressive episode (MDE).
B. More than one manic episode.
C. At least two manic episodes and one MDE.
D. At least one manic episode.
E. At least one manic or hypomanic episode.

The correct response is option D: At least one manic episode.

Patients with bipolar I disorder have experienced at least one manic episode (option D). A single hypomanic episode is insufficient for making a diagnosis of either bipolar I or bipolar II disorder (option E), and having multiple manic episodes is not necessary to establish a diagnosis of bipolar I disorder (option B). Mood episodes in bipolar I disorder (and in bipolar II disorder) are not permitted to be better accounted for by schizoaffective disorder or superimposed on schizophrenia, schizophreniform disorder, delusional disorder, or other specified or unspecified schizophrenia spectrum and other psychotic disorder. It is noteworthy that although the vast majority of patients with bipolar I disorder also experience major depressive episodes, such episodes are not required for the diagnosis of bipolar I disorder (options A, C). Less than 10% of patients with bipolar I disorder only experience a single manic episode (with no other manic episodes or major depressive episodes); the vast majority of patients with bipolar I disorder experience recurrent episodes. DSM-5 (American Psychiatric Association 2013) differs from DSM-IV-TR (American Psychiatric Association 2000) in that the diagnosis of bipolar I disorder, single manic episode is no longer included. Diagnostic codes for bipolar I disorder are based on type of current or most recent episode and its status with respect to current severity, presence of psychotic features, and remission status. These are followed by as many of the following specifiers without codes as apply to the current or most recent episode: with anxious distress (presence of at least two of the following five symptoms: feeling keyed up/tense, feeling unusually restless, difficulty concentrating due to worry, fear of something awful happening, fear of loss of control); with mixed features; with rapid cycling (if there have been at least four syndromal major depressive, manic, or hypomanic episodes in the prior 12 months); with melancholic features (for depression); with atypical features (for depression); with mood-congruent or mood-incongruent psychotic features; with catatonia; with peripartum onset; and with seasonal pattern. **(Hales RE, Yudofsky SC, Roberts LW [eds]: APP Textbook of Psychiatry, 6th Edition, Chapter 10, pp. 318–319)**

3.2   To receive a diagnosis of bipolar II disorder, a patient must have experienced which of the following?

    A. At least one hypomanic episode and one MDE.
    B. At least one hypomanic episode.
    C. At least two hypomanic episodes and one MDE.
    D. More than one hypomanic episode.
    E. At least one manic or hypomanic episode.

The correct response is option A: At least one hypomanic episode and one MDE.

Patients with bipolar II disorder have experienced at least one hypomanic episode as well as at least one MDE (option A), but no manic episode (option E). Having only hypomanic episodes in the absence of depressive episodes is insufficient for establishing a diagnosis of bipolar II disorder (options B, D). It is not necessary to have multiple episodes of either hypomania or depression to make a diagnosis of bipolar II disorder; one episode of each type is adequate (option C). Bipolar II disorder has only one diagnostic code. Its status with respect to current severity, presence of psychotic features, course, and other specifiers cannot be coded but should be indicated in writing. Thus, current or most recent episode is specified as hypomanic or depressed. This is followed by as many of the following specifiers as apply to the current or most recent episode: with anxious distress, rapid cycling, mood-congruent or mood-incongruent psychotic features, catatonia, peripartum onset, and seasonal pattern (for depressive episodes). These are followed by either a course specifier (in partial remission or in full remission) if full criteria for a mood episode are not met, or by a severity specifier (mild, moderate, or severe) if full criteria for a mood episode are met. **(Hales RE, Yudofsky SC, Roberts LW [eds]: APP Textbook of Psychiatry, 6th Edition, Chapter 10, p. 320)**

3.3   A mood episode that meets full criteria for both mania and depression would be diagnosed as which of the following in DSM-5?

    A. A depressive episode, yielding a diagnosis of major depressive disorder.
    B. A manic episode, yielding a diagnosis of bipolar I disorder.
    C. A hypomanic episode, yielding a diagnosis of bipolar II disorder.

D. A mixed episode, yielding a diagnosis of bipolar II disorder.

E. A mixed episode, yielding a diagnosis of major depressive disorder with mixed features.

The correct response is option B: A manic episode, yielding a diagnosis of bipolar I disorder.

In DSM-5, the DSM-IV-TR diagnosis of "mixed episode" has been replaced with a "with mixed features" specifier for MDEs (options D, E). This specifier is applied if at least three mood-elevation symptoms (including elevated/expansive mood, inflated self-esteem/grandiosity, overtalkativeness, racing thoughts, increased energy/goal-directed activity, impulsivity, and decreased need for sleep; but excluding distractibility, irritability, and psychomotor agitation, which may occur in either pole) occur concurrently with at least five depressive symptoms. DSM-5 indicates that episodes that meet full criteria for both mania and depression simultaneously should be labeled as manic episodes as opposed to depressive episodes (option A) "due to the marked impairment and clinical severity of full mania," yielding a diagnosis of bipolar I disorder (option B). In contrast, DSM-5 is silent regarding episodes that meet full criteria for both hypomania and depression simultaneously, neither prohibiting nor endorsing simultaneously diagnosing hypomanic and depressive episodes (as opposed to selecting one pole for the episode and adding a "with mixed features" specifier), although such patients would have a diagnosis of bipolar II disorder (option C). It is important to note that MDEs with mixed features can occur in both bipolar and depressive disorders, consistent with a unitary mood disorders model. **(Hales RE, Yudofsky SC, Roberts LW [eds]: APP Textbook of Psychiatry, 6th Edition, Chapter 10, pp. 314–315)**

3.4   To receive a DSM-5 diagnosis of cyclothymic disorder, an adult patient must have experienced which of the following?

A. Chronic subsyndromal symptoms of mood elevation and depression for at least 1 year.

B. Chronic subsyndromal symptoms of mood elevation and depression for at least 6 months.

C. Chronic subsyndromal symptoms of mood elevation and depression for at least 2 years.

D. At least one manic episode interposed with subsyndromal symptoms of mood elevation and depression.

E. At least one depressive episode and at least one manic episode interposed with subsyndromal symptoms of mood elevation and depression.

The correct response is option C: Chronic subsyndromal symptoms of mood elevation and depression for at least 2 years.

Patients with cyclothymic disorder have a chronic pattern of subsyndromal mood elevation and depression symptoms lasting at least 2 years in adults (option C) and at least 1 year in children and adolescents (option A), without a 2-month interruption. Subsyndromal symptoms of mood elevation and depression of at least 6 months' duration is insufficient for establishing a diagnosis of cyclothymic disorder in either adults or children and adolescents (option B). Cyclothymic disorder may not be diagnosed if there has been any major depressive, manic, or hypomanic episode during the first 2 years of the disturbance (1 year in children and adolescents); if such an episode occurs during this time period, the chronic subsyndromal mood swings may be considered to be residual symptoms of bipolar I disorder or bipolar II disorder (options D, E). However, after the initial 2-year period (1 year in children and adolescents) of cyclothymic disorder, there may be superimposed manic episodes (in which case both bipolar I disorder and cyclothymic disorder may be diagnosed), hypomanic episodes (in which case both other specified bipolar and related disorder and cyclothymic disorder may be diagnosed), or MDEs (in which case both major depressive disorder and cyclothymic disorder may be diagnosed). **(Hales RE, Yudofsky SC, Roberts LW [eds]: APP Textbook of Psychiatry, 6th Edition, Chapter 10, p. 321)**

3.5   A patient with a history of bipolar disorder reports experiencing 1 week of elevated and expansive mood. Evidence of which of the following would suggest that the patient is experiencing a hypomanic, rather than manic, episode?

A. Irritability.
B. Decreased need for sleep.
C. Increased productivity at work.
D. Psychotic symptoms.
E. Good insight into the illness.

The correct response is option C: Increased productivity at work.

The primary factor that differentiates manic and hypomanic episodes is that manic episodes cause marked impairment in social or occupational functioning or necessitate hospitalization to prevent harm to self or others, or there are psychotic features (Criterion C of bipolar I disorder). In hypomania, "The episode is not severe enough to cause marked impairment in social or occupational functioning or to necessitate hospitalization" (Criterion E of bipolar II disorder) (option C). If psychotic features are present, the episode is, by definition, manic (option D).

Both types of episodes can cause irritability (option A) or decreased need for sleep (option B). Insight is not included in the diagnostic criteria (option E). **(DSM-5, Bipolar and Related Disorders, pp. 123–136)**

3.6   How do the depressive episodes associated with bipolar II disorder differ from those associated with bipolar I disorder?

A. They are less frequent than those associated with bipolar I disorder.
B. They are lengthier than those associated with bipolar I disorder.

C. They are less disabling than those associated with bipolar I disorder.

D. They are less severe than those associated with bipolar I disorder.

E. They are rarely a reason for the patient to seek treatment.

The correct response is option B: They are lengthier than those associated with bipolar I disorder.

The recurrent MDEs associated with bipolar II disorder are typically more frequent (option A) and lengthier than those associated with bipolar I disorder (option B). The depressive episodes can be very severe and disabling; because of this, DSM-5 stresses that bipolar II disorder should not be considered a "milder" form of bipolar I disorder (options C, D). Bipolar II patients are more likely to seek treatment when depressed than during hypomanic episodes (option E). **(DSM-5, Bipolar and Related Disorders, pp. 135–136)**

3.7   A 29-year-old woman with no prior psychiatric history is placed on prednisone for a flare of systemic lupus erythematosus. Several days later she develops pressured speech, sleeplessness, irritability, and paranoid ideation. Prednisone is stopped, and the patient's symptoms persist for 2 weeks before resolving. Neurological evaluation and imaging do not demonstrate any evidence of central nervous system lupus. Which of the following is the most likely DSM-5 diagnosis?

A. Substance-induced bipolar disorder.

B. Bipolar disorder due to another medical condition.

C. Other specified bipolar and related disorder.

D. Bipolar II disorder.

E. Cyclothymic disorder.

The correct response is option A: Substance-induced bipolar disorder.

Substance/medication-induced bipolar and related disorder is associated with the ingestion of a substance (e.g., a drug of abuse, a medication, or another treatment) or the withdrawal of that substance. Substances and treatments associated with secondary mood disorders include general medications such as endocrine agents (e.g., corticosteroids, hormonal contraceptives) (option A).

      Bipolar and related disorder due to another medical condition in DSM-5 is a function of the direct physiological effects of another medical condition (option B). Although neurological manifestations of lupus may be associated with manic, hypomanic, and psychotic signs or symptoms, this patient's overall presentation does not suggest the presence of neurological lupus. Other specified bipolar and related disorder applies to individuals experiencing significant manic or hypomanic and depressive symptoms that do not meet diagnostic criteria for any other disorder from the "Bipolar and Related Disorders" chapter of DSM-5 and are not attributable to the direct physiological effects of a substance (option C). To meet criteria for a diagnosis of bipolar II disorder or cyclothymic disorder, symptoms cannot be attributable to the physiological effects of a substance or another medical condition (options D, E). **(Hales RE, Yudofsky SC, Roberts LW [eds]: APP Textbook of Psychiatry, 6th Edition, Chapter 10, pp. 318–325 and Table 10–1, p. 323)**

References

American Psychiatric Association: Diagnostic and Statistical Manual of Mental Disorders, 4th Edition, Text Revision. Washington, DC, American Psychiatric Association, 2000

American Psychiatric Association: Diagnostic and Statistical Manual of Mental Disorders, 5th Edition. Arlington, VA, American Psychiatric Association, 2013

CHAPTER 4

Dangerousness

4.1   How should a psychiatrist assess for homicidality during the psychiatric interview?

A. By asking the patient about ideation, intent, and plan, as well as access to any weapons.
B. Cautiously so as not to agitate the patient and cause him or her to act on these impulses.
C. By threatening the patient with involuntary hospitalization.
D. By relying on the patient's close friends and family rather than directly asking the patient.
E. By asking the patient about perceptual disturbances.

The correct response is option A: By asking the patient about ideation, intent, and plan, as well as access to any weapons.

Suicidality and homicidality are integral to the evaluation of thought content. For both, the interviewer should assess for ideation, intent, and plan, as well as access to weapons (option A). Interviewers will sometimes shy away from such exploration, perhaps fearing that introduction of the topic will cause the patient to become irritable, offended, or destructive or that any mention of suicidality or homicidality will inevitably lead to psychiatric admission. Such concerns are generally unwarranted (option B). Passive suicidal and homicidal thoughts are common, and discussion can often lead to a deepening of the alliance, so the psychiatrist should not rely exclusively on family or friends (option D). Furthermore, most such thoughts do not lead to involuntary treatment (option C). More importantly, people who do eventually kill themselves or others have often sent out clear warnings beforehand. Although assessments are imperfect, the psychiatric interview is a crucial time to identify people at risk (Fowler 2012). Perceptual disturbances do not have a direct correlation with homicidality (option E). **(Hales RE, Yudofsky SC, Roberts LW [eds]: APP Textbook of Psychiatry, 6th Edition, Chapter 1, pp. 24–25)**

4.2   A 32-year-old man presents with a history of frequent angry and impulsive outbursts. Which of the following instruments would be the most appropriate choice for assessing this patient's ability to control his anger?

A. Overt Aggression Scale—Modified.
B. Buss-Durkee Hostility Inventory.
C. State-Trait Anger Expression Inventory—2.
D. Anger, Irritability, and Assault Questionnaire.
E. Overcontrolled Hostility Scale.

The correct response is option D: Anger, Irritability, and Assault Questionnaire.

The Anger, Irritability, and Assault Questionnaire (Coccaro et al. 1991) is a 42-item self-report questionnaire designed to assess several aspects of impulsive aggression putatively related to serotonergic function; it focuses primarily on the inability to control aggression (option D). The Overt Aggression Scale—Modified (Coccaro et al. 1991) is a semi-structured clinician interview that assesses aggression, irritability, and suicidality in the past week (option A). The Buss-Durkee Hostility Inventory (Buss and Durkee 1957) is a self-report questionnaire that measures different aspects of hostility and aggression (option B). The State-Trait Anger Expression Inventory—2 (option C) (Spielberger 1999) divides behavior into state anger (current feelings) and trait anger (disposition to angry feelings). Megargee et al. (1967) developed an overcontrolled hostility scale using Minnesota Multiphasic Personality Inventory items (option E). **(Hales RE, Yudofsky SC, Roberts LW [eds]: APP Textbook of Psychiatry, 6th Edition, Chapter 3, p. 70)**

4.3   The landmark *Tarasoff* case (*Tarasoff v. Regents of the University of California* 1976) defined a therapist's duty to protect third parties. Which of the following is true of this ruling or the interpretation of the ruling?

A. It is a federal ruling that sets a universal standard applicable in all states.
B. There must be a threat of imminent danger.
C. The only permissible action is to immediately warn the threatened individual.
D. It may apply to failure to warn a patient about the risks of driving while psychotic.
E. It can only be used if the patient is not psychotic.

The correct response is option B: There must be a threat of imminent danger.

As a general rule, absent a special relationship, one person has no duty to control the conduct of a second person to prevent that person from harming a third person (Restatement [Second] of Torts 1965). Applying this rule to psychiatric care, psychiatrists traditionally have had only a limited duty owed to third persons to control their patients. Included in this limited class of duty to third persons for the acts of their patients are negligent discharge of a dangerous patient who harms a third person and failure to warn a patient about the risks of driving while taking certain medications, resulting in injury to others (Felthous 1990). There is no mention of warning psychotic patients (option D). In *Tarasoff*, the California Supreme Court reasoned that a duty to protect third parties was imposed when a special relationship existed between the individual whose conduct created the danger and the defendant. Finding this special relationship requirement met in this setting, the court concluded "the single relationship of a doctor to his patient is sufficient to support the duty to exercise reasonable care to protect others [from the violent acts of patients]." There has never been a federal ruling; the psychiatrist's duty has been decided by individual states (option A). Some states have adopted the *Tarasoff* holding, whereas others have limited or extended its scope and reach. In most states, psychotherapists have a duty, established by case law or statute, to act affirmatively to protect an endangered third party from a patient's violent or dangerous acts. A few courts have declined to find a *Tarasoff* duty in a specific case, whereas some courts have simply rejected the *Tarasoff* duty (*Evans v. United States* 1995; *Green v. Ross* 1997). In *Thapar v. Zezulka* (1999), the Texas Supreme Court ruled that the state statute on confidentiality *permits* but does not require disclosures by therapists of threats of harm to endangered third parties by their patients. When courts have found a duty to protect, they have required an "imminent" threat of serious harm to a foreseeable victim (option B). In some jurisdictions, courts have held that the need to safeguard the public well-being overrides all other considerations, including confidentiality. Despite the fact that the *Tarasoff* duty is still not law in some jurisdictions and is subject to different interpretations by individual courts, the duty to protect is, in effect, a national standard of practice. The duty-to-protect language stated in some statutes allows for a greater variety of clinical interventions than does warning alone (option C). Diagnosis of the patient does not have an impact on application of the ruling (option E). **(Hales RE, Yudofsky SC, Roberts LW [eds]: APP Textbook of Psychiatry, 6th Edition, Chapter 6, pp. 186–187)**

4.4   Which of the following factors was a predictor of violence in schizophrenic patients in the Clinical Antipsychotic Trials of Intervention Effectiveness (CATIE)?

A. Living alone.
B. History of victimization.
C. History of substance abuse absent.
D. Preponderance of negative symptoms.
E. High socioeconomic status.

The correct response is option B: History of victimization.

In the CATIE study (Lieberman et al. 2005; Swartz et al. 2006), 19% of patients exhibited violent behavior at some point prior to the study. Predictors of violence were childhood conduct problems, substance misuse (option C), a history of victimization (option B), economic deprivation, and living with other people, rather than living alone (option A). Economic deprivation, not affluence, is a predictor of violence (option E). Patients with a history of violence were more likely to discontinue their medication. A history of violence was a predictor of violence over the next 6 months (Swanson et al. 2008). Increased positive symptoms were associated with increased rates of violent behaviors, whereas negative symptoms were protective (option D). A history of an eating disorder has not been found to be related to violence in patients with schizophrenia (option C). **(Hales RE, Yudofsky SC, Roberts LW [eds]: APP Textbook of Psychiatry, 6th Edition, Chapter 9, p. 278)**

4.5   Patients with a history of violent behavior are more likely to have a lesion in which area of the brain?

A. Dorsal prefrontal cortex.
B. Prefrontal cortex.
C. Cingulate gyrus.
D. Left posterior middle temporal gyrus.
E. Superior temporal gyrus.

The correct response is option B: Prefrontal cortex.

The prefrontal cortex modulates limbic and hypothalamic activity and is associated with the social and judgment aspects of aggression. The frontal cortex coordinates timing of social cues, often before the expression of associated emotions. Lesions in this area give rise to disinhibited anger after minimal provocation, characterized by an individual showing little regard for the consequences of affect and behavior. Weiger and Bear (1988) suggest that whereas patients with temporal lobe epilepsy may express deep remorse over an aggressive act, patients with prefrontal lesions often indicate indifference. Patients with violent behavior have been found to have a high frequency of prefrontal lobe lesions (option B), and orbitofrontal cortex lesions, in particular, tend to result in antisocial behaviors (Blair 2004; Séguin 2004). Prefrontal damage may cause aggression by a secondary process involving lack of inhibition of the limbic area. Dorsal lesions of the prefrontal cortex are associated with impairment in long-term planning and increased apathy (option A). Orbital lesions of the prefrontal cortex are associated with increases in reflexive emotional responses to environmental stimuli (Luria 1980). The cingulate gyrus has consistently been implicated in the pathogenesis of depression and mood regulation (option C). Anomic aphasia may be related to lesions of the left angular or left posterior middle temporal gyrus and is common in Alzheimer's disease. (option D), and the superior temporal gyrus contains the primary auditory cortex (option E). **(Hales RE, Yudofsky SC, Roberts LW [eds]: APP Textbook of Psychiatry, 6th Edition, Chapter 24, p. 840; Chapter 28, p. 1014; Yudofsky SC, Hales RE [eds]: APP Textbook of Neuropsychiatry and Behavioral Neuroscience, 5th Edition, Chapter 13, p. 541)**

4.6   The diagnostic criteria of recurrent suicidal or self-injurious behaviors are included in which of the following DSM-5 diagnoses?

A. Paranoid personality disorder.
B. All personality disorders.

C. Antisocial personality disorder.
D. Borderline personality disorder.
E. Narcissistic personality disorder.

The correct response is option D: Borderline personality disorder.

Personality disorders (PDs) are associated with a relatively high prevalence of suicidal behavior and death by suicide. One psychological autopsy study (Schneider et al. 2006) of suicide completers using semistructured interviews with informants indicated that 72.3% of men and 66.7% of women met criteria for at least one PD. Another study of completed suicides (Isometsä et al. 1996) concluded that 29.3% of the sample met criteria for at least one PD. Although research evidence supports an association between a number of PD diagnoses and death by suicide, only borderline PD (option D), the best studied of the PDs, has a diagnostic criterion in DSM-5 ("recurrent suicidal behavior, gestures, or threats, or self-mutilating behavior") specifically describing suicidal behavior (American Psychiatric Association 2013). DSM-5 diagnostic criteria for paranoid PD, antisocial PD, and narcissistic PD (options A–C, E) do not include suicidality. **(Oldham JM, Skodol AE, Bender DS [eds]: APP Textbook of Personality Disorders, 2nd Edition, Chapter 18, pp. 385–389)**

References

American Psychiatric Association: Diagnostic and Statistical Manual of Mental Disorders, 5th Edition. Arlington, VA, American Psychiatric Association, 2013

Blair RJ: The roles of orbital frontal cortex in the modulation of antisocial behavior. Brain Cogn 55(1):198–208, 2004 15134853

Buss AH, Durkee A: An inventory for assessing different kinds of hostility. J Consult Psychol 21(4):343–349, 1957 13463189

Coccaro EF, Harvey PD, Kupsaw-Lawrence E, et al: Development of neuropharmacologically based behavioral assessments of impulsive aggressive behavior. J Neuropsychiatry Clin Neurosci 3(2):S44–S51, 1991 1821222

Evans v United States, 883 F.Supp. 124 (SD Miss 1995)

Felthous AR: The duty to warn or protect to prevent automobile accidents, in American Psychiatric Press Review of Clinical Psychiatry and the Law, Vol 1. Edited by Simon RI. Washington, DC, American Psychiatric Press, 1990, pp 221–238

Fowler JC: Suicide risk assessment in clinical practice: pragmatic guidelines for imperfect assessments. Psychotherapy (Chic) 49(1):81–90, 2012 22369082

Green v Ross, 691 So.2d 542 (Fla. 2d DCA 1997)

Isometsä ET, Henriksson MM, Heikkinen ME, et al: Suicide among subjects with personality disorders. Am J Psychiatry 153(5):667–673, 1996 8615412

Lieberman JA, Stroup TS, McEvoy JP, et al; Clinical Antipsychotic Trials of Intervention Effectiveness (CATIE) Investigators: Effectiveness of antipsychotic drugs in patients with chronic schizophrenia. N Engl J Med 353(12):1209–1223, 2005 16172203

Luria AR: Higher Cortical Functions in Man. New York, Basic Books, 1980

Megargee EI, Cook PE, Mendelsohn GA: Development and validation of an MMPI scale of assaultiveness in overcontrolled individuals. J Abnorm Psychol 72(6):519–528, 1967 4383844

Restatement [Second] of Torts 315(a) (1965)

Schneider B, Wetterling T, Sargk D, et al: Axis I disorders and personality disorders as risk factors for suicide. Eur Arch Psychiatry Clin Neurosci 256(1):17–27, 2006 16133739

Séguin JR: Neurocognitive elements of antisocial behavior: Relevance of an orbitofrontal cortex account. Brain Cogn 55(1):185–197, 2004 15134852

Spielberger CD: State-Trait Anger Expression Inventory–2. Odessa, FL, Psychological Assessment Resources, 1999

Swanson JW, Swartz MS, Van Dorn RA, et al; CATIE investigators: Comparison of antipsychotic medication effects on reducing violence in people with schizophrenia. Br J Psychiatry 193(1):37–43, 2008 18700216

Swartz MS, Wagner HR, Swanson JW, et al: Substance use in persons with schizophrenia: baseline prevalence and correlates from the NIMH CATIE study. J Nerv Ment Dis 194(3):164–172, 2006 16534433

Tarasoff v Regents of the University of California, 17 Cal.3d 425, 551 P.2d 334; 131 Cal. Rptr. 14 (1976)

Thapar v Zezulka, 944 S.W.2d 635 (Tex. 1999)

Weiger WA, Bear DM: An approach to the neurology of aggression. J Psychiatr Res 22(2):85–98, 1988 3042990

CHAPTER 5

Depressive Disorders

5.1 What is the most likely DSM-5 (American Psychiatric Association 2013) diagnosis for a child presenting with persistent, chronic irritability and frequent episodes of extreme behavioral dyscontrol?

A. Pediatric bipolar disorder.
B. Disruptive mood dysregulation disorder.
C. Oppositional defiant disorder.
D. Attention-deficit/hyperactivity disorder.
E. Major depressive disorder.

The correct response is option B: Disruptive mood dysregulation disorder.

Disruptive mood dysregulation disorder (DMDD) is a disorder with acute temperamental outbursts on a background of chronic irritability (option B). In contrast, pediatric bipolar disorder is characterized by discrete episodic periods of mood disturbance with euphoria, grandiosity, racing thoughts, and lack of need for sleep in a sustained energized state (option A). Oppositional defiant disorder is frequently found in children with DMDD; however, the presence of chronic symptoms of irritability suggests DMDD as opposed to oppositional defiant disorder (option C). Attention-deficit/hyperactivity disorder may frequently coexist with DMDD but is not characterized by the profound outbursts of temper (option D). Major depressive disorder and dysthymia often have irritability as a prominent clinical symptom but also lack frequent episodes of extreme behavioral dyscontrol (option E). **(Hales RE, Yudofsky SC, Roberts LW [eds]: APP Textbook of Psychiatry, 6th Edition, Chapter 11, pp. 361–362)**

5.2 Which of the following agents is most likely to cause substance-induced depressive disorder in the context of withdrawal?

A. Interferon.
B. Reserpine.
C. Propranolol.

D. Dextroamphetamine.

E. Prednisone.

The correct response is option D: Dextroamphetamine.

Depression has been clearly associated with the *use* of various substances, such as interferon (option A), reserpine (option B), β-blockers (option C), and steroids (option E). The *withdrawal* of substances may precipitate a depression; in particular, the stimulant substances are notorious for contributing to a depressive crash after a period of heavy use and bingeing (option D). **(Hales RE, Yudofsky SC, Roberts LW [eds]: APP Textbook of Psychiatry, 6th Edition, Chapter 11, pp. 380–381)**

5.3   Which of the following symptoms would suggest the presence of a major depressive episode *in addition to* a normal and expected response to a significant loss (e.g., bereavement, financial ruin, natural disaster)?

A. Intense sadness.

B. Ruminations about the loss.

C. Insomnia.

D. Poor appetite.

E. Feelings of worthlessness.

The correct response is option E: Feelings of worthlessness.

Symptoms resembling a major depressive episode, including intense sadness (option A), ruminations about the loss (option B), insomnia (option C), poor appetite (option D), and weight loss, can be part of a normal and expected response to a loss. Other symptoms are less commonly associated with bereavement, including feelings of worthlessness (option E), suicidal ideation (distinct from wanting to join a deceased loved one), psychomotor retardation, and severe impairment in overall functioning. Bereavement is no longer considered an exclusion to a depressive disorder diagnosis within the first 2 months of the loss. **(Hales RE, Yudofsky SC, Roberts LW [eds]: APP Textbook of Psychiatry, 6th Edition, Chapter 11, pp. 363–366)**

5.4   Which of the following symptoms should alert the physician to the possible presence of depression in a patient with a serious medical condition?

A. Anhedonia.

B. Weight loss.

C. Fatigue.

D. Hypersomnia.

E. Insomnia.

The correct response is option A: Anhedonia.

The diagnostic formulation of the symptoms of a major depressive episode is especially difficult when they occur in an individual who also has a general medical condition (e.g., cancer, stroke, myocardial infarction, diabetes, pregnancy). Some of the criterion signs and symptoms of a major depressive episode are identical to those of general medical conditions (e.g., weight loss with untreated diabetes [option B], fatigue with cancer [option C], hypersomnia early in pregnancy [option D], insomnia later in pregnancy or during the postpartum period [option E]). Such symptoms count toward a major depressive diagnosis except when they are clearly and fully attributable to a general medical condition. Nonvegetative symptoms of dysphoria, anhedonia, guilt or worthlessness, impaired concentration or indecision, and suicidal thoughts should be assessed with particular care in such cases (option A). **(Hales RE, Yudofsky SC, Roberts LW [eds]: APP Textbook of Psychiatry, 6th Edition, Chapter 11, p. 369)**

5.5　A 30-year-old woman reports 2 years of persistently depressed mood, accompanied by loss of pleasure in all activities, ruminations that she would be better off dead, feelings of guilt about "bad things" she has done, and thoughts about quitting work because of her inability to make decisions. Although she has never been treated for depression, she feels so distressed at times that she wonders if she should be hospitalized. She experiences an increased need for sleep but still feels fatigued during the day. Her overeating has led to a 12-kg weight gain. She denies drug or alcohol use, and her medical workup is completely normal, including laboratory tests of vitamins. The consultation was prompted by her worsened mood for the past several weeks. What is the most appropriate DSM-5 diagnosis?

A. Major depressive disorder.
B. Persistent depressive disorder (dysthymia), with persistent major depressive episode.
C. Cyclothymia.
D. Bipolar II disorder.
E. Major depressive disorder, with melancholic features.

The correct response is option B: Persistent depressive disorder (dysthymia), with persistent major depressive episode.

The essential feature of persistent depressive disorder (dysthymia) is a depressed mood that occurs for most of the day, for more days than not, for at least 2 years. This disorder represents a consolidation of DSM-IV–defined chronic major depressive disorder and dysthymic disorder (American Psychiatric Association 1994). Major depression may precede persistent depressive disorder, and major depressive episodes may occur during persistent depressive disorder. Individuals whose symptoms meet major depressive disorder criteria for 2 years should be given a diagnosis of persistent depressive disorder as well as major depressive disorder.

If there is a depressed mood plus two or more symptoms meeting criteria for a persistent depressive episode for 2 years or more, then the diagnosis of persistent depressive disorder is made. The diagnosis depends on the 2-year duration, which distinguishes it from episodes of depression that do not last 2 years (option A). If the symptom criteria are sufficient for a diagnosis of major depressive episode at any time during this period, then the diagnosis of major depression should be noted; however, it is coded not as a separate diagnosis but rather as a specifier with the diagnosis of persistent depressive disorder. If the individual's symptoms currently meet full criteria for a major depressive episode, then the specifier "with intermittent major depressive episodes, with current episode" would be applied. If—as in the patient described in the above vignette—the major depressive episode has persisted for at least a 2-year duration and remains present, then the specifier "with persistent major depressive episode" is used (option B). When full major depressive episode criteria are not currently met but there has been at least one previous episode of major depression in the context of at least 2 years of persistent depressive symptoms, then the specifier "with intermittent major depressive episodes, without current episode" is used. If the individual has not experienced an episode of major depression in the past 2 years, then the specifier "with pure dysthymic syndrome" is used.

The patient described in the vignette does not provide a history of having had prior hypomanic episodes or episodes of subsyndromal mood elevation, making diagnoses of bipolar II disorder (option D) and cyclothymia (option C), respectively, unlikely. In addition to the diagnosis of major depressive disorder being insufficient for capturing the chronicity of the symptoms, the symptoms described in the vignette of hypersomnia, overeating, and weight gain are more consistent with an "atypical features" specifier than with a "melancholic features" specifier (option E). **(DSM-5, Depressive Disorders, pp. 168–171, 184–186)**

5.6   Which of the following is one of the core symptoms required to meet DSM-5 criteria for premenstrual dysphoric disorder?

A. Marked affective lability.
B. Decreased interest in usual activities.
C. Physical symptoms such as breast tenderness.
D. Marked change in appetite.
E. A sense of feeling overwhelmed or out of control.

The correct response is option A: Marked affective lability.

Of the 11 symptoms listed in the DSM-5 premenstrual dysphoric disorder diagnostic criteria, the patient must have a total of at least five symptoms. One of the five must be one of the following symptoms: 1) marked affective lability (option A); 2) marked irritability or anger or increased interpersonal conflicts; 3) marked depressed mood, feelings of hopelessness, or self-deprecating thoughts; and 4) marked anxiety, tension, and/or feelings of being keyed up or on edge. Decreased interest in usual activities (option B); subjective difficulty in concentration; lethargy, easy fatigability, or marked lack of energy; marked change in appetite (option D); hypersomnia or insomnia; a sense of being overwhelmed or out of control (option E); and physical symptoms such as breast tenderness (option C) may also be included among the five symptoms but are not among the core symptoms required to make the diagnosis. **(DSM-5, Depressive Disorders, pp. 171–172)**

References

American Psychiatric Association: Diagnostic and Statistical Manual of Mental Disorders, 4th Edition. Washington, DC, American Psychiatric Association, 1994

American Psychiatric Association: Diagnostic and Statistical Manual of Mental Disorders, 5th Edition. Arlington, VA, American Psychiatric Association, 2013

CHAPTER 6

Development: Adulthood

6.1 Socioemotional selectivity theory explains how older adults experience life events differently than younger adults, which may explain the lower frequency of major depression in the older adult community. Which of the following is a tenet of that theory?

A. Younger adults are motivated by the pursuit of pleasure.
B. Younger adults have much to learn and too little time to learn.
C. Younger adults pursue knowledge augmented with emotional well-being.
D. Older adults ruminate on their negative life experiences.
E. Older adults prioritize emotionally meaningful goals.

The correct response is option E: Older adults prioritize emotionally meaningful goals.

Socioemotional selectivity theory may explain differences across the life cycle in the experience of events that lead to depression (Carstensen et al. 2000). The theory focuses on the perception by older persons of time left in life, rather than on past experiences. Younger adults have much to learn and relatively long futures over which to learn (option B). They are motivated by pursuit of knowledge, even when this requires that they suppress emotional well-being (option C). In contrast, elders perceive that they have lived longer than they should live and therefore deemphasize negative experience (option D) and prioritize emotionally meaningful goals (option E). In one study, negative emotional experiences (e.g., the perception of stressors) declined from young adulthood until around age 60 (Carstensen et al. 2000). Periods of highly positive emotional experience endured as meaningful among older adults compared with younger adults. Option A may be true but is not part of socioemotional selectivity theory. **(Steffens DC, Blazer DG, Thakur ME [eds]: The APP Textbook of Geriatric Psychiatry, 5th Edition, Chapter 9, p. 257)**

6.2   Which of the following best describes the age at which individuals become aware of their sexual or gender identity?

A. Childhood.
B. Adolescence.
C. Young adults.
D. Midlife.
E. It varies among different patients.

The correct response is option E: It varies among different patients.

People become aware of sexual or gender identity at different times in life (option E). Some individuals become aware of this identity in childhood (option A), others in adolescence (option B), still others as young adults (option C), and some in midlife or later (option D). There also are differing ages at onset in individuals experiencing gender dysphoria. **(Hales RE, Yudofsky SC, Roberts LW [eds]: APP Textbook of Psychiatry, 6th Edition, Chapter 37, p. 1296)**

6.3   What is the name of the developmental stage when people transition from home to college, reflecting a shift in relationship to family and sense of autonomy and self-determination?

A. Adolescence proper.
B. Early adolescence.
C. Middle adolescence.
D. Late adolescence.
E. Emerging adulthood.

The correct response is option D: Late adolescence.

Late adolescence begins with the transition from home to college and marks a significant shift in adolescents' relationship to family and their sense of autonomy and self-determination (option D). Beginning in the senior year of high school, particularly after college applications are in, there is increasing anticipation of college life, which portends release from parental supervision and the opportunity to make independent choices about the future. *Adolescence proper* (option A) involves three major intrapsychic developments: integration of the sexual self and romantic longings into the self-representation, the second individuation, and the identity crisis. *Early adolescence* (age 11 or 12 through 14 years; option B), is centered on transformation of the body with prepubertal growth spurt and secondary sexual characteristics. *Middle adolescence* (age 14 or 15 through 18 years; option C) is a peak conflictual moment in parent-child relationships as teenagers' increasing independence makes the task of knowing how and when to intervene, set limits, and guide behavior a tremendous challenge for parents. *Emerging adulthood* (option E) reflects a notable generational shift in the achievement of adult markers. **(Hales RE, Yudofsky SC, Roberts LW [eds]: APP Textbook of Psychiatry, 6th Edition, Chapter 5, pp. 158–166)**

6.4 James Arnett coined the term *emerging adulthood*, referring to a postponement of traditional adulthood markers such as marriage, starting a family, and independent living. Which of the following items is a criterion of this stage?

A. Financial explorations.
B. Stability.
C. Outward focus.
D. Feeling in-between.
E. Narrowing of possibilities.

The correct response is option D: Feeling in-between.

Arnett (2000) proposed five criteria for this stage: identity explorations (option A), instability (option B), self-focus (option C), feeling in-between (option D), and a widening of possibilities (option E). **(Hales RE, Yudofsky SC, Roberts LW [eds]: APP Textbook of Psychiatry, 6th Edition, Chapter 5, p. 166)**

6.5 According to James Arnett, which risky behavior peaks in emerging adulthood?

A. Alcohol abuse.
B. Amphetamine abuse.
C. Benzodiazepine abuse.
D. Cannabis abuse.
E. Cocaine abuse.

The correct response is option A: Alcohol abuse.

For emerging adults in twenty-first-century Western society, after a period of exploration in college, identity is extended, revisited, and resized for the adult world. Some risky behaviors actually peak in emerging adulthood, especially alcohol consumption (option A) (Arnett 2000). Options B–E occur but do not peak in this developmental period. **(Hales RE, Yudofsky SC, Roberts LW [eds]: APP Textbook of Psychiatry, 6th Edition, Chapter 5, p. 167)**

6.6 After a therapy session during which a patient expressed frustration at his job, the therapist relates to these feelings at her own workplace. This feeling of counter-transference, or emotional reaction of the therapist to the patient, may be affected by how the therapist hears the patient. Which of the following is the most likely to exert such an influence on the therapist?

A. The patient's transference to the therapist.
B. The therapist's conscious conflicts.
C. The increased clarity of the therapist's judgment.
D. The developmental period of the therapist's life.
E. The lack of intensity of the transference.

The correct response is option D: The developmental period of the therapist's life.

Countertransference is the emotional reaction of the therapist to the patient. Historically, countertransference was limited in meaning to the therapist's transference onto the patient. This was felt to be a response to the patient's transference (option A). Like all transferences, the therapist's countertransference was the result of unconscious conflicts (option B); however, these unresolved conflicts were those of the therapist rather than those of the patient. This countertransference was thought to obscure the therapist's judgment (option C) in conducting the therapy (Gabbard 1995; Gabbard and Wilkinson 2001). Countertransferences are many and varied. Often, they are the result of events occurring in the therapist's life that may make him or her more sensitive to certain themes in the patient's associations. The developmental period (option D) of the therapist's life—involving issues of intimacy, achievement, or old age, for example—may also affect how the therapist hears the patient. Intense transferences (option E) of all kinds—erotic, aggressive, devaluing, idealizing, and others—are ripe for serving as stimuli to awaken in the therapist elements of his or her own past. **(Hales RE, Yudofsky SC, Roberts LW [eds]: APP Textbook of Psychiatry, 6th Edition, Chapter 30, p. 1085)**

6.7   In some Asian cultures, women who graduate from college typically move back home while working in their first job after graduation. It is a cultural expectation that they live with their parents until they get married, and while living at home, they do not pay rent and remain somewhat dependent on their parents. This situation reflects which developmental phase?

   A. Adolescence proper.
   B. Early adolescence.
   C. Middle adolescence.
   D. Late adolescence.
   E. Emerging adulthood.

The correct response is option E: Emerging adulthood.

The existence of the emerging adulthood phase reflects a notable generational shift in terms of the achievement of adult markers (option E). In twenty-first-century Western society, the typical markers of adulthood—the concrete accomplishments of independent living, marriage, starting a family, and career—have been postponed. For example, in 1960, about 44% of male and 68% of female 25-year-olds had accomplished all of the traditional indicators of adulthood (employment, marriage, parenthood, financial independence), whereas in 2000, only 13% of males and 25% of females had done so (Furstenberg 2010).

   Adolescence proper (option A) involves three major intrapsychic developments: integration of the sexual self and romantic longings into the self-representation, the second individuation, and the identity crisis. *Early adolescence* (age 11 or 12 through 14 years; option B) is centered on transformation of the body with prepubertal growth spurt and secondary sexual characteristics. *Middle adolescence* (age 14 or 15 through 18 years; option C) is a peak conflictual moment in parent-child relationships as teenagers' increasing independence makes the task of knowing how and when to intervene, set limits, and guide behavior a tremendous challenge for parents. *Late adolescence* (option D) begins with the transition from home to college and marks a significant shift in adolescents' relationship to family and their sense of autonomy and self-determination. **(Hales RE, Yudofsky SC, Roberts LW [eds]: APP Textbook of Psychiatry, 6th Edition, Chapter 5, pp. 158–166)**

6.8   Which of the following is a task of emerging adulthood?

A. Disregard the accepted path toward autonomous living.
B. Move back to the family to reassess the value of career achievements.
C. Complete identity exploration in the adult world.
D. Renegotiate family relationships toward inequality.
E. Postpone the capacity to love, commit to, and depend on a significant other.

The correct response is option C: Complete identity exploration in the adult world.

The following are key tasks of emerging adulthood: to complete identity exploration in the adult world (option C); to negotiate the path toward achievement of the so-called adult milestones, including autonomous living, career, marriage, and child rearing (options A, B); to renegotiate family relationships toward equality (option D); and to develop the capacity to love, commit to, and depend on a significant other (option E). **(Hales RE, Yudofsky SC, Roberts LW [eds]: APP Textbook of Psychiatry, 6th Edition, Chapter 5, p. 167 and Table 5–8, p. 167)**

6.9   Erik Erikson's stage theory of late-life development indicates that the major developmental task of older age is to look back and seek meaning across the lifespan, rather than looking forward. The task is to maintain more integrity than despair about one's life. Each earlier life stage conflict must be reconciled and integrated with the current stage, allowing resolution of earlier conflicts. Which of the following describes what might occur for persons with personality disorders in late life?

A. Have an easier time in accomplishing this resolution compared with others.
B. Have a similar path of accomplishing this resolution compared with others.
C. Have accomplished this resolution completely or not at all.
D. Have some conflict resolution and mellowing in their personality disorder.
E. Have no change since the factors that affect healthy adjustment do not change.

The correct response is option D: Have some conflict resolution and mellowing in their personality disorder.

Erikson was a strong proponent of the interaction of the psychosocial environment with development across the lifespan. Erikson et al. (1986) proposed that the major developmental task of older age is to look back and seek meaning across the lifespan. The goal of this task, as discussed by Erikson, is to maintain more integrity than despair about one's life. In this process, as at previous life stages, each earlier life stage conflict must be reconciled and integrated with the current stage, allowing resolution of earlier conflicts. Persons with personality disorders might be expected to have greater difficulty in accomplishing this resolution than other individuals (options A, B). However, this resolution is not an all-or-nothing phenomenon (option C). The achievement of even some resolution may contribute to the mellowing of a personality disorder (option D). As Vaillant (2012) has pointed out through his extended involvement with longitudinal research, "If you follow lives long enough, they change as do the factors that affect healthy adjustment" (option E). **(Steffens DC, Blazer DG, Thakur ME [eds]: The APP Textbook of Geriatric Psychiatry, 5th Edition, Chapter 18, p. 496)**

6.10 Adults acquire more wisdom as they age. Baltes and Staudinger (2000) consider wisdom to be an expert knowledge system concerning the fundamental pragmatics of life. Which of the following statements is most consistent with this definition of wisdom?

A. Factual knowledge is unrelated to wisdom.
B. Procedural knowledge is the only measure of wisdom.
C. Wise people have difficulty integrating life experiences.
D. Tolerance for differences in society is relatively unimportant.
E. Wise individuals can recognize and manage uncertainty.

The correct response is option E: Wise individuals can recognize and manage uncertainty.

Wisdom is an expert knowledge system concerning the fundamental pragmatics of life, including knowledge and judgment about the meaning and conduct of life and the orchestrating of human development toward excellence while attending conjointly to personal and collective well-being. Five criteria can be used to assess wisdom: rich factual knowledge (option A); rich procedural knowledge (e.g., the ability to develop strategies for addressing problems) (option B, not the *only* measure of wisdom); lifespan contextualization (e.g., integrating life experiences) (option C); relativism of values and life priorities (e.g., tolerance for differences in society) (option D); and recognition and management of uncertainty (accepting that the future cannot be known with certainty and that the ability to assess one's sociocultural environment is inherently constrained) (option E). **(Steffens DC, Blazer DG, Thakur ME [eds]: APP Textbook of Geriatric Psychiatry, 5th Edition, Chapter 9, p. 257)**

References

Arnett JJ: Emerging adulthood. A theory of development from the late teens through the twenties. Am Psychol 55(5):469–480, 2000 10842426

Baltes PB, Staudinger UM: Wisdom. A metaheuristic (pragmatic) to orchestrate mind and virtue toward excellence. Am Psychol 55(1):122–136, 2000 11392856

Carstensen LL, Pasupathi M, Mayr U, Nesselroade JR: Emotional experience in everyday life across the adult life span. J Pers Soc Psychol 79(4):644–655, 2000 11045744

Erikson EH, Erikson JM, Kivnick HQ: Vital Involvement in Old Age. New York, WW Norton, 1986

Furstenberg FF Jr: On a new schedule: transitions to adulthood and family change. Future Child 20(1):67–87, 2010 20364622

Gabbard GO: Countertransference: the emerging common ground. Int J Psychoanal 76(Pt 3):475–485, 1995 7558607

Gabbard GO, Wilkinson SM: Management of Countertransference With Borderline Patients. Washington, DC, American Psychiatric Press, 2001

Vaillant GE: Triumphs of Experience: The Men of the Harvard Grant Study. Cambridge, MA, London, England, 2012

CHAPTER 7

Development: Infancy Through Adolescence

7.1 Mary Ainsworth's "Strange Situation" research on patterns of attachment examined the quality of the mother-child relationship in children of what age?

A. Age 2 months.
B. Age 6 months.
C. Age 12 months.
D. Age 2 years.
E. Age 3 years.

The correct response is option C: Age 12 months.

Ainsworth's seminal research on patterns of attachment examined the secure base behaviors in 12- to 18-month-old children in order to assess the quality of the mother-infant relationship (option C is correct; options A, B, D, E are incorrect) (Ainsworth et al. 1978). In the widely replicated Strange Situation experiment, mother and child are observed in a laboratory playroom as they are exposed to a sequence of 3-minute events that stress the infant's sense of security. After a period of playing and acclimating to the new environment, the dyad is joined by a stranger (stranger anxiety). Then the mother departs (separation anxiety). The mother reenters and then both adults exit, leaving the baby briefly alone. When the mother returns to the baby, particular attention is paid to the quality of their reunion; this is considered the most potent indicator of the quality of attachment security. **(Hales RE, Yudofsky SC, Roberts LW [eds]: APP Textbook of Psychiatry, 6th Edition, Chapter 5, p. 144)**

7.2 At what age do most children begin to develop a gendered sense of self?

A. Age 14 months.
B. Age 2 years.
C. Age 3 years.

D. Age 4 years.

E. Age 5 years.

The correct response is option B: Age 2 years.

By around the age of 2 years, most children begin to acquire a gendered sense of self (option B is correct; options A, C–E are incorrect). Children accurately label themselves as boy or girl; positive and negative self-feelings accrue to the toddler's notion of male and female. A full understanding of gender concepts—that is, of the link between one's sex and genitalia, the stability of one's sex, and the idiosyncratic but shared meanings of gender—is not grasped until several years later, toward the close of the oedipal phase (De Marneffe 1997). **(Hales RE, Yudofsky SC, Roberts LW [eds]: APP Textbook of Psychiatry, 6th Edition, Chapter 5, p. 146)**

7.3   Using puppets, the following scenario is presented to a normally developing 5-year-old child: "Jane is playing with a doll in the bedroom she shares with her sister, Eliza. She places the doll on her bed, then leaves to go into the kitchen. While she is gone, her sister Eliza enters, plays with the doll, places it in the toy chest, and leaves the room. When Jane returns to the bedroom, where will she look first for the doll—on the bed or in the toy chest?" How would one expect this child to answer?

A. "On the bed."

B. "In the toy chest."

C. "In the kitchen."

D. A child would be unable to comprehend this question at 5 years of age.

E. "Sister Eliza has the toy."

The correct response is option A: "On the bed."

The acquisition of a theory of mind, or understanding of mental states, is a transformational process in development, usually demonstrable by the age of 4 years. In the numerous studies that have investigated theory of mind development, false belief tests are often used to assess whether children can successfully discern another person's point of view and then predict behavior based on that individual's knowledge. Typically, 3-year-olds have trouble with the puppet task described and tend to reach faulty conclusions: they assume that Jane knows what they know and respond that she will look in the chest (option B). Four- and 5-year-olds, however, answer correctly (option D) that Jane will look on the bed (option A) because she has no knowledge of Eliza's activities (options C, E); moreover, older children grasp a fundamental principle of mental state knowledge—that is, that people's private beliefs, even when false, nonetheless guide their behavior. **(Hales RE, Yudofsky SC, Roberts LW [eds]: APP Textbook of Psychiatry, 6th Edition, Chapter 5, pp. 149–150)**

7.4   Which of the following is an innate behavior exhibited by newborns that elicits caregiver responsiveness and engagement?

A. Social referencing.
B. Separation anxiety.
C. Joint attention.
D. Stranger anxiety.
E. Sucking.

The correct response is option E: Sucking.

The newborn is innately equipped for social responsiveness. Behaviors that are available at or soon after birth, such as sucking (option E), crying, and smiling, help the baby seek and maintain proximity to the parent. These are manifestations of a biologically based attachment system (Bowlby 1969) that ensures the infant's physical and emotional survival. Social referencing, joint attention, separation anxiety, and stranger anxiety (options A–D) are all capacities that develop later in infancy. **(Hales RE, Yudofsky SC, Roberts LW [eds]: APP Textbook of Psychiatry, 6th Edition, Chapter 5, pp. 141–144)**

7.5   In the "still-face" experiment, the sudden loss of an affectively reciprocal interaction with the parent would likely cause a healthily attached infant to exhibit which of the following?

A. Acute distress, crying, and averting the gaze.
B. A mirrored impassive, unresponsive expression.
C. Social smiling with playful affect.
D. No change in affect or behavior.
E. Cooing and babbling.

The correct response is option A: Acute distress, crying, and averting the gaze.

Beginning at 2–3 months with the emergence of social smiling, the infant enters a period of intense social interest and availability. Dyadic face-to-face exchanges with the parent bring tremendous pleasure and excitement to both; these affectively reciprocal interactions are comprised of continuous, largely unconscious processes of mutual self-regulating shifts and gestures (Beebe 2000). Young infants' sensitivity to their parents' interactive style is illustrated in the still-face experiment, wherein mothers are instructed to engage in normal face-to-face behavior, followed by a "still-face" (i.e., an impassive, unresponsive expression). When confronted with a nonreactive parent, babies exhibit acute distress, frequently crying and averting their gazes (option A) (Tronick et al. 1978). Positive reactions such as social smiling and cooing would not be expected (options C, E), and no change in behavior or mirrored impassive reactions (i.e., the baby's affect becomes flat and unresponsive) would trigger concern for the lack of a healthy attachment (options B, D). **(Hales RE, Yudofsky SC, Roberts LW [eds]: APP Textbook of Psychiatry, 6th Edition, Chapter 5, p. 143)**

7.6   At around what age do children begin to look at and attempt to "read" the facial expressions of others to obtain emotional clues to guide their own behavior?

   A. Between 0 and 2 months.
   B. Between 4 and 6 months.
   C. Between 8 and 10 months.
   D. Between 12 and 14 months.
   E. Between 16 and 18 months.

The correct response is option C: Between 8 and 10 months.

A momentous shift in the baby's social and emotional capacities becomes evident at 8–10 months of age as he or she actively begins to seek shared mental experience with the parent (option C). For the first time, the infant engages in *joint attention,* gazing back and forth from the mother's face to a toy of mutual focus. An emerging propensity for *social referencing,* the deliberate soliciting and use of the parent's emotional state (referenced in the question stem), is demonstrated in the visual cliff experiment: in this paradigm, crawling infants are placed on an apparent visual drop-off; when their mothers smile and beckon, the children cross the "cliff," but when their mothers manifest fear or alarm, the babies refuse to move (Sorce and Emde 1981). This remarkable capacity to use the mother's expression as a guide serves as an extension of the attachment system into more complex, distal exchanges. **(Hales RE, Yudofsky SC, Roberts LW [eds]: APP Textbook of Psychiatry, 6th Edition, Chapter 5, p. 143)**

7.7   In Mary Ainsworth's "Strange Situation," a child with secure attachment would be expected to behave in which of the following ways?

   A. Exhibit minimal observable distress when the parent departs.
   B. Show difficulty reuniting with the parent after the brief separation.
   C. Display no distress when alone with the stranger.
   D. Display difficult-to-control anger even before the mother has left the room.
   E. Explore the environment comfortably while the mother is near.

The correct response is option E: Explore the environment comfortably while the mother is near.

Ainsworth's original Strange Situation research yielded three distinct types of attachment (Ainsworth et al. 1978). Secure babies acclimate to the unfamiliar room and explore comfortably while the mother is near (option E), evidence distress during separation, and are easily comforted by the parent's return. The absence of observable distress with separation (option A) and a difficult reunification with the parent (option B) are not observed with a securely attached baby. In contrast to secure babies, avoidant children appear less connected, and their expression of emotionality is muted (option C); they pay little overt attention to the mother's comings and goings despite less observable somatic evidence of distress. Ambivalent/resistant babies—not securely attached babies—manifest angry, upset, poorly regulated reactions: they are hard to settle even before the mother has left the room (option D) and fail to use her proximity for soothing and self-regulation (including upon reunification; option B). More recently, Main and Solomon (1990) identified children with disorganized/disoriented attachments whose inconsistent and incoherent reactions to separation indicated a particular vulnerability to poor self-regulation. **(Hales RE, Yudofsky SC, Roberts LW [eds]: APP Textbook of Psychiatry, 6th Edition, Chapter 5, pp. 143–144)**

7.8   At around what age do children become able to recognize themselves in a mirror?

A. Age 6 months.
B. Age 12 months.
C. Age 18 months.
D. Age 24 months.
E. Age 36 months.

The correct response is option C: Age 18 months.

As the baby enters the toddler period, he or she begins to acquire knowledge about the self as a separate, objective entity. Empirically, this major leap of self-awareness is illustrated via mirror self-recognition, a clever experiment wherein children are placed in front of a mirror after their noses are surreptitiously rouged; beginning at around 18 months (option C), toddlers tend to smile and attempt to remove the marks from their own noses rather than merely pointing toward their reflections (Lewis and Brooks-Gunn 1979). **(Hales RE, Yudofsky SC, Roberts LW [eds]: APP Textbook of Psychiatry, 6th Edition, Chapter 5, p. 145)**

7.9   Which of the following is a major developmental goal of late adolescence?

A. Exclusion of sexuality from the self-representation.
B. Dependence on parental values and morals.
C. Establishment of peer relationships and group activities.
D. Revision/reworking of the superego.
E. Use of sublimation to deal with feelings and impulses.

The correct response is option D: Revision/reworking of the superego.

Late adolescence begins with the transition from home to college and marks a significant shift in adolescents' relationships to family and their sense of autonomy and self-determination. The search for self-selected "new developmental objects" (i.e., adults available for idealization and identification) is guided in the college or employment setting by the young person's more conscious and deliberate interests and beliefs: the choice of a mentor facilitates the gradual revision of the superego that is the work of late adolescence (option D). In contrast to the youngster's earlier dependence on parental values and morals (option B), the grip of parental values diminishes as the older adolescent is exposed to a vastly expanded world; with this loosening, new identifications develop that are at least in part directed by self-selected interests and ideals. Another task of this period is containment and integration—not exclusion (option A)—of sexuality to facilitate intimate relationships. Establishment of peer relationships and group activities and the use of sublimation to deal with feelings and impulses (options C, E) are both tasks of the latency period (ages 6–10 years) and not of late adolescence. **(Hales RE, Yudofsky SC, Roberts LW [eds]: APP Textbook of Psychiatry, 6th Edition, Chapter 5, pp. 164–165 and Table 5–7, p. 166)**

7.10 A 2-year-old mimics his mother vacuuming around the house. Which of the following describes this behavior?

A. Social fantasy play.
B. Basic early pretend play.
C. Parallel play.
D. Social referencing.
E. Joint attention.

The correct response is option B: Basic early pretend play.

Pretend play is a natural, growth-promoting developmental capacity that provides a window into the child's inner life. Vygotsky (1978) noted that in play, "the child is always behaving beyond his age": narrative building, dialogue creation, social perspective taking, and elaborate planning are in evidence as the child acts out deeply satisfying imaginary roles and plots (option B). By age 4 or 5 years, a particular type of play—*social fantasy play* (also known as *dual symbolic play*)—is a core feature of peer relationships, encouraging the need to collaborate, verbally share intentions, and incorporate others' ideas and desires (option A) (Howe et al. 2005). *Parallel play* is a particular form of play in which each child engages in independent activities adjacent to one another, but they do not try to influence or share each other's behaviors (option C). *Social referencing* is the deliberate soliciting and use of the parent's emotional state (option D). *Joint attention* emerges at 8–10 months of age and is exemplified by an infant's gazing back and forth from the mother's face to an object of mutual focus (e.g., a toy) (option E). **(Hales RE, Yudofsky SC, Roberts LW [eds]: APP Textbook of Psychiatry, 6th Edition, Chapter 5, pp. 143–144, 150)**

7.11 What does the play of a 5-year-old boy with an imaginary companion suggest?

A. He is among a significant minority of children 5–12 years of age who report sharing such experiences.
B. He is likely psychotic and responding to hallucinations.
C. He may have exemplary communication skills.
D. He has never experienced any unwanted psychodynamic urges or impulses.
E. He inevitably will experience conflict with his parents regarding this companion.

The correct response is option C: He may have exemplary communication skills.

Imaginary companions are a commonly observed phenomenon in normally developing children that begins during the oedipal years and, as such, does not suggest inherent pathology (option B); a survey of children 5–12 years of age reported that 46% of children acknowledged an imaginary companion currently or in the past (option A) (Pearson et al. 2001). These invented creatures often serve as the repository of the child's unwanted impulses while providing their creators with a sense of control and power (option D). For example, a preschooler wrestling with self-control and fears of bodily injury may find consolation in a friendly, domesticated, but nonetheless invincible lion or tiger that requires frequent admonishments and behavioral restrictions. Interestingly, children with access to this imaginary vehicle show richer narratives and greater communication skills (option C). As is true with the transitional objects of infancy, parents instinctively tend to tolerate the companion's existence and refrain from challenging its basis in reality (option E). **(Hales RE, Yudofsky SC, Roberts LW [eds]: APP Textbook of Psychiatry, 6th Edition, Chapter 5, p. 151)**

7.12   As part of a school project, a 12-year-old girl designs a science experiment, beginning with the formulation of an initial hypothesis that she plans to test. This cognitive ability marks a transition to which of Piaget's stages?

A. Concrete operational stage.
B. Formal operational stage.
C. Preoperational stage.
D. Sensorimotor stage.
E. Presensorimotor stage.

The correct response is option B: Formal operational stage.

In the *sensorimotor* stage (birth to 18 months of age; option D), the child actively constructs information about the world via physical explorations and actions (Piaget and Inhelder 1969). The *preoperational* stage (from 18 months to 7 years of age; option C) is marked by *object permanence* and more abstract symbolic functions, such as word combinations, deferred imitation, and early forms of pretense. Children enter the *concrete operational* stage at around age 7 years (option A) (Piaget and Inhelder 1969). This stage brings an increasing orientation to the reality-based world, and more organized, coherent mental structures allow for internal, rather than action-oriented, problem solving. However, it is not until the *formal operational stage* (option B), which typically begins between the ages of 10 and 12 years, that the cognitive ability outlined in the question develops. Piaget and Inhelder (1969) and Ryan and Kuczkowski (1994) observed this shift to higher-level abstract thinking and hypothetico-deductive reasoning. Piaget did not define a *presensorimotor* stage (option E). **(Hales RE, Yudofsky SC, Roberts LW [eds]: APP Textbook of Psychiatry, 6th Edition, Chapter 5, pp. 143, 146, 154, 161 and Tables 5–3, 5–6, pp. 148, 159)**

7.13   What does a teenage girl's expression of disgust for her mother's professional career while idolizing a notorious drug abusing and sexually audacious celebrity
suggest?

A. Second individuation.
B. Contingent response.
C. Decentering.
D. Sublimation.
E. Rapprochement crisis.

The correct response is option A: Second individuation.

The *second individuation,* beginning in the preadolescent phase, refers to the young
teenager's growing need to reconfigure and renegotiate his or her relationship to
parents in order to establish a sense of autonomous identity and self-responsibility
and to achieve "object removal"—in effect, a shift in the focus from the primary
objects of childhood (mother and father) toward appropriate nonincestuous objects (option A). In Blos's formulation, the process is ideally neither fraught with
conflict nor hinged on a physical separation or rejection of parental supports and
values (Blos 1967). However, psychosocial regression (as the teen grapples with
the threat of sexual impulses and the demands of greater responsibility) can result
in occasional "violent ruptures": the adolescent attempts to avoid the backward
pull toward childish dependency by battling with parents. This teenager's behavior can be understood as a regressive attempt to disengage from the mother by a
childish, contrarian idealization. A *contingent response* is a concept that typically
pertains to infancy and is a behavior (frequently that of a caretaker) that closely
corresponds to an individual's (frequently a baby's) signal (option B). *Decentering*
is characteristic of the latency period and represents a shift away from highly subjective, egocentric thinking toward awareness of multiple perspectives, making it
possible to engage in abstract reasoning (option C). *Sublimation* is the transformation of socially unacceptable impulses and feelings into more socially acceptable behaviors or actions, often in the form of structured activities such as
academics and competitive sports (option D). *Rapprochement crisis* (Mahler 1972)
refers to a period during toddlerhood of relative negativity and contradictory behaviors (e.g., shadowing the parent and then darting away), which encompasses
the toddler's competing urges to reestablish the proximity with parents that a toddler typically experienced during infancy and, alternatively, to move toward autonomy, exploration, and mastery (option E). **(Hales RE, Yudofsky SC, Roberts
LW [eds]: APP Textbook of Psychiatry, 6th Edition, Chapter 5, pp. 142–143, 146,
153–155, 160)**

7.14   A child is first asked to make sure that the amounts of water in two identical beakers are the same. The water from one of the beakers is then transferred into a tall, narrow cylinder. The child is asked whether the remaining beaker contains the same amount of water as the tall, narrow cylinder. In which one of Piaget's stages of cognitive maturation would the child insist that because the tall, narrow cylinder is "higher," it must contain more liquid?

A. Preoperational stage.
B. Formal operational stage.
C. Concrete operational stage.
D. Sensorimotor stage.
E. Presensorimotor stage.

The correct response is option A: Preoperational stage.

This question illustrates Piaget's Tests of Conservation, a series of experiments assessing children's abilities to think beyond highly conspicuous physical features. A child's entry into the cognitive period of *concrete operations* (Piaget and Inhelder 1969) at around age 7 years brings an increasing orientation to the reality-based world. Time and money concepts are mastered; collecting, sorting, and classifying materials are favored activities. More organized, coherent mental structures allow for internal, rather than action-oriented, problem solving; this momentous change has huge implications for the child's capacity to substitute thought for behavior and avoid impulsive reactions. Thinking becomes more logical, and the child is less likely to be deceived by the appearance of things; the process of decentering—that is, the shift away from highly subjective, egocentric thinking toward awareness of multiple perspectives—makes it possible to engage in abstract reasoning. Unlike the child's response described in the question, the youngster in the concrete operational stage (option C) grasps that the volumes of water in both the remaining original beaker and the tall, narrow cylinder are the same despite appearances. Given the response of the child described in the question stem, this youngster does not yet understand conservation of quantity and most likely remains in the *preoperational* stage (option A). The preoperational stage (from 18 months to 7 years of age) is marked by *object permanence* and more abstract symbolic functions, such as word combinations, deferred imitation, and early forms of pretense. In the *sensorimotor* stage (birth to 18 months of age), the child actively constructs information about the world via physical explorations and actions. A child in the sensorimotor stage (option D) would not be able to engage or participate in Piaget's Tests of Conservation. In the *formal operational* stage (which typically begins between 10 and 12 years of age), there is higher-level abstract thinking and hypothetico-deductive reasoning. An adolescent in the formal operational stage (option B) would not make the cognitive error described in the question. Finally, Piaget did not define a *presensorimotor* stage (option E). **(Hales RE, Yudofsky SC, Roberts LW [eds]: APP Textbook of Psychiatry, 6th Edition, Chapter 5, pp. 143, 146, 154, 161 and Table 5–3, p. 148)**

References

Ainsworth MD, Blehar MC, Waters E, et al: Patterns of Attachment: A Psychological Study of the Strange Situation. Hillsdale, NJ, Erlbaum, 1978

Beebe B: Co-constructing mother-infant distress: the microsynchrony of maternal impingement and infant avoidance in the face-to-face encounter. Psychoanal Inq 20:421–440, 2000

Blos P: The second individuation process of adolescence. Psychoanal Study Child 22:162–186, 1967 5590064

Bowlby J: Attachment and Loss, Vol I. New York, Basic Books, 1969

De Marneffe D: Bodies and words: a study of young children's genital and gender knowledge. Gender and Psychoanalysis 2:3–33, 1997

Howe N, Petrakos H, Rinaldi CM, LeFebvre R: "This is a bad dog, you know...": constructing shared meanings during sibling pretend play. Child Dev 76(4):783–794, 2005 16026496

Lewis M, Brooks-Gunn J: Social Cognition and the Acquisition of Self. New York, Plenum, 1979

Mahler MS: On the first three subphases of the separation-individuation process. Int J Psychoanal 53(Pt 3):333–338, 1972 4499978

Main M, Solomon J: Procedures for identifying infants as disorganized/disoriented during the Ainsworth Strange Situation, in Attachment in the Preschool Years: Theory, Research, and Intervention. Edited by Greenberg MT, Cicchetti D, Cummings EM. Chicago, University of Chicago Press, 1990, pp 121–160

Pearson D, Rouse H, Doswell S, et al: Prevalence of imaginary companions in a normal child population. Child Care Health Dev 27(1):13–22, 2001 11136338

Piaget J, Inhelder B: The Psychology of the Child. New York, Basic Books, 1969

Ryan RM, Kuczkowski R: The imaginary audience, self-consciousness and public individuation in adolescence. J Pers 62(2):219–238, 1994 8046574

Sorce J, Emde R: Mother's presence is not enough: the effect of emotional availability on infant experience. Dev Psychol 17:737–745, 1981

Tronick E, Als H, Adamson L, et al: The infant's response to entrapment between contradictory messages in face-to-face interaction. J Am Acad Child Psychiatry 17(1):1–13, 1978 632477

Vygotsky L: Mind in Society: The Development of Higher Psychological Processes. Cambridge, MA, Harvard University Press, 1978

CHAPTER 8

Developmental Issues in Older Adults

8.1   Which of the following is a characteristic sleep change occurring in later life?

A. Increased total sleep time.
B. Fewer nighttime arousals.
C. Increased Stage 1 and Stage 2 sleep.
D. Increased Stage 3 and Stage 4 sleep.
E. Increased rapid eye movement (REM) sleep latency.

The correct response is option C: Increased Stage 1 and Stage 2 sleep.

Sleep changes characteristic in late life include decreased total sleep time (option A), frequent arousals (option B), increased percentages of Stage 1 and Stage 2 sleep (option C), decreased percentages of Stage 3 and Stage 4 sleep (option D), decreased REM sleep latency (option E), decreased absolute amounts of REM sleep, and a tendency to exhibit a redistribution of sleep across the 24-hour day (e.g., napping during the day). Many of these sleep changes are similar to those that occur in depression and dementing disorders, although not as severe. Older persons are also more likely to phase-advance in the sleep-wake cycle, with a phase tendency toward "morningness." **(Hales RE, Yudofsky SC, Roberts LW [eds]: APP Textbook of Psychiatry, 6th Edition, Chapter 35, pp. 1242–1243)**

8.2   When prescribing benzodiazepines for anxiety in geriatric patients, which of the following is an important consideration?

A. Benzodiazepine half-life is often decreased in older individuals; therefore, longer-acting agents are preferred.
B. Withdrawal symptoms are usually not a problem when older individuals are prescribed short-acting benzodiazepines.
C. Older individuals are more susceptible than younger adults to the side effects of fatigue, motor dysfunction, and memory impairment.

D. In some older patients, long-acting benzodiazepines may lead to withdrawal episodes and a rebound of anxiety.

E. Side-effect profiles of benzodiazepines tend to be relatively consistent across age groups.

The correct response is option C: Older individuals are more susceptible than younger adults to the side effects of fatigue, motor dysfunction, and memory impairment.

The benzodiazepines (e.g., alprazolam, oxazepam, lorazepam) are the cornerstone of pharmacological therapy for the anxiety disorders. These drugs repeatedly have been demonstrated to be effective for the control of anxiety when compared with a placebo and are relatively free of side effects. They are generally well tolerated by persons of all ages but present unique problems when prescribed to older persons (option E). For example, the half-life of the benzodiazepines may be increased dramatically in late life (option A), with diazepam (2.5–5.0 mg) having a half-life nearing 4 days in persons in their 80s. Older persons are also more susceptible to benzodiazepines' potential side effects, such as fatigue, drowsiness, motor dysfunction, and memory impairment (option C). Clinicians must be especially careful when prescribing benzodiazepines to older individuals who drive. Therefore, the shorter-acting benzodiazepines, such as alprazolam (0.25 mg), oxazepam (15 mg), and lorazepam (0.5 mg), given two to three times a day, have been preferred agents in late life. Nevertheless, short-acting drugs in some older patients may lead to brief withdrawal episodes during the day and a rebound of anxiety (options B, D). **(Hales RE, Yudofsky SC, Roberts LW [eds]: APP Textbook of Psychiatry, 6th Edition, Chapter 35, pp. 1247–1248)**

8.3 Older adults have elevated levels of which of the following hormones?

A. Thyroid-stimulating hormone (TSH).
B. Corticotropin.
C. Epinephrine.
D. Dehydroepiandrosterone (DHEA).
E. Growth hormone.

The correct response is option A: Thyroid-stimulating hormone (TSH).

In aging adults, the level of TSH increases, while the thyroxine (T_4) level remains the same and the triiodothyronine (T_3) level decreases (option A). The basal corticotropin, its pulse frequency, and its circadian rhythm of secretion remain unaltered with age (option B). While the norepinephrine levels increase, both the secretion and the clearance of epinephrine increase, leaving the levels remaining the same (option C). DHEA production peaks at age 20 years and then declines with age (option D). Growth hormone levels peak at puberty and then decrease by 14% per decade (option E). The decline in growth hormone with age may result in a decrease in both lean body mass and bone mass. **(Steffens DC, Blazer**

DG, Thakur ME [eds]: APP Textbook of Geriatric Psychiatry, 5th Edition, Chapter 2, pp. 38–39, 41)

8.4 Which of the following changes is seen in the elderly that could affect drug pharmacokinetics?

A. Decreased hepatic conjugation.
B. Increased protein binding.
C. Decreased hepatic blood flow.
D. Increased body water.
E. Decreased gastric acid transit time.

The correct response is option C: Decreased hepatic blood flow.

Although acid secretion, gastrointestinal perfusion, and membrane transport all may decrease and thereby *lower* absorption, gastrointestinal transit time is prolonged and *increases* absorption, and thus no net change occurs (option E). Older patients, with decreased lean body mass and total body water, have a smaller volume of distribution (option D). This is particularly relevant when choosing proper dosages for drugs, such as antibiotics or lithium that are primarily distributed in water. Protein binding also can affect the volume of distribution; it is generally unaffected by age (option B). Hepatic drug clearance is decreased by an age-related decline in hepatic blood flow (option C); oxidative metabolism in the cytochrome P450 system is slower, thereby affecting elimination, but conjugation is not slower (option A). **(Steffens DC, Blazer DG, Thakur ME [eds]: APP Textbook of Geriatric Psychiatry, 5th Edition, Chapter 2, p. 44)**

8.5 Personality in older adults is characterized by higher levels of which of the following?

A. Depression.
B. Vulnerability to stress.
C. Openness.
D. Agreeableness.
E. Sociability.

The correct response is option D: Agreeableness.

The most frequently used model in research on aging-related personality traits uses the five-factor model consisting of neuroticism, extraversion, openness, agreeableness, and conscientiousness (Digman 1990). In nonclinical samples, younger persons are somewhat higher on traits of extraversion (being more outgoing and sociable [option E]), neuroticism (having more anxiety, depression, and vulnerability to stress [options A, B]), and openness (option C), whereas older persons are higher on agreeableness (option D) and conscientiousness, with most of the change occurring in young adulthood rather than later life (Roberts et al. 2006). **(Steffens**

DC, Blazer DG, Thakur ME [eds]: APP Textbook of Geriatric Psychiatry, 5th Edition, Chapter 18, p. 495)

8.6 Personality development in healthy elderly is characterized by which of the following?

A. Increase in neurotic defenses.
B. Looking forward to meaning in life ahead.
C. Denial of one's mortality.
D. Tendency to remember more negative events.
E. Expectation of death of loved ones.

The correct response is option E: Expectation of death of loved ones.

Erik Erikson's stage theory of late-life development (Erikson et al. 1986) proposed that the major developmental task of older age is to look back and seek meaning across the lifespan, rather than looking forward as in previous developmental modes that are now in decline (option B). George Vaillant (1993) established that mature defenses were more consistently identified primarily in Erikson's later developmental stages (option A). People expect to experience the death of loved ones (option E) and anticipate their own declining health as they age and have time to mentally rehearse how they will respond to these "on-time losses" (option C). The improvement in coping skills with aging is also accompanied by socioemotional selectivity—that is, the tendency of elderly persons to remember more pleasant events and positive emotions rather than unpleasant ones (option D). **(Steffens DC, Blazer DG, Thakur ME [eds]: APP Textbook of Geriatric Psychiatry, 5th Edition, Chapter 18, pp. 496–497)**

8.7 Which of the following cognitive functions is the most likely to remain intact in healthy older adults?

A. Divergent thinking.
B. Attentional capacity.
C. Executive skills.
D. Visual integration.
E. Verbal abilities.

The correct response is option E: Verbal abilities.

Compared with young adults, older individuals show selective losses in functions related to speed and efficiency of information processing. Particularly vulnerable are memory retrieval abilities, attentional capacity (option B), executive skills (option C), and divergent thinking (option A) such as working memory and multitasking (Salthouse 1996; Samson and Barnes 2013; van Hooren et al. 2007). One explanation posits that the profile of cognitive change in normal aging is the result of a loss in fluid abilities—that is, skills that require novel problem solving and flexible thought (Botwinick 1977; Horn 1982); by contrast, well-rehearsed verbal abilities—so-called crystallized skills—are less susceptible to age-associated change (option E). Normal older adults also show some decrements compared with younger cohorts on tests of visuoperceptual, visuospatial, and constructional functions (Eslinger et al. 1985; Howieson et al. 1993; Park and Schwarz 1999). These modest declines are seen on tests involving visual analysis and integration (option D), such as the Block Design subtest of the Wechsler Adult Intelligence Scale, 4th Edition (WAIS-IV), and similar integrative tests involving visual processing. **(Steffens DC, Blazer DG, Thakur ME [eds]: APP Textbook of Geriatric Psychiatry, 5th Edition, Chapter 6, pp. 132–133)**

8.8   Which of the following memory abilities most likely remains intact in healthy older adults?

A. Working memory.
B. Cued recall.
C. Delayed free recall.
D. Memory retrieval.

The correct response is option B: Cued recall.

Compared with young adults, older individuals show selective losses in functions related to speed and efficiency of information processing. Particularly vulnerable are memory retrieval abilities (option D), attentional capacity, executive skills, and divergent thinking such as working memory (option A) and multitasking (Salthouse 1996; Samson and Barnes 2013; van Hooren et al. 2007). On formal neuropsychological testing, memory measures involving delayed free recall are typically affected (option C) (Craik and Rose 2012), although not to the pronounced extent found in Alzheimer's disease (AD) (Welsh et al. 1991). Unlike individuals with neurocognitive disorder due to AD, older adults without neurocognitive disorders typically demonstrate intact memory ability on tests such as cued recall and delayed recognition (option B). This profile of performance suggests different mechanisms underlying the memory loss of normal aging and AD. In AD, the problem appears to involve the consolidation or storage of new information into long-term memory stores. In normal aging, the principal problem appears to be primarily in the efficient accessing of recently stored information. **(Steffens DC, Blazer DG, Thakur ME [eds]: APP Textbook of Geriatric Psychiatry, 5th Edition, Chapter 6, p. 132)**

8.9   Which of the following best characterizes sexual activity in old age?

A. The frequency of sex decreases with age equally in both men and women.
B. Only a minority of women without partners masturbate.
C. Physical health is the most important factor in determining levels of sexual activity in women.
D. Past levels of sexual activity do not affect later levels of activity.
E. Single individuals are more sexually active than those with steady partners.

The correct response is option B: Only a minority of women without partners masturbate.

Several major studies have shown that a majority of middle-aged and older individuals continue to be sexually active, although with modest decreases in activity, determined in part by gender and the availability of partners. These studies have indicated that older men are more sexually active than older women (option A) and that individuals with steady partners are more active than single individuals (option E). In general, sexual interest and activity in late life depend on the previous level of sexual activity (option D); the availability, health, and sexual interest of the partner; and the individual's overall physical health. Physical health appears to be the most important factor for older men, whereas the quality of the relationship is most influential for older women (option C). In an AARP 1999 mail survey, researchers gathered responses from 1,384 men and women ages 45 years and older (Jacoby 1999). Of the respondents, the majority of men without partners said they masturbated, whereas the majority of the women said they did not (option B). **(Steffens DC, Blazer DG, Thakur ME [eds]: APP Textbook of Geriatric Psychiatry, 5th Edition, Chapter 14, pp. 389–390)**

8.10   Normal age-related change in sexual functioning of women includes which of the following?

A. Libido may decrease due to decreased testosterone levels.
B. Vaginal size increases.
C. Blood supply to the pelvic region is increased.
D. Orgasm remains as intense.
E. Sexual arousal may occur faster due to increased vaginal congestion.

The correct response is option A: Libido may decrease due to decreased testosterone levels.

The decline and eventual cessation of ovarian estrogen production during menopause leads to important changes in sexual function, including atrophy of urogenital tissue. Blood supply to the pelvic region is reduced (option C), the vagina shortens and narrows (option B), and vaginal mucosa is thinner and less lubricated. As a result, sexual desire may decrease, sexual arousal may require more time (option E), sexual intercourse may be more uncomfortable because of reduced lubrication of vaginal and clitoral tissue, and orgasms may be felt as less intense (option D). During menopause, women also experience decreases in testosterone production that may lead to diminished sensitivity of erogenous tissue and reduced libido (option A). **(Steffens DC, Blazer DG, Thakur ME [eds]: APP Textbook of Geriatric Psychiatry, 5th Edition, Chapter 14, p. 393 and Table 14–1, p. 394)**

8.11   Which of the following differentiates bereavement in women compared with men after the death of their spouse?

A. Greater death rate in the next few years.
B. Greater risk of depression.
C. Greater life satisfaction.
D. Experience more personal growth.
E. Focus on restoration of their life pattern.

The correct response is option D: Experience more personal growth.

Widowers appear to be at relatively higher risk of death than widows (option A). A study of elderly widows and widowers for 6 years after their loss found that men age 75 or older had excessive mortality compared with men of the same age in the general population (Bowling 1988–1989). Another study found that widowers who died within the first year of spousal bereavement had reported more often than survivors that their wives were their main confidants and that they had minimal involvement in activities with other persons after their wives' deaths (Gallagher-Thompson et al. 1993). Several studies (van Groothcest et al. 1999; Williams 2003) have found that bereavement has a greater impact on depression scores in men than in women (option B). However, women have been found to have less life satisfaction than men following the loss of a spouse (option C) (Lichtenstein et al. 1996; Williams 2003), but they may also experience more personal growth after the loss (option D) (Carr 2004). Women appear to be more focused on psychological aspects of coping with the loss, whereas men are more focused on restoring their life pattern without the loved one (option E) (Stroebe et al. 2001). **(Steffens DC, Blazer DG, Thakur ME [eds]: APP Textbook of Geriatric Psychiatry, 5th Edition, Chapter 15, pp. 421–422)**

8.12   A recently retired 63-year-old woman with a history of depression, currently in remission, says that now that she has retired she is interested in an exercise routine. She has not exercised much before and is moderately overweight. She stresses that her primary motivation is preventing cognitive loss, which she greatly fears. She asks the psychiatrist's opinion regarding popular news items regarding preventing cognitive loss with exercise. Which of the following statements by the psychiatrist would be the most accurate reply?

A. Although unlikely to be helpful for preventing cognitive loss, exercise confers many other benefits, including preventing depression.
B. Positive studies show that only those who have been exercising for many years have benefited from exercise, and there is no evidence supporting later-life adoption.
C. Exercise has been shown to be primarily effective in men only, and studies in women have been more equivocal.

D. Evidence suggests that physical activity is associated with lower risk of cognitive decline compared with a sedentary lifestyle.

E. Early open trials showed a positive effect of exercise on cognitive loss; however, more rigorous studies do not support any effect of exercise on any prevention of cognitive loss.

The correct response is option D: Evidence suggests that physical activity is associated with lower risk of cognitive decline compared with a sedentary lifestyle.

Physical activity in older adults has been associated with numerous cognitive benefits (options A–C), including delayed onset of dementia (Larson et al. 2006), higher Mini-Mental State Examination scores (Almeida et al. 2006), and increased brain volumes (Colcombe et al. 2006). A Cochrane review on the impact of aerobic exercise on cognition in adults ages 55 and older found positive association on cognitive speed (option D) and auditory and visual attention (Angevaren et al. 2008). Furthermore, in a meta-analysis of prospective studies of healthy older adults, low to moderate physical activity was associated with a reduced risk of cognitive decline compared with sedentary individuals (option E) (Sofi et al. 2011). Mental health is also associated with physical activity; studies have found that those older adults who were significantly less likely to report depressive symptoms were more physically active (Hamer et al. 2014). **(Steffens DC, Blazer DG, Thakur ME [eds]: APP Textbook of Geriatric Psychiatry, 5th Edition, Chapter 22, p. 624)**

References

Almeida OP, Norman P, Hankey G, et al: Successful mental health aging: results from a longitudinal study of older Australian men. Am J Geriatr Psychiatry 14(1):27–35, 2006 16407579

Angevaren M, Aufdemkampe G, Verhaar HJ, et al: Physical activity and enhanced fitness to improve cognitive function in older people without known cognitive impairment. Cochrane Database Syst Rev 2:CD005381, 2008

Botwinick J: Intellectual abilities, in The Handbook of the Psychology of Aging. Edited by Birren JE, Schaie KW. New York, Van Nostrand Reinhold, 1977, pp 508–605

Bowling A: Who dies after widow(er)hood? A discriminant analysis. Omega 19:135–153, 1988–1989

Carr D: Gender, preloss marital dependence, and older adults' adjustment to widowhood. J Marriage Fam 66:220–235, 2004

Colcombe SJ, Erickson KI, Scalf PE, et al: Aerobic exercise training increases brain volume in aging humans. J Gerontol A Biol Sci Med Sci 61(11):1166–1170, 2006 17167157

Craik FIM, Rose NS: Memory encoding and aging: a neurocognitive perspective. Neurosci Biobehav Rev 36(7):1729–1739, 2012 22155274

Digman JM: Personality structure: emergence of the five-factor model. Annu Rev Psychol 41:417–440, 1990

Erikson EH, Erikson JM, Kivnick HQ: Vital Involvement in Old Age. New York, WW Norton, 1986

Eslinger PJ, Damasio AR, Benton AL, Van Allen M: Neuropsychologic detection of abnormal mental decline in older persons. JAMA 253(5):670–674, 1985 3968802

Gallagher-Thompson D, Futterman A, Farberow N, et al: The impact of spousal bereavement on older widows and widowers, in Handbook of Bereavement. Edited by Stroebe MS, Stroebe W, Hansson R. Cambridge, United Kingdom, Cambridge University Press, 1993, pp 227–239

Hamer M, Lavoie KL, Bacon SL: Taking up physical activity in later life and healthy ageing: the English longitudinal study of ageing. Br J Sports Med 48(3):239–243, 2014 24276781

Horn J: The theory of fluid and crystallized intelligence in relation to concepts of cognitive psychology and aging in adulthood, in Aging and Cognitive Processes. Edited by Craik F, Trehub S. New York, Plenum, 1982, pp 237–278

Howieson DB, Holm LA, Kaye JA, et al: Neurologic function in the optimally healthy oldest old. Neuropsychological evaluation. Neurology 43(10):1882–1886, 1993 8413942

Jacoby S: Great sex: what's age got to do with it? Modern Maturity Sept/Oct:43–48, 1999

Larson EB, Wang L, Bowen JD, et al: Exercise is associated with reduced risk for incident dementia among persons 65 years of age and older. Ann Intern Med 144(2):73–81, 2006 16418406

Lichtenstein P, Gatz M, Pedersen NL, et al: A co-twin–control study of response to widowhood. J Gerontol B Psychol Sci Soc Sci 51(5):279–289, 1996 8809004

Park DC, Schwarz N: Cognitive Aging: A Primer. Philadelphia, PA, Psychology Press, 1999

Roberts BW, Walton KE, Viechtbauer W: Patterns of mean-level change in personality traits across the life course: a meta-analysis of longitudinal studies. Psychol Bull 132(1):1–25, 2006 16435954

Salthouse TA: The processing-speed theory of adult age differences in cognition. Psychol Rev 103(3):403–428, 1996 8759042

Samson RD, Barnes CA: Impact of aging brain circuits on cognition. Eur J Neurosci 37(12):1903–1915, 2013 23773059

Sofi F, Valecchi D, Bacci D, et al: Physical activity and risk of cognitive decline: a meta-analysis of prospective studies. J Intern Med 269(1):107–117, 2011 20831630

Stroebe MS, Stroebe W, Schut H: Gender differences in adjustment to bereavement: an empirical and theoretical review. Rev Gen Psychol 5:62–83, 2001

Vaillant GE: The Wisdom of the Ego. Cambridge, MA, Harvard University Press, 1993

van Grootheest DS, Beekman ATF, Broese van Groenou MI, Deeg DJ: Sex differences in depression after widowhood. Do men suffer more? Soc Psychiatry Psychiatr Epidemiol 34(7):391–398, 1999 10477960

van Hooren SA, Valentijn AM, Bosma H, et al: Cognitive functioning in healthy older adults aged 64–81: a cohort study into the effects of age, sex, and education. Neuropsychol Dev Cogn B Aging Neuropsychol Cogn 14(1):40–54, 2007 17164189

Welsh K, Butters N, Hughes J, et al: Detection of abnormal memory decline in mild cases of Alzheimer's disease using CERAD neuropsychological measures. Arch Neurol 48(3):278–281, 1991 2001185

Williams K: Has the future of marriage arrived? A contemporary examination of gender, marriage, and psychological well-being. J Health Soc Behav 44(4):470–487, 2003 15038144

CHAPTER 9

Diagnostic Procedures

Diagnostic Assessment and Rating Scales

9.1   Which of the following self-report assessment tools takes the least amount of time to administer?

A. Symptom Checklist-90—Revised.
B. Brief Symptom Inventory.
C. Minnesota Multiphasic Personality Inventory—2.
D. Personality Assessment Inventory.
E. Positive and Negative Syndrome Scale.

The correct response is option B: Brief Symptom Inventory.

The Symptom Checklist-90—Revised (SCL-90-R; Derogatis 1994) is a revision of a much-used self-report instrument designed to provide information about a broad range of complaints typical of individuals with psychological symptomatic distress. The Brief Symptom Inventory (Derogatis 1993) is a 53-item self-report form of the SCL-90-R that assesses the same nine symptom dimensions and three global indices. The psychometric properties of the Brief Symptom Inventory are comparable with those of the SCL-90-R (option A), and the Brief Symptom Inventory has the advantage of increased ease of administration, taking only 8–10 minutes to complete (option B). The Minnesota Multiphasic Personality Inventory—2 (Hathaway and McKinley 1989) is also an efficient self-report assessment tool but with 567 items would take longer to complete (option C). The Personality Assessment Inventory (Morey 1991), which focuses on personality disorders, has 344 items (option D). The Positive and Negative Syndrome Scale (Kay et al. 1987), which assesses symptoms of disordered thinking, is a semistructured interview, not a self-report instrument (option E). **(Hales RE, Yudofsky SC, Roberts LW [eds]: APP Textbook of Psychiatry, 6th Edition, Chapter 3, p. 64 and Tables 3–1 and 3–2, pp. 65, 68)**

9.2   Which of the following descriptions correctly matches the assessment tool with its targeted area of symptomatology?

   A. Alcohol Use Disorders and Associated Disabilities Interview Schedule, DSM-IV Version, assesses a patient's readiness to change in relation to the use of alcohol.
   B. Thematic Apperception Test assesses personality disorders.
   C. Reasons for Living Inventory assesses suicidal behavior.
   D. Eating Disorder Examination diagnoses binge-eating disorder.
   E. University of Rhode Island Change Assessment measures dependence-related symptoms.

The correct response is option D: Eating Disorder Examination diagnoses binge-eating disorder.

The Eating Disorder Examination, 16th Edition (Fairburn et al. 2008), includes a module to diagnose binge-eating disorder (option D). The Alcohol Use Disorders and Associated Disabilities Interview Schedule, DSM-IV Version (Grant et al. 2001), assesses dependence-related symptoms (e.g., withdrawal, craving, tolerance), familial and medical risk factors, and amount of drug and alcohol consumption (option A). The Thematic Apperception Test (Murray 1943) has its origins in the efforts of clinical psychologists to provide an assessment of such psychodynamic factors as drives, unconscious wishes, conflicts, and defenses (option B). It is a widely used projective process for assessing the patient's self-concept in relation to others. The Reasons for Living Inventory (Linehan et al. 1983) does not directly assess suicidal behavior (option C) but does examine the beliefs and expectations that lead a person to refrain from committing suicide. The University of Rhode Island Change Assessment (McConnaughy et al. 1983) is a measure developed to assess a patient's readiness to change in relation to the use of substances (option E). **(Hales RE, Yudofsky SC, Roberts LW [eds]: APP Textbook of Psychiatry, 6th Edition, Chapter 3, pp. 64–69, 74)**

9.3   Which of the following is the most widely used self-report inventory of depression?

   A. Positive and Negative Syndrome Scale.
   B. Schedule for Affective Disorders and Schizophrenia.
   C. Beck Depression Inventory—II.
   D. Beck Hopelessness Scale.
   E. Reasons for Living Inventory.

The correct response is option C: Beck Depression Inventory—II.

The Beck Depression Inventory—II (Beck et al. 1996) is probably the most widely used self-report inventory of depression (option C). The inventory includes 21 items to assess mood, pessimism, crying spells, guilt, self-hate and accusations, irritability, social withdrawal, work inhibition, sleep and appetite disturbance, and loss of libido. The Positive and Negative Syndrome Scale (Kay et al. 1987) is a commonly used measure of disordered thinking (option A). The Schedule for Affective Disorders and Schizophrenia (Endicott and Spitzer 1978) is a semistructured interview that can assist with assessment of cognition and thought disorder (option B). The Beck Hopelessness Scale (Beck et al. 1974) is a suicide assessment instrument (option D). The Reasons for Living Inventory (Linehan et al. 1983) does not directly assess suicidal behavior but examines the beliefs and expectations that lead a person to refrain from committing suicide (option E). **(Hales RE, Yudofsky SC, Roberts LW [eds]: APP Textbook of Psychiatry, 6th Edition, Chapter 3, pp. 65, 70–71 and Table 3–2, pp. 66–69)**

9.4   Which of the following instruments can be used to assess psychodynamic factors such as drives, unconscious wishes, conflicts, and defenses?

A. Anger, Irritability, and Assault Questionnaire.
B. Thematic Apperception Test.
C. Wisconsin Card Sorting Test.
D. Brief Psychiatric Rating Scale.
E. Beck Depression Inventory—II.

The correct response is option B: Thematic Apperception Test.

Part of the "standard battery" used by clinical psychologists, the Thematic Apperception Test is a widely used projective process for assessing the patient's self-concept in relation to others. Originally developed by Murray (1943), the test consists of a set of 30 pictures depicting one or more individuals. The patient is asked to make up a story based on each picture. The stories generated are then scored for the individual's needs as reflected in the feelings and impulses attributed to the major character in each story and the interactions with the environment leading to a resolution (option B). The Anger, Irritability, and Assault Questionnaire (Coccaro et al. 1991) is a 42-item self-report questionnaire designed to assess several aspects of impulsive aggression putatively related to serotonergic function; the instrument focuses primarily on the inability to control aggression (option A). The Wisconsin Card Sorting Test (Grant and Berg 1948) is used to measure cognitive flexibility and concept formation (option C). The Brief Psychiatric Rating Scale (Overall and Gorham 1962) assesses a broad range of psychiatric symptoms (option D) most relevant to inpatient populations. The Beck Depression Inventory—II (Beck et al. 1996) is a widely used self-report inventory of depression (option E). **(Hales RE, Yudofsky SC, Roberts LW [eds]: APP Textbook of Psychiatry, 6th Edition, Chapter 3, pp. 70, 74 and Table 3–4, p. 76)**

9.5   The Global Assessment of Functioning Scale is useful for which of the following purposes?

A. Rating patients on a hypothetical continuum from psychological sickness to mental health.
B. Measuring the construct of quality of life.

C. Assessing the patient's degree of social adjustment.

D. Tracking the progress and impact of treatment.

E. Assessing activity limitations and participation restrictions.

The correct response is option A: Rating patients on a hypothetical continuum from psychological sickness to mental health.

Several widely used scales of overall psychosocial functioning (i.e., symptoms, social and occupational functioning) that rate patients on a hypothetical continuum from psychological sickness to mental health are the Global Assessment Scale (Endicott et al. 1976), the Global Assessment of Functioning Scale (American Psychiatric Association 2000) (option A), and the Social and Occupational Functioning Assessment Scale (Goldman et al. 1992). All three rating scales are extremely easy to use, are appropriate for use in numerous contexts, and have been shown to be reliable.

The construct of *quality of life* (option B) is multidimensional in nature and includes the psychological, social functioning, and physical domains (and their combinations). Quality-of-life measures include the Quality of Life Interview (Lehman 1988), the Quality of Life Scale (Heinrichs et al. 1984), and the Wisconsin Quality of Life Index (Becker et al. 1993).

The concept of *social adjustment* (option C) indicates the skill of the individual in handling interpersonal situations. Notable assessment instruments in this area include the Katz Adjustment Scale—Relative's Form (Katz and Lyerly 1963), the Social Adjustment Scale—Self-Report (Weissman and Bothwell 1976), and the Dyadic Adjustment Scale (Spanier 1976).

Many efficient, easy-to-administer omnibus measures have been developed that can quickly assess changes in patients' symptoms, behaviors, quality of life, and functional levels during the treatment process (option D). Instruments typical of this type include the Clinical Outcomes in Routine Evaluation Outcome Measure (Barkham et al. 2001), Outcome Questionnaire—45 (Lambert et al. 2004), and Partners for Change Outcome Management System (Miller et al. 2005). Activity limitations and participation restrictions (option E) are assessed by the World Health Organization Disability Assessment Schedule 2.0 (Üstün et al. 2010). **(Hales RE, Yudofsky SC, Roberts LW [eds]: APP Textbook of Psychiatry, 6th Edition, Chapter 3, pp. 80–82)**

9.6   Which of the following instruments could provide information about the adequacy of the support system available to a 34-year-old schizophrenic man who lives alone?

A. World Health Organization Disability Assessment Schedule 2.0.

B. Independent Living Scale.

C. Brief Psychiatric Rating Scale.

D. Social Support Questionnaire.

E. Positive and Negative Syndrome Scale.

The correct response is option D: Social Support Questionnaire.

The Social Support Questionnaire (Sarason et al. 1983) is an efficient method for assessing social satisfaction. This instrument provides information about available resources of support and the patient's level of satisfaction with this support system (option D). The World Health Organization Disability Assessment Schedule 2.0 (Üstün et al. 2010) is a 36-item self-report questionnaire used to assess the individual's activity limitations and participation restrictions for the prior month (option A). The Independent Living Scale (Loeb 1996) is a self-report measure of an individual's competency to perform daily activities and self-care (option B). The Brief Psychiatric Rating Scale (Overall and Gorham 1962) assesses a broad range of psychiatric symptoms most relevant to inpatient populations (option C). The Positive and Negative Syndrome Scale (Kay et al. 1987) is a commonly used measure of disordered thinking (option E). **(Hales RE, Yudofsky SC, Roberts LW [eds]: APP Textbook of Psychiatry, 6th Edition, Chapter 3, pp. 64, 80–82)**

Laboratory Monitoring

9.7   Which of the following screening tests is correctly matched to the clinical picture for recommended screening prior to initiating pharmacotherapy and at regular intervals during maintenance treatment?

A. Potassium level in a 25-year-old man being started on carbamazepine.
B. Complete blood count (CBC) for a 48-year-old woman being treated with fluoxetine.
C. Electrocardiogram (ECG) for a 30-year-old man without any medical history being started on nortriptyline.
D. Blood urea nitrogen (BUN) and creatinine for a 68-year-old man being treated with valproate.
E. Follow-up CBC for a 13-year-old girl with bipolar disorder being treated with carbamazepine.

The correct response is option E: Follow-up CBC for a 13-year-old girl with bipolar disorder being treated with carbamazepine.

Carbamazepine treatment screening tests initially include a CBC with platelets (option E), liver function tests (LFTs), and BUN/creatinine. These tests are repeated once a maintenance dose is achieved. Potassium is not specifically monitored for patients treated with carbamazepine (option A). A CBC is not needed for a patient treated with fluoxetine (option B). Nortriptyline, like all tricyclic antidepressants, requires an ECG in a patient older than 40 years or with preexisting cardiac disease prior to initiation of treatment (option C). Before a patient is treated with valproate, a CBC with platelets, LFTs, and beta–human chorionic gonadotropin, if appropriate, should be obtained (option D). For follow-up in patients taking valproate, LFTs and a CBC are recommended every 6 months. **(Hales RE,**

Yudofsky SC, Roberts LW [eds]: APP Textbook of Psychiatry, 6th Edition, Chapter 4, pp. 102–106 and Table 4–8, pp. 104–105)

9.8   In which of the following options is the recommended laboratory test correctly matched to the medication scenario?

A. LFT for monitoring lithium therapy.
B. Renal function panel for monitoring valproate therapy.
C. Serum level for assessing clinical response to nortriptyline therapy.
D. Serum level for assessing clinical response to risperidone therapy.
E. ECG for monitoring carbamazepine therapy.

The correct response is option C: Serum level for assessing clinical response to nortriptyline therapy.

Nortriptyline is one of the tricyclic antidepressants for which the relationship of drug levels to therapeutic response is known (option C). Nortriptyline appears to have a specific therapeutic window between 50 and 150 ng/mL, and poor clinical response occurs both above and below that window. At initiation of treatment, lithium requires laboratory values for sodium, potassium, calcium, phosphate, BUN, creatinine, thyroid-stimulating hormone, thyroxine (T_4), CBC, urinalysis, beta-human chorionic gonadotropin if appropriate, and an ECG in a patient older than 50 years or with a preexisting cardiac condition, but LFTs are not required (option A). Renal function does not need to be monitored for patients taking valproate (option B). The monitoring of blood levels for antipsychotics, including risperidone, is not routine in clinical practice (option D). An ECG is not required for carbamazepine monitoring (option E). **(Hales RE, Yudofsky SC, Roberts LW [eds]: APP Textbook of Psychiatry, 6th Edition, Chapter 4, pp. 102–106 and Table 4–8, pp. 104–105)**

9.9   In which of the following options is the appropriate laboratory test matched to the medication scenario?

A. CBC monitoring during carbamazepine treatment.
B. Fasting serum glucose before initiating a tricyclic antidepressant.
C. Echocardiogram before initiating a tricyclic antidepressant.
D. LFT monitoring during lithium treatment.
E. Electroencephalogram before starting valproate.

The correct response is option A: CBC monitoring during carbamazepine treatment.

A CBC screen is necessary in monitoring carbamazepine treatment because of the possible side effect of leukopenia (option A). There is no indication for fasting serum glucose before initiating a tricyclic antidepressant (option B), an echocardiogram before starting a tricyclic antidepressant (option C), LFT monitoring during lithium treatment (option D), or an electroencephalogram prior to starting valproate (option E). **(Hales RE, Yudofsky SC, Roberts LW [eds]: APP Textbook of Psychiatry, 6th Edition, Chapter 4, pp. 102–106 and Table 4–8, pp. 104–105)**

9.10 Which of the following tests is routinely recommended as part of the initial diagnostic workup of a patient presenting with an altered mental status?

A. Ceruloplasmin.
B. Lead level.
C. Electromyogram.
D. Positron emission tomography scan.
E. HIV test.

The correct response is option E: HIV test.

HIV is one of the tests in an initial workup of a patient with altered mental status (option E). Options A–D are not indicated unless and until further evaluation suggests their necessity. **(Hales RE, Yudofsky SC, Roberts LW [eds]: APP Textbook of Psychiatry, 6th Edition, Chapter 4, pp. 97–99 and Table 4–5, p. 99)**

9.11 A 48-year-old British man is admitted to the inpatient unit for progressive cognitive decline and abnormal jerky movements in his left leg over the last 2 months. The clinician suspects Creutzfeldt-Jakob disease. Which of the following laboratory studies could be helpful in confirming the diagnosis?

A. Lumbar puncture and cerebrospinal fluid biomarkers.
B. Serum iron level.
C. Liver function tests.
D. Lumbar puncture and culture.
E. Urinalysis.

The correct response is option A: Lumbar puncture and cerebrospinal fluid biomarkers.

The cerebrospinal fluid 14-3-3 protein is useful for confirmation of Creutzfeldt-Jakob disease in a patient with rapidly progressive dementia and pathognomonic neurological symptoms (i.e., myoclonic jerks) (option A). Options B–E are not helpful in the diagnosis of Creutzfeldt-Jakob disease. **(Hales RE, Yudofsky SC, Roberts LW [eds]: APP Textbook of Psychiatry, 6th Edition, Chapter 4, p. 100)**

Other Tests

9.12 Which of the following is a true statement about use of electroencephalography (EEG) in psychiatric diagnosis?

A. EEG is essential in evaluating a first episode of depression.
B. EEG is useful in the diagnosis of bipolar disorder.
C. EEG can always diagnose epilepsy.

D. EEG can be helpful in diagnosing sleep disorders.

E. EEG can help in differentiating types of dementias.

The correct response is option D: EEG can be helpful in diagnosing sleep disorders.

An abnormal electroencephalogram will consist of one or more of the following: 1) paroxysmal activity indicative of transient, episodic neuronal discharges as seen in epilepsy; 2) nonparoxysmal slowing of activity, as seen in delirium; 3) asymmetric activity as observed with mass lesions or infarction; or 4) sleep abnormalities consistent with sleep-wake disorders including sleep apneas, narcolepsy, and parasomnias such as rapid eye movement sleep behavior disorder (option D). EEG is not an essential test in the evaluation of a first episode of depression (option A). It would be prudent to obtain an electroencephalogram in a patient with new-onset psychosis, episodic behavioral disturbance, or altered mental status. A normal electroencephalogram does not rule out the possibility of epilepsy (option C); 20% of patients with epilepsy will have a normal electroencephalogram, and 2% of patients without epilepsy will have spike and wave formations. EEG has fairly limited utility in the differentiation of psychiatric disorders and dementias (options B, E) in spite of the fact that EEG is widely available, noninvasive, inexpensive, and useful for diagnosing neurological disorders. **(Hales RE, Yudofsky SC, Roberts LW [eds]: APP Textbook of Psychiatry, 6th Edition, Chapter 4, pp. 111–112)**

9.13 Which of the following statements correctly describes an advantage of computed tomography (CT) over magnetic resonance imaging (MRI)?

A. CT can acquire images in the axial, coronal, and sagittal planes, whereas MRI can acquire them only in the coronal and axial planes.

B. CT has superior visualization of brain tissue compared to MRI.

C. CT can be used in patients with pacemakers, whereas MRI is contraindicated in such patients.

D. There is less radiation exposure with CT than with MRI.

E. CT provides better visualization of the posterior fossa than does MRI.

The correct response is option C: CT can be used in patients with pacemakers, whereas MRI is contraindicated in such patients.

MRI has many advantages over CT. First and foremost, it has superior visualization of brain tissue (option B), providing enhanced gray/white matter discrimination compared with that of CT and allowing quantitative or volumetric measurement of brain regions. Deep brain structures, including those of the posterior fossa (option E) such as the cerebellum and brain stem, are better visualized with MRI. Furthermore, axial, coronal, and sagittal images may be acquired by MRI (option A). MRI image acquisition is complex and, depending on parameters, can produce T1- (or longitudinal relaxation), T2- (or transverse relaxation), or PD (proton density)-weighted images, spin-echo, and inversion-recovery images. Patients with pacemakers cannot have MRIs (option C). A brain CT scan involves some radiation exposure (option D). **(Hales RE, Yudofsky SC, Roberts LW [eds]: APP Textbook of Psychiatry, 6th Edition, Chapter 4, pp. 114–115 and Table 4–12, p. 117)**

9.14   In which of the following options is the appropriate imaging study matched to the clinical presentation?

A. MRI of the brain in a 60-year-old man with new-onset dementia.
B. A head CT scan in a 25-year-old man with new-onset depression.
C. Magnetic resonance spectroscopy in a 35-year-old woman with a first psychotic episode.
D. A head CT scan with contrast in a 45-year-old woman with a suspected infarct.
E. Diffusion tensor imaging in the evaluation of depression.

The correct response is option A: MRI of the brain in a 60-year-old man with new-onset dementia.

The clinical utility of MRI in the evaluation of adult psychiatric patients was studied by Hollister and Shah (1996). In their study of CT and MRI scans ordered in a psychiatric hospital over a 2-year period, 17% (12 of 68) of scans were abnormal. The authors concluded that brain imaging scans are indicated for psychiatric patients with cognitive impairment (to evaluate for neurocognitive disorder; option A), a first psychotic break, personality change in a patient older than 50 years, or new or unexplained focal neurological signs. Routine screening with a head CT scan is unlikely to be helpful for the evaluation of psychiatric patients without neurological signs on clinical examination (option B) (Agzarian et al. 2006). Magnetic resonance spectroscopy has been used extensively to research numerous psychiatric disorders and is even used to assess pharmacokinetics and pharmacodynamics of psychotropic medications. Its clinical use is currently somewhat limited for primary psychiatric disorders (option C). Diffusion tensor imaging, a fairly new imaging technique, is the subject of intense psychiatric and neurological research, including in neurocognitive disorders, schizophrenia, mood and anxiety disorders, substance-related disorders, and brain injury. At this time, the clinical utility of diffusion tensor imaging is limited (option E). Non-contrast head CT is used in patients with suspected trauma or acute stroke (option D). **(Hales RE, Yudofsky SC, Roberts LW [eds]: APP Textbook of Psychiatry, 6th Edition, Chapter 4, pp. 115–119)**

9.15   In which of the following options is the appropriate neuroimaging test ordered for the clinical presentation?

A. Single positron emission computed tomography (SPECT) scan for a 55-year-old man with hypertension and signs of a stroke.
B. MRI for a 30-year-old man with mild traumatic brain injury.
C. SPECT for a 23-year-old woman with mild traumatic brain injury.

D. Head CT scan with contrast for a 46-year-old woman with a history of chronic renal failure and a suspected brain hemorrhage after a hypertensive crisis.

E. PET scan for a 60-year-old man with a history of diabetes mellitus and suspected frontotemporal dementia.

The correct response is option E: PET scan for a 60-year-old man with a history of diabetes mellitus and suspected frontotemporal dementia.

Frontotemporal dementia is generally associated with reduced perfusion of the frontal and/or lateral temporal lobes bilaterally on PET scan (option E). A SPECT scan is an extremely sensitive test for stroke: it is able to visualize perfusion defects and define the size of the stroke; however, a head CT scan is still used in the acute setting because it is quick and easy to obtain (option A). In addition, CT is superior to SPECT in differentiating between hemorrhagic and nonhemorrhagic stroke, which is essential to know prior to starting thrombolytic medications. Using contrast material in a patient with chronic renal failure is contraindicated (option D). Patients with mild traumatic brain injuries often complain of persistent neuropsychiatric symptoms despite having normal CT or MRI scans (option B); because of its increased sensitivity, SPECT may show regional cerebral blood flow hypoperfusion despite normal CT or MRI scans. However, the prognosis of patients with an abnormal SPECT scan is unclear. It may be further complicated by difficulties in recognizing which specific SPECT abnormalities are attributable to brain injury as opposed to motion artifact, normal variation, and processing errors. Thus, the clinical utility of the SPECT scan in mild traumatic brain injury is not clear and requires further investigation (option C). **(Hales RE, Yudofsky SC, Roberts LW [eds]: APP Textbook of Psychiatry, 6th Edition, Chapter 4, pp. 122, 124–126)**

9.16 In which of the following options is the screening test correctly matched to the clinical presentation?

A. Thyroid-stimulating hormone screening for a 27-year-old man with anhedonia, suicidal ideation, and newly diagnosed major depressive disorder.

B. Chest radiograph for a 55-year-old woman with first-episode delusions of jealousy.

C. Electrocardiogram for a 39-year-old woman starting on citalopram for anxiety.

D. Electroencephalogram for a 22-year-old woman with recurrent mania.

E. Head CT scan for a 70-year-old woman with a first episode of atypical depression.

The correct response is option E: Head CT scan for a 70-year-old woman with a first episode of atypical depression.

A screening head CT scan is very easy to perform, takes only a few minutes, produces little discomfort, and has a fairly high resolution and sensitivity. It can thus be easily performed on any psychiatric patient admitted with clinical features that do not appear to be classic for the disorder diagnosed. For example, if a patient has late-onset depression or mood disorder, then a head CT scan can be useful for screening for vascular disease, demyelinating disease, subdural hematoma, and subarachnoid hemorrhage (option E). Thyroid screening of female psychiatric patients older than 50 years, especially those with mood symptoms, may be justified because of a high prevalence of hypothyroidism in these patients. Thyroid screening of men and younger women, among whom the prevalence of thyroid dysfunction is estimated to be 0.1%, should be limited to patients with two or more clinical signs of hypothyroidism (option A) (Anfinson and Stoudemire 2000). A routine screening chest radiograph is not indicated for a person being evaluated for the presence of a psychiatric disorder (option B). Several studies have shown that routine screening ECGs are unnecessary in young, medically healthy psychiatric patients who do not have cardiovascular symptoms (option C). An electroencephalogram can be very useful when a patient has altered mental status, such as delirium or encephalopathy (option D), but not in this case of recurrent mania (option D). **(Hales RE, Yudofsky SC, Roberts LW [eds]: APP Textbook of Psychiatry, 6th Edition, Chapter 4, pp. 92–94)**

References

Agzarian MJ, Chryssidis S, Davies RP, Pozza CH: Use of routine computed tomography brain scanning of psychiatry patients. Australas Radiol 50(1):27–28, 2006 16499723

American Psychiatric Association: Diagnostic and Statistical Manual of Mental Disorders, 4th Edition, Text Revision. Washington, DC, American Psychiatric Association, 2000

Anfinson TJ, Stoudemire A: Laboratory and neuroendocrine assessment in medical-psychiatric patients, in Psychiatric Care of the Medical Patient, 2nd Edition. Edited by Stoudemire AS, Fogel BS, Greenberg D. New York, Oxford University Press, 2000, pp 119–145

Barkham M, Margison F, Leach C, et al; Clinical Outcomes in Routine Evaluation-Outcome Measures: Service profiling and outcomes benchmarking using the CORE-OM: toward practice-based evidence in the psychological therapies. J Consult Clin Psychol 69(2):184–196, 2001 11393596

Beck AT, Weissman A, Lester D, Trexler L: The measurement of pessimism: the hopelessness scale. J Consult Clin Psychol 42(6):861–865, 1974 4436473

Beck AT, Steer RA, Brown GK: Beck Depression Inventory Manual, 2nd Edition. San Antonio, TX, Psychological Corporation, 1996

Becker M, Diamond R, Sainfort F: A new patient focused index for measuring quality of life in persons with severe and persistent mental illness. Qual Life Res 2(4):239–251, 1993 8220359

Coccaro EF, Harvey PD, Kupsaw-Lawrence E, et al: Development of neuropharmacologically based behavioral assessments of impulsive aggressive behavior. J Neuropsychiatry Clin Neurosci 3(2):S44–S51, 1991 1821222

Derogatis LR: Brief Symptom Inventory (BSI): Administration, Scoring, and Procedures Manual, 3rd Edition. Minneapolis, MN, National Computer Systems, 1993

Derogatis LR: Symptom Checklist 90-R: Administration, Scoring, and Procedures Manual, 3rd Edition. Minneapolis, MN, National Computer Systems, 1994

Endicott J, Spitzer RL: A diagnostic interview: the schedule for affective disorders and schizophrenia. Arch Gen Psychiatry 35(7):837–844, 1978 678037

Endicott J, Spitzer RL, Fleiss JL, Cohen J: The global assessment scale. A procedure for measuring overall severity of psychiatric disturbance. Arch Gen Psychiatry 33(6):766–771, 1976 938196

Fairburn CG, Cooper Z, O'Connor ME: Eating Disorder Examination (16.0D), in Cognitive Behavior Therapy and Eating Disorders. Edited by Fairburn CG. New York, Guilford, 2008, pp 265–308

Goldman HH, Skodol AE, Lave TR: Revising axis V for DSM-IV: a review of measures of social functioning. Am J Psychiatry 149(9):1148–1156, 1992 1386964

Grant BF, Dawson DA, Hasin DS: The Alcohol Use Disorder and Associated Disabilities Interview Schedule, DSM-IV Version. Bethesda, MD, National Institute on Alcohol Abuse and Alcoholism, 2001

Grant DA, Berg EA: A behavioral analysis of degree of reinforcement and ease of shifting to new responses in a Weigl-type card-sorting problem. J Exp Psychol 38(4):404–411, 1948 18874598

Hathaway SR, McKinley JC: Minnesota Multiphasic Personality Inventory 2. Minneapolis, University of Minnesota Press, 1989

Heinrichs DW, Hanlon TE, Carpenter WT Jr: The Quality of Life Scale: an instrument for rating the schizophrenic deficit syndrome. Schizophr Bull 10(3):388–398, 1984 6474101

Hollister LE, Shah NN: Structural brain scanning in psychiatric patients: a further look. J Clin Psychiatry 57(6):241–244, 1996 8666560

Katz MM, Lyerly SB: Methods for measuring adjustment and social behavior in the community, I: rationale, description, discriminative validity and scale development. Psychol Rep Monogr 13:503–535, 1963

Kay SR, Fiszbein A, Opler LA: The positive and negative syndrome scale (PANSS) for schizophrenia. Schizophr Bull 13(2):261–276, 1987 3616518

Lambert MJ, Morton JJ, Hatfield D, et al: Administration and Scoring Manual for the Outcome Questionnaire-45. Orem, UT, America Professional Credentialing Services, 2004

Lehman AF: Quality of Life Interview for the chronically mentally ill. Eval Program Plann 11:51–62, 1988

Linehan MM, Goodstein JL, Nielsen SL, Chiles JA: Reasons for staying alive when you are thinking of killing yourself: the reasons for living inventory. J Consult Clin Psychol 51(2):276–286, 1983 6841772

Loeb PA: Independent Living Scales (ILS) Manual. San Antonio, TX, Psychological Corporation, 1996

McConnaughy EA, Prochaska JO, Velicer WF: Stages of change in psychotherapy: measurement and sample profiles. Psychotherapy 20:368–375, 1983

Miller SD, Duncan BL, Sorrell R, Brown GS: The partners for change outcome management system. J Clin Psychol 61(2):199–208, 2005 15609362

Morey LC: Personality Assessment Inventory: Professional Manual. Odessa, FL, Psychological Assessment Resources, 1991

Murray HA: Thematic Apperception Test Manual. Cambridge, MA, Harvard University Press, 1943

Overall JE, Gorham DR: The Brief Psychiatric Rating Scale. Psychol Rep 10:799–812, 1962

Sarason IG, Levine HM, Basham RB, et al: Assessing social support: the Social Support Questionnaire. J Pers Soc Psychol 44:127–139, 1983

Spanier GB: Measuring dyadic adjustment: new scales for assessing the quality of marriage and similar dyads. J Marriage Fam 38:15–28, 1976

Ustün TB, Kostanjsek N, Chatterji S, et al: Measuring Health and Disability: Manual for WHO Disability Assessment Schedule (WHODAS 2.0). Geneva, World Health Organization, 2010

Weissman MM, Bothwell S: Assessment of social adjustment by patient self-report. Arch Gen Psychiatry 33(9):1111–1115, 1976 962494

CHAPTER 10

Disruptive Behavior Disorders

10.1   Which of the following disorders is most commonly comorbid with oppositional defiant disorder (ODD)?

A. Attention-deficit/hyperactivity disorder (ADHD).
B. Major depressive disorder.
C. Conduct disorder (CD).
D. Bipolar disorder.
E. Specific learning disorder.

The correct response is option A: Attention-deficit/hyperactivity disorder (ADHD).

The most common disorder that coexists with ODD is ADHD (option A), with comorbidity rates reportedly reaching up to 39% (Speltz et al. 1999). Other disorders that frequently co-occur with ODD include anxiety and depressive disorders (option B) (Angold et al. 1999). Whether ODD can manifest with CD has been a question of debate (option C). A concurrent diagnosis of CD with ODD was prohibited in DSM-IV-TR (American Psychiatric Association 2000) because ODD typically encompasses the features present in CD; however, research suggests that the presence of ODD is an important predictor of future clinical outcomes such as depression, anxiety, and CD (Rowe et al. 2010; Stringaris and Goodman 2009), as well as substance use, ADHD, peer rejection, and family impairment (Nock et al. 2007). The implications of knowing that a child with ODD is at risk for developing other conditions propelled DSM-5 (American Psychiatric Association 2013) to allow for the diagnosis of both ODD and CD concurrently (i.e., an individual can now be diagnosed with ODD even if the criteria for CD are also met). Other important disorders that are associated with ODD include specific learning disorder (option E) and communication disorders. A mood episode in the context of bipolar disorder during which symptoms occurred must be ruled out in the diagnosis

223

of ODD (option D). **(Hales RE, Yudofsky SC, Roberts LW [eds]: APP Textbook of Psychiatry, 6th Edition, Chapter 22, pp. 706–708)**

10.2   The presence of ODD with emotional symptoms predicts the future development of which of the following?

A. Anxiety disorders.
B. Personality disorders.
C. Psychotic disorders.
D. Eating disorders.
E. Substance abuse disorders.

The correct response is option A: Anxiety disorders.

DSM-5 now categorizes ODD symptoms based on whether they have an emotional component (e.g., angry, irritable, resentful), a behavioral element (e.g., argumentative, defiant), or a spiteful/vindictive aspect to them. This classification structure is important because recent research suggests that the emotional symptoms are linked to the development of future mood and anxiety disorders (option A), whereas the spiteful and vindictive behaviors are predictive of conduct disorder and delinquent behaviors (Rowe et al. 2010; Stringaris and Goodman 2009). Signs and symptoms of ODD must not occur exclusively during the course of a psychotic disorder (option C) or a substance use disorder (option E). Personality disorders (option B) and eating disorders (option D) are related disorders of emotional and/or behavioral dysregulation but are not predicted by ODD. **(Hales RE, Yudofsky SC, Roberts LW [eds]: APP Textbook of Psychiatry, 6th Edition, Chapter 22, pp. 706–707)**

10.3   A 21-year-old man with a history of oppositional defiant disorder presents with frequent impulsive behavioral outbursts that are grossly out of proportion to the stressor. He reports that he is unable to control himself and is worried that he might lose his job if his behavior continues. What is the most likely diagnosis?

A. Bipolar disorder.
B. Attention-deficit/hyperactivity disorder (ADHD).
C. Intermittent explosive disorder (IED).
D. Conduct disorder (CD).
E. Adjustment disorder.

The correct response is option C: Intermittent explosive disorder (IED).

IED is a disorder characterized by recurrent episodes of inability to control aggressive impulses, reflected by verbal and/or physical aggression (option C). Acts of aggression in IED are not premeditated, are greatly disproportionate to precipitating stressors, and are not targeted toward specific ends. Aggressive acts may be dystonic in that they bring distress to the perpetrating individual. The diagnosis of IED must rule out existing psychopathology that better accounts for displays of aggressive behavior and use of substances with psychotropic properties. Diagnosis of IED cannot be made before age 6. The diagnosis of IED can be made in addition to the diagnosis of ADHD (option B), CD (option D), oppositional defiant disorder, or autism spectrum disorder when recurrent impulsive aggressive outbursts are in excess of those usually seen in these disorders and warrant independent clinical attention. His lack of major stressors would argue against an adjustment disorder as the cause of his behavior (option E), and his relatively intact insight and judgment would argue against a manic, hypomanic, or mixed episode in bipolar disorder (option A). **(Hales RE, Yudofsky SC, Roberts LW [eds]: APP Textbook of Psychiatry, 6th Edition, Chapter 22, pp. 709–710)**

10.4   Which of the following is true regarding the incidence and course of ODD?

A. Symptoms of oppositional defiant disorder (ODD) usually emerge first in the school setting.
B. The majority of patients with ODD will not develop conduct disorder (CD).
C. The number of ODD symptoms is not positively correlated with the development of CD.
D. Typical age at onset of ODD is between 10 and 12 years of age.
E. Boys are twice as likely as girls to meet criteria for ODD at all ages.

The correct response is option B: The majority of patients with ODD will not develop conduct disorder (CD).

Although CD is usually preceded by ODD, the majority of children with ODD do not go on to develop CD or antisocial behaviors in adulthood (Loeber et al. 2000) (option B). Symptoms more commonly first materialize in the home setting (option A), with the typical age of onset between 6 and 8 years of age (option D). A high number of ODD symptoms are associated with the development of CD (option C). Slightly more boys than girls have been reported to have ODD, with data from the National Comorbidity Survey showing a prevalence of 11.2% in boys and 9.2% in females (Nock et al. 2007) (option E). This gender difference appears to even out after puberty (Loeber et al. 2000). **(Hales RE, Yudofsky SC, Roberts LW [eds]: APP Textbook of Psychiatry, 6th Edition, Chapter 22, pp. 707–708)**

10.5   Which of the following has been shown to be more effective for aggression in patients with Cluster B personality disorders than in patients with IED?

A. Fluoxetine.
B. Divalproex.
C. Risperidone.
D. Lithium.
E. Propranolol.

The correct response is option B: Divalproex.

Divalproex has shown promise as an option for the treatment of aggression, performing better than placebo in treating impulsive aggression in borderline personality disorder. Higher baseline trait impulsivity and state aggression symptoms may be solid candidate markers for divalproex treatment. Divalproex, however, did not have antiaggressive effects in IED patients, although it did have such effects in patients with Cluster B personality disorders (option B). The drug may be preferentially effective in highly aggressive subjects with personality disorders (Hollander et al. 2003, 2005).

Symptoms of IED may respond to selective serotonin reuptake inhibitors (SSRIs) (option A), anticonvulsants, antipsychotics (option C), phenytoin, β-blockers (option E), and α_2-adrenergic agonists (Dell'Osso et al. 2006). SSRIs typically fail to produce long-term remission of aggressive symptoms. Temperamental factors, including neuroticism and harm avoidance, may be indicators for SSRI treatment response (Phan et al. 2011). If aggression is within the context of mood episode in bipolar disorder, lithium (option D) may reduce aggression with treatment of the episode; however, there is less evidence that it would be helpful for aggression in patients with a Cluster B personality disorder (Comai et al. 2012). **(Hales RE, Yudofsky SC, Roberts LW [eds]: APP Textbook of Psychiatry, 6th Edition, Chapter 22, p. 712; *Journal of Clinical Psychopharmacology* 32(2):237–260, 2012)**

10.6 Which of the following is characteristic of pyromania?

A. Fire setting for monetary gain.
B. Fire setting for revenge.
C. Fascination with fire.
D. Fire setting due to impaired judgment.
E. Delusional thinking.

The correct response is option C: Fascination with fire.

Motives for arson include delusional thinking, revenge, property damage, and excitement from fire setting. However, not all individuals with fire-setting behavior or who have committed arson meet the criteria for pyromania. The essential feature of pyromania is multiple instances of deliberate and purposeful fire setting that is unrelated to the following: another psychiatric state (option E) or ideology, vengeance (option B), criminality (option A), impaired judgment (e.g., dementia or mental retardation) (option D), or arson to communicate a desire or need (commonly seen in arsonists with mental or personality disorders). Individuals with pyromania have a fascination with fire (option C) and are commonly "watchers" at fires, or they may seek employment or volunteer as firefighters. Although the fire setting results from a failure to resist an impulse, significance may also lie in the preparation of the fire. Pyromania, however, is considered an uncontrolled and impulsive behavior (Hollander et al. 2008). **(Hales RE, Yudofsky SC, Roberts LW [eds]: APP Textbook of Psychiatry, 6th Edition, Chapter 22, pp. 719–721)**

References

American Psychiatric Association: Diagnostic and Statistical Manual of Mental Disorders, 4th Edition, Text Revision. Washington, DC, American Psychiatric Association, 2000

American Psychiatric Association: Diagnostic and Statistical Manual of Mental Disorders, 5th Edition. Arlington, VA, American Psychiatric Association, 2013

Angold A, Costello EJ, Erkanli A: Comorbidity. J Child Psychol Psychiatry 40(1):57–87, 1999 10102726

Comai S, Tau M, Pavlovic Z, Gobbi G: The psychopharmacology of aggressive behavior: a translational approach: part 2: clinical studies using atypical antipsychotics, anticonvulsants, and lithium. J Clin Psychopharmacol 32(2):237–260, 2012 22367663

Dell'Osso B, Altamura AC, Allen A, et al: Epidemiologic and clinical updates on impulse control disorders: a critical review. Eur Arch Psychiatry Clin Neurosci 256(8):464–475, 2006 16960655

Hollander E, Tracy KA, Swann AC, et al: Divalproex in the treatment of impulsive aggression: efficacy in cluster B personality disorders. Neuropsychopharmacology 28(6):1186–1197, 2003 12700713

Hollander E, Swann AC, Coccaro EF, et al: Impact of trait impulsivity and state aggression on divalproex versus placebo response in borderline personality disorder. Am J Psychiatry 162(3):621–624, 2005 15741486

Hollander E, Berlin HA, Stein DJ: Impulse-control disorders not elsewhere classified, in The American Psychiatric Publishing Textbook of Psychiatry, 5th Edition. Edited by Hales RE, Yudofsky SC, Gabbard GO. Washington, DC, American Psychiatric Publishing, 2008, pp 777 820

Loeber R, Green SM, Lahey BB, et al: Findings on disruptive behavior disorders from the first decade of the Developmental Trends Study. Clin Child Fam Psychol Rev 3(1):37–60, 2000 11228766

Nock MK, Kazdin AE, Hiripi E, Kessler RC: Lifetime prevalence, correlates, and persistence of oppositional defiant disorder: results from the National Comorbidity Survey Replication. J Child Psychol Psychiatry 48(7):703–713, 2007 17593151

Phan KL, Lee R, Coccaro EF: Personality predictors of antiaggressive response to fluoxetine: inverse association with neuroticism and harm avoidance. Int Clin Psychopharmacol 26(5):278–283, 2011 21795983

Rowe R, Costello EJ, Angold A, et al: Developmental pathways in oppositional defiant disorder and conduct disorder. J Abnorm Psychol 119(4):726–738, 2010 21090876

Speltz ML, McClellan J, DeKlyen M, Jones K: Preschool boys with oppositional defiant disorder: clinical presentation and diagnostic change. J Am Acad Child Adolesc Psychiatry 38(7):838–845, 1999 10405501

Stringaris A, Goodman R: Longitudinal outcome of youth oppositionality: irritable, headstrong, and hurtful behaviors have distinctive predictions. J Am Acad Child Adolesc Psychiatry 48(4):404–412, 2009 19318881

CHAPTER 11

Dissociative Disorders

11.1 Which of the following conditions is characterized by an inability to recall important personal information (including traumatic memories) that cannot be explained by ordinary forgetfulness, overt brain pathology, or substance use?

A. Dissociative amnesia.
B. Dissociative fugue.
C. Forgetfulness.
D. Derealization.
E. Posttraumatic stress disorder.

The correct response is option A: Dissociative amnesia.

As detailed in Criterion A in the DSM-5 diagnostic criteria, the hallmark of dissociative amnesia is the inability to recall important personal information, usually of a traumatic or stressful nature, that cannot be explained by ordinary forgetfulness (option C), in the absence of overt brain pathology or substance use (option A) (American Psychiatric Association 2013). The dissociative disorders involve a disturbance in the integrated organization of consciousness, memory, identity, emotion, perception, body representation, motor control, and behavior. Events normally experienced on a smooth continuum are isolated from the other mental processes with which they would ordinarily be associated. This discontinuity results in a variety of dissociative disorders, depending on the primary cognitive process affected. When memories are poorly integrated, the resulting disorder is *dissociative amnesia*. No longer its own diagnosis, in DSM-5 *dissociative fugue* exists as a specifier ("with dissociative fugue") if the amnesia also includes aimless wandering (option B). *Derealization* describes experiences of unreality or detachment with respect to surroundings (option D). Derealization often, but not always, co-occurs with *depersonalization* (i.e., persistent feelings of unreality, detachment, or estrangement from oneself or one's body, usually with the feeling that one is an outside observer of one's own mental processes). When this happens, individuals experience an altered perception of their surroundings in which the world seems unreal or dreamlike. Disordered perception yields *depersonalization/derealization disorder* and, in conjunction with the symptoms of posttraumatic stress disorder (PTSD), produces its dissociative subtype (option E). **(Hales RE, Yudofsky SC, Roberts LW [eds]: APP Textbook of Psychiatry, 6th Edition, Chapter 15, pp. 499, 517–518, 521)**

11.2   Which of the following conditions is characterized by persistent feelings of unreality, detachment, or estrangement from oneself?

A. Dissociative amnesia.
B. Dissociative fugue.
C. Depersonalization/derealization disorder.
D. Acute stress disorder.
E. Peritraumatic dissociation.

The correct response is option C: Depersonalization/derealization disorder.

As specified in the DSM-5 diagnostic criteria, the essential feature of depersonalization/derealization disorder is the presence of *depersonalization* (i.e., persistent feelings of unreality, detachment, or estrangement from oneself or one's body, usually with the feeling that one is an outside observer of one's own mental processes), *derealization* (i.e., experiences of unreality or detachment with respect to surroundings), or both (option C). Of note, Criterion A allows for the presence of either or both phenomena. Clinically, depersonalization is characterized by a profound disruption of self-awareness, mainly involving feelings of disembodiment and subjective emotional numbing (Sierra and David 2011; Spiegel et al. 2011). When derealization co-occurs with depersonalization, individuals experience an altered perception of their surroundings in which the world seems unreal or dreamlike. Affected individuals often will ruminate about this alteration and be preoccupied with their own somatic and mental functioning. Depersonalization/derealization disorder is thus primarily a disturbance in the integration of perceptual experiences. Individuals with the disorder have intact reality testing, and are distressed by their symptoms.

The hallmark of *dissociative amnesia* is the inability to recall important personal information, usually of a traumatic or stressful nature, that cannot be explained by ordinary forgetfulness, in the absence of overt brain pathology or substance use (option A). If the amnesia also includes aimless wandering, the specifier "with dissociative fugue" is used (option B). Acute stress disorder in DSM-5 includes—but does not require—dissociative symptoms (Bryant et al. 2011) (option D). Peritraumatic dissociation has been found to be a strong predictor for later development of posttraumatic stress disorder, dissociation, and depression (option E). **(Hales RE, Yudofsky SC, Roberts LW [eds]: APP Textbook of Psychiatry, 6th Edition, Chapter 14, p. 480; Chapter 15, pp. 499, 503–504, 517, 521–522, and Table 15–2, p. 506)**

11.3 Recall of a personal experience identified with the self, such as attending a base-ball game, involves which of the following types of memory?

A. Episodic memory.
B. Implicit memory.
C. Procedural memory.
D. Semantic memory.
E. Nondeclarative memory.

The correct response is option A: Episodic memory.

Modern research on memory shows that there are at least two broad categories of memory, variously described as *explicit* (*episodic*) and *implicit* (*semantic*). These two memory systems serve different functions. Explicit/episodic memory involves recall of personal experience identified with the self (e.g., going to the ball game last week) (option A). *Implicit/semantic memory* involves the execution of routine operations (e.g., riding a bicycle or typing) (options B, D); this is sometimes referred to as *procedural memory* or nondeclarative memory (options C, E). Unlike declarative memory, nondeclarative memory cannot be considered a system. Rather, the term is simply a general classification for a disparate group of tasks (and presumably memory processes) whose performance is not mediated by conscious recall. One unifying feature of nondeclarative memory tasks is that they demand implicit recall, in which there is no need for conscious storage or recall of material. The term procedural memory is typically applied to tasks that assess the acquisition of motor or cognitive skills. One can describe procedural memory as "knowing how" as opposed to declarative memory's "knowing that" (Cohen and Squire 1980). Such operations may be carried out with a high degree of proficiency with little conscious awareness of either their current execution or the learning episodes on which the skill is based. Indeed, these two types of memory have different neuroanatomical localizations: the limbic system, especially the hippocampal formation, and mammillary bodies for episodic memory, and the basal ganglia and cortex for semantic memory (Mishkin and Appenzeller 1987). The distinction between these two types of memory may account for certain dissociative phenomena. The automaticity observed in certain dissociative disorders may be a reflection of the separation of self-identification in certain kinds of explicit memory from routine activity in implicit or semantic memory. **(Hales RE, Yudofsky SC, Roberts LW [eds]: APP Textbook of Psychiatry, 6th Edition, Chapter 15, pp. 502–503; Yudofsky SC, Hales RE [eds]: APP Textbook of Neuropsychiatry and Behavioral Neurosciences, 5th Edition, Chapter 14, pp. 568–569)**

11.4 Which of the following statements best characterizes the nature of memory loss in dissociative amnesia?

A. The memory loss is procedural.
B. The memory loss is permanent.

C. The memory deficit typically involves an inability to lay down new episodic memories.
D. The amnesia is typically anterograde.
E. The memory loss is generally for traumatic or stressful events.

The correct response is option E: The memory loss is generally for traumatic or stressful events.

Dissociative amnesia is the most common of the dissociative disorders. It is the classical functional disorder of memory and involves difficulty in retrieving discrete components of autobiographical-episodic memory (Kritchevsky et al. 2004; Spiegel et al. 2011). Dissociative amnesia has three primary characteristics: 1) The memory loss is episodic; the first-person recollection of certain events is lost, but procedural knowledge is not (option A). 2) The memory loss is for a discrete period of time, ranging from minutes to years. 3) The memory loss is generally for events of a traumatic or stressful nature (option E). Because dissociative amnesia primarily involves difficulties in retrieval rather than encoding or storage, the memory deficits are usually reversible (option B). There is usually no difficulty in learning new episodic information; thus the amnesia is typically retrograde rather than anterograde (options C, D). **(Hales RE, Yudofsky SC, Roberts LW [eds]: APP Textbook of Psychiatry, 6th Edition, Chapter 15, pp. 518–519)**

11.5   Experiencing of others as unreal, dreamlike, or foggy is an example of which of the following?

A. Delusional disorder.
B. Depersonalization.
C. Dissociative amnesia.
D. Impaired reality testing.
E. Derealization.

The correct response is option E: Derealization.

As defined in Criterion A of the DSM-5 definition of depersonalization/derealization disorder, *derealization* refers to experiences of unreality or detachment with respect to surroundings (e.g., individuals or objects are experienced as unreal, dreamlike, foggy, lifeless, or visually distorted [option E]). *Depersonalization* refers to experiences of unreality, detachment, or being an outside observer with respect to one's thoughts, feelings, sensations, body, or actions. Experiences of depersonalization can include experiencing an unreal self, perceptual alterations, emotional numbing, or a distorted sense of time (option B). The hallmark of *dissociative amnesia* is the inability to recall important personal information, usually of a traumatic or stressful nature, that cannot be explained by ordinary forgetfulness, in the absence of overt brain pathology or substance use (option C). Reality testing remains intact in depersonalization/derealization disorder (option D). Patients are aware of some distortion in their perceptual experience and therefore are not delusional (option A). Their intact reality testing often leads to symptomatic distress. **(Hales RE, Yudofsky SC, Roberts LW [eds]: APP Textbook of Psychiatry, 6th Edition, Chapter 15, pp. 521–522)**

11.6   Which of the following statements regarding the treatment of dissociative identity disorder (DID) is most correct?

A. Hypnosis is the gold standard for diagnosis and treatment.
B. In psychotherapy, alters should be addressed by name rather than as identity states.
C. The goal of psychotherapeutic treatment is to facilitate integration of disparate elements.
D. It is unusual for a negative transference to develop between patients with DID and their therapists.
E. Short-acting barbiturates (e.g., sodium amobarbital) remain the pharmacological treatment of choice in treating DID.

The correct response is option C: The goal of psychotherapeutic treatment is to facilitate integration of disparate elements.

Psychotherapy can help patients with DID gain control over the dissociative process underlying their symptoms. The fundamental psychotherapeutic stance should involve meeting patients halfway in the sense of acknowledging that they experience themselves as fragmented, yet the reality is that the fundamental problem is a failure of integration of disparate memories and aspects of the self. Therefore, the goal in therapy is to facilitate the integration of disparate elements (option C). Hypnosis can be helpful in therapy as well as in diagnosis, but it is not the gold standard of treatment (option A). The simple structure of hypnotic induction may elicit dissociative phenomena. The capacity to elicit such symptoms on command provides the first hint of the ability to control these symptoms. Hypnosis can also be helpful in facilitating access to dissociated personalities. After some training, a therapist may simply call up a given "identity state" (e.g., "the part of you that felt hurt") as opposed to a specific "person" (e.g., an alter who identifies herself as "Lucy" when the patient's given name is Barbara). The reason for using a particular identity state rather than a specific name to address an alter (option B) is that fostering a relationship with each personality state (which the patient identifies as a distinctive "person" or entity) serves to promote integration of these dissociated or fragmented personality states. During psychotherapy, patients with DID may develop traumatic transferences (option D). Although their reality testing is good enough that they can perceive genuine caring, these patients face significant challenges. Patients with DID may expect therapists to exploit them, with the patients viewing the working through of traumatic memories as a reinflicting of the trauma with the therapists' taking sadistic pleasure in their suffering. Patients may also expect their therapists to be excessively passive, identifying them with some uncaring family figure who knew abuse was occurring but did little or nothing to stop it. To date, no good evidence shows that medication of any type has a direct therapeutic effect on the dissociative process manifested by patients with DID (Loewenstein 2006; Putnam 1989). Pharmacological treatment has been limited to the control of signs and symptoms afflicting patients with DID or comorbid conditions, rather than the treatment of dissociation per se. Whereas in the past, short-acting barbiturates such as sodium amobarbital were used intravenously to reverse functional amnesias, this technique is no longer used, largely because of poor results (option E). **(Hales RE, Yudofsky SC, Roberts LW [eds]: APP Textbook of Psychiatry, 6th Edition, Chapter 15, pp. 510–513, 516)**

References

American Psychiatric Association: Diagnostic and Statistical Manual of Mental Disorders, 5th Edition. Arlington, VA, American Psychiatric Association, 2013

Bryant RA, Friedman MJ, Spiegel D, et al: A review of acute stress disorder in DSM-5. Depress Anxiety 28(9):802–817, 2011 21910186

Cohen NJ, Squire LR: Preserved learning and retention of pattern-analyzing skill in amnesia: dissociation of knowing how and knowing that. Science 210(4466):207–210, 1980 7414331

Kritchevsky M, Chang J, Squire LR: Functional amnesia: clinical description and neuropsychological profile of 10 cases. Learn Mem 11(2):213–226, 2004 15054137

Loewenstein RJ: DID 101: a hands-on clinical guide to the stabilization phase of dissociative identity disorder treatment. Psychiatr Clin North Am 29(1):305–332, xii, 2006 16530599

Mishkin M, Appenzeller T: The anatomy of memory. Sci Am 256(6):80–89, 1987 3589645

Putnam FW: Diagnosis and Treatment of Multiple Personality Disorder. New York, Guilford Press, 1989

Sierra M, David AS: Depersonalization: a selective impairment of self-awareness. Conscious Cogn 20(1):99–108, 2011 21087873

Spiegel D, Loewenstein RJ, Lewis-Fernández R, et al: Dissociative disorders in DSM-5. Depress Anxiety 28(12):E17–E45, 2011 22134959

CHAPTER 12

Elimination Disorders

12.1   What is the earliest age at which a child can be diagnosed with enuresis according to DSM-5 criteria?

A. 3 years.
B. 4 years.
C. 5 years.
D. 6 years.
E. 7 years.

The correct response is option C: 5 years.

There is considerable variation in the age at which urinary continence is achieved in youngsters. Children ages 3 and 4 years (options A, B) may frequently exhibit inappropriate elimination as they learn to control their bladders consistently. At age 5 years, which is the minimum age at which enuresis can be diagnosed according to DSM-5 (American Psychiatric Association 2013) criteria (option C), approximately 5%–15% of children will have nocturnal enuresis, and this number declines to 1%–2% by adulthood. Individuals who have never attained continence are said to have primary enuresis, whereas the term secondary enuresis is used to describe children who experience incontinence following at least 6 months of continence. Older children (options D, E) are more likely to present with comorbid diagnoses; therefore, a comprehensive medical and psychiatric evaluation is indicated for these children. **(DSM-5, Elimination Disorders, pp. 355–357; Dulcan MK [ed]: Dulcan's Textbook of Child and Adolescent Psychiatry, 2nd Edition, Chapter 22, pp. 479–481; Hales RE, Yudofsky SC, Roberts LW [eds]: APP Textbook of Psychiatry, 6th Edition, Chapter 18, pp. 588–590)**

12.2   What is the most common cause of encopresis?

A. Intellectual disability.
B. Obsessive-compulsive disorder.
C. Sexual abuse.

D. Attention-deficit/hyperactivity disorder (ADHD).

E. Constipation.

The correct response is option E: Constipation.

Etiology of encopresis is divided into retentive and nonretentive factors. Retentive encopresis occurs more commonly than nonretentive encopresis, and chronic constipation is the physiological mechanism (option E). Encopresis can occur in cases of intellectual disability (option A), but not all children with intellectual disability have encopresis; evaluation for constipation in these children is especially important given frequent impairment in communication. Nonretentive encopresis due to sexual abuse has been described (option C), although constipation is a more common cause. Children with obsessional traits (option B) may develop encopresis due to fears of using bathrooms outside the home, but these children should also be evaluated for constipation. Although a failure to recognize the need to defecate secondary to attentional problems may contribute to encopresis, ADHD as a causal factor of encopresis has not been definitively documented (option D). **(Hales RE, Yudofsky SC, Roberts LW [eds]: APP Textbook of Psychiatry, 6th Edition, Chapter 18, pp. 597–598 and Table 18–1, p. 590)**

12.3   What factors do enuresis and encopresis have in common?

A. Both enuresis and encopresis will not remit without treatment in most children.

B. Both enuresis and encopresis have a similar longitudinal trajectory.

C. Both enuresis and encopresis share the same treatment modality.

D. Both enuresis and encopresis are strongly associated with ADHD.

E. Both enuresis and encopresis have approximately the same incidence rate.

The correct response is option B: Both enuresis and encopresis have a similar longitudinal trajectory.

Overall, the incidence of encopresis is much lower than that of enuresis (option E). There is a strong association with ADHD that is seen with enuresis that has not been documented with encopresis (option D). The longitudinal trajectory of encopresis is similar to that of enuresis; both disorders usually resolve over time, and their incidence in adolescence is extremely low (option B). Although the literature reviewed in this chapter indicates that both enuresis and encopresis will eventually remit without treatment in almost all children (option A), the symptoms of these disorders are so psychologically distressing that active treatment is justified to limit their duration. There is no single treatment modality that will be appropriate for every child who presents with an elimination disorder (option C). **(Hales RE, Yudofsky SC, Roberts LW [eds]: APP Textbook of Psychiatry, 6th Edition, Chapter 18, pp. 597–598, 600)**

Reference

American Psychiatric Association: Diagnostic and Statistical Manual of Mental Disorders, 5th Edition. Arlington, VA, American Psychiatric Association, 2013

CHAPTER 13

Epidemiology and Public Policy: Health Care Economics/ Public Policy Issues

13.1 The American Psychiatric Association principles of medical ethics prohibit serious boundary violations such as sexual contact with patients. Which of the following sets of physician risk factors are associated with sexual contact with patients?

A. Intense transference, isolation from colleagues, and narcissistic pathology.
B. Inadequate training, isolation from colleagues, and borderline personality.
C. Inadequate training, isolation from colleagues, and narcissistic pathology.
D. Intense transference, isolation from colleagues, and borderline personality.
E. Intense transference, inadequate training, and narcissistic pathology.

The correct response is option C: Inadequate training, isolation from colleagues, and narcissistic pathology.

A review of qualitative and quantitative studies of therapists who had sexual relations with their patients suggests that risk factors for such behavior include inadequate training, isolation from colleagues, and narcissistic pathology (option C) (Epstein 1994) rather than borderline personality pathology (option B) and intense transference (options A, D, E). The American Psychiatric Association's principles of medical ethics have prohibited sexual contact between patients and physicians since 1973 (American Psychiatric Association 2001), and such contact is illegal in many states (Milne 2002). **(Hales RE, Yudofsky SC, Roberts LW [eds]: APP Textbook of Psychiatry, 6th Edition, Chapter 7, p. 210)**

13.2   A cardiology resident is obtaining consent from a 65-year-old woman for cardiac catheterization and stent placement. The patient agrees to have the procedure because "whatever the doctor says is probably best." When asked about the procedure, the patient states, "I'm a homemaker and I can't really understand these things; it's something to do with the heart. I guess it will make me better. It'll probably be fine." Why would this patient's agreement *not* meet the standard for informed consent?

A. The patient's level of education does not provide for a thorough understanding of the procedure.
B. All that was needed was to present the patient with important information necessary to make a decision.
C. The patient cannot articulate an understanding of the procedure or of its risks, benefits, and alternatives.
D. The physician does not have an overall therapeutic relationship with the patient.
E. Informed consent is not important in this case, because the procedure is clearly in the patient's best interests.

The correct response is option C: The patient cannot articulate an understanding of the procedure or of its risks, benefits, and alternatives.

Informed consent is the process by which individuals make free, knowledgeable decisions about whether to accept a proposed plan for assessment and/or treatment. Informed consent is thus a cornerstone of ethical practice. An adequate process of informed consent reflects and promotes the ethical principle of *autonomy*. The principle of *beneficence* is also crucial in this context. This requires the clinician, regardless of whether he or she has an overall therapeutic relationship with the patient (option D), to thoroughly appraise the degree to which the consent process meets the patient's needs for information (option A) and for the opportunity to make a choice consistent with his or her authentic preferences and values (Roberts 2002).

It is important to remember that patients who *accept* recommended treatment that is in their best interest may do so while lacking adequate capacity for that decision (option E). Thus, even in cases where a patient is accepting treatment, an inability to articulate an understanding of the risks, benefits, and alternatives to the proposed treatment may signal an absence of intact decision-making capacity (option C). In such cases, a surrogate decision maker should be sought to provide consent for the treatment in order to ensure that the informed consent process respects the patient's diminished autonomy. Informed consent is an ethically and legally important practice by which individuals make free, knowledgeable decisions about their care; however, this patient was not making a knowledgeable decision (option B). **(Hales RE, Yudofsky SC, Roberts LW [eds]: APP Textbook of Psychiatry, 6th Edition, Chapter 7, pp. 212–214, 222)**

13.3 Medical trainees often provide care beyond their current capabilities in order to learn skills that will ultimately benefit future patients. Which of the following safeguards is required to handle this ethical dilemma?

A. Safeguards to ensure that trainees practice only marginally beyond their current capabilities, with adequate supervision and informed consent of patients.
B. Safeguards to ensure that trainees practice only marginally beyond their current capabilities after a thorough orientation.
C. Safeguards to ensure that trainees practice only marginally beyond their current capabilities, with adequate supervision and thorough evaluations.
D. Safeguards to ensure that trainees practice well beyond their current capabilities, with adequate supervision and informed consent of patients.
E. Safeguards to ensure that trainees practice well beyond their current capabilities, with adequate supervision and thorough evaluations.

The correct response is option A: Safeguards to ensure that trainees practice only marginally beyond their current capabilities, with adequate supervision and informed consent of patients.

Medical school and residency training give rise to specific ethical issues because of the need for trainees to provide care that is beyond their current level of expertise. Handling this ethical dilemma requires the informed consent of patients as willing participants in the educational setting as well as safeguards to ensure that trainees practice only marginally beyond their current capabilities and with adequate supervision (option A) (Fry 1991; Hoop 2004; Roberts and Dyer 2004; Vinicky et al. 1991). Practicing only marginally beyond current capabilities (options D, E) and informed patient consent (options B, C) are crucial. **(Hales RE, Yudofsky SC, Roberts LW [eds]: APP Textbook of Psychiatry, 6th Edition, Chapter 7, p. 221)**

13.4 What is collaborative care?

A. Primary care physicians getting psychiatric consultations for depressed patients.
B. Psychiatrists getting medical consultations for patients.
C. An informal interaction between primary care physicians and psychiatrists.
D. An evidence-based, systematic approach in which primary care and behavioral health providers work closely together to deliver effective treatment.
E. Nonpsychiatrists providing mental health care to patients with serious mental illness.

The correct response is option D: An evidence-based, systematic approach in which primary care and behavioral health providers work closely together to deliver effective treatment.

Collaborative care is an evidence-based, systematic approach in which primary care and behavioral health providers work closely together to deliver effective treatment for depression and other common mental disorders in primary care settings (option D). It represents one opportunity for psychiatrists to "leverage" their unique skills and reach a larger share of the millions of people living with mental health and substance use problems who are in need of quality care. The interaction of behavioral and physical health problems at an individual and population level (Katon 2003; Moussavi et al. 2007) suggests that when psychiatrists (option E) collaborate more closely (options A–C) with their medical colleagues, they have a greater chance of providing care that addresses the whole spectrum of behavioral and medical health needs. **(Raney LE [ed]: Integrated Care: Working at the Interface of Primary Care and Behavioral Health, Chapter 1, p. 4)**

13.5   Which of the following best describes the interaction between serious mental illness (SMI) and medical disorders?

A. People with SMI have lower rates of medical disorders than people in the general population.
B. Rates of disease in people with SMI are only increased for diabetes.
C. Cardiovascular disease is increased 2–3 times for people with schizophrenia.
D. Medical disorders are uncommon in adults with mental illness.
E. Cardiovascular disease occurs, but at an older age in persons with SMI.

The correct response is option C: Cardiovascular disease is increased 2–3 times for people with schizophrenia.

Medical illness is highly prevalent in individuals with psychiatric disorders: greater than 68% of adults with mental illness were found to have at least one medical disorder in the 2001–2003 National Comorbidity Survey Replication (Alegria et al. 2003) (option A). Rates of disease in those with SMI exceed those of the general population in every disease category (Parks et al. 2006) (option B). Specifically, patients with SMI display greater rates of obesity, diabetes, metabolic syndrome, chronic obstructive pulmonary disease, HIV, viral hepatitis, and tuberculosis than the general population (option D). Cardiovascular disease is also common, with prevalence increased twofold to threefold in patients with bipolar disorder and schizophrenia (option C). Cardiovascular disease also occurs at a younger age in persons with SMI (option E) (De Hert et al. 2011). **(Raney LE [ed]: Integrated Care: Working at the Interface of Primary Care and Behavioral Health, Chapter 7, p. 142)**

13.6   Which of the following best describes a "health home"?

A. A living facility where persons with severe mental illness are housed.
B. A short-term service model of health care delivery.
C. Delivery of the full array of required services.
D. A cost-effective way to facilitate access to an interdisciplinary array of care.
E. Services that are only provided to adults.

The correct response is option D: A cost-effective way to facilitate access to an interdisciplinary array of care.

The 2010 Patient Protection and Affordable Care Act established a "health home" option under Medicaid to serve enrollees with chronic conditions by building a person-centered system of care that achieves improved outcomes for beneficiaries and better services and value for state Medicaid programs (Mann 2012). The health home service delivery model is intended to provide a cost-effective, longitudinal "home" (option B) to facilitate access to an interdisciplinary array of medical care (option D), behavioral health care, and community-based social services and supports for both children and adults (option E) with chronic conditions. Health homes are designed to improve the health care delivery system for individuals with chronic conditions by employing a whole-person approach—caring not just for an individual's behavioral and physical condition, but providing linkages to long-term community care services and supports, social services, and family services. It is not merely housing (option A). The integration of primary care and behavioral health services is critical to the achievement of enhanced outcomes. The health home service delivery model is expected to result in lower rates of emergency room use, reduction in hospital admissions and readmissions, reduction in health care costs, less reliance on long-term-care facilities, and improved experience of care and quality-of-care outcomes for the individual. The guidance from the Centers for Medicare and Medicaid Services (CMS) regarding the Medicaid health home option indicates that health homes do not need to provide the full array of required services themselves (option C) but must ensure such services are available and coordinated (Centers for Medicare and Medicaid Services 2010). **(Centers for Medicare and Medicaid Services: Health Homes for Enrollees with Chronic Conditions (Letter to State Medicaid Directors and State Health Officials, SMDL# 10-024, ACA# 12). Baltimore, MD, Department of Health and Human Services, November 16, 2010; Raney LE [ed]: Integrated Care: Working at the Interface of Primary Care and Behavioral Health, Chapter 9, pp. 193–194)**

13.7   What prompted Congress to enact the Nursing Home Reform Act as part of the Omnibus Budget Reconciliation Act of 1987?

A. Attempt to shift costs for patients' care to the federal government.
B. Attempt to put more elderly patients with mental health problems into nursing homes.
C. The misuse of physical and chemical restraints in nursing homes.
D. Patients with chronic psychiatric problems needing the type of care provided in nursing homes.
E. Overregulation of nursing facilities by the government.

The correct response is option C: The misuse of physical and chemical restraints in nursing homes.

The misuse of physical and chemical restraints was a rallying point for advocacy groups that urged the federal government to institute a process of nursing home reform (option C). In addition, the U.S. General Accounting Office was concerned that states were admitting patients with chronic and severe psychiatric problems to Medicaid-certified nursing homes not because patients needed this type of care (options B, D) but because admission would shift a substantial portion of the costs of patients' care from the state to the federal government (options A). Apparently in response to both sets of concerns, Congress enacted the Nursing Home Reform Act as part of the Omnibus Budget Reconciliation Act of 1987 (P.L. 100-203). This legislation provided for government regulation of the operation of nursing facilities and of the care that they provide (option E) (Elon and Pawlson 1992). **(Steffens DC, Blazer DG, Thakur ME [eds]: APP Textbook of Geriatric Psychiatry, 5th Edition, Chapter 25, pp. 719–720)**

13.8   What led Congress to the Mental Retardation Facilities and Community Mental Health Centers Construction Act in 1963?

A. Too many state-level child mental health systems.
B. The child guidance movement with a shift from a punishment model to a corrective model.
C. The underutilization of institutionalized care for children and adolescents.
D. Excessive reimbursement for school consultations.
E. Too many community mental health centers providing children's services.

The correct response is option B: The child guidance movement with a shift from a punishment model to a corrective model.

An early progenitor of systems of care is the child guidance movement, which emerged at the turn of the nineteenth century and led a shift from a punishment model to a corrective model ("guiding" children) that emphasized advocacy in multiple life domains (option B) (Jones 1999). Congress passed the Mental Retardation Facilities and Community Mental Health Centers (CMHCs) Construction Act in 1963 in order to create a national network of community mental health centers. Because the act did not specifically address children, only half of the centers had children's services (option E). The indirect costs of child services, such as consultation with schools, were poorly reimbursed, if at all (option D). Once the planned transition of the responsibility for managing CMHCs moved to the states, few states had a child mental health system or expertise (option A) (Lourie 2003). The book *Unclaimed Children* (Knitzer 1982), which described the inadequacies of the national response to children with serious emotional disturbances and their families, served as a rallying point for advocates. This concern, coupled with philosophical and financial concerns about the overutilization of institutionalized care (option C), ultimately facilitated congressional funding of the Child and Adolescent Service System Program in 1984 and later the Comprehensive Community Mental Health Services for Children and Their Families Program. These programs, along with state and foundation funding, led to the development of community-based services for youth with significant emotional disturbances. **(Dulcan M [ed]: Dulcan's Textbook of Child and Adolescent Psychiatry, 2nd Edition, Chapter 46, pp. 1007–1008)**

13.9   Which of the following would fall into the "social" component of a biopsychosocial patient interview?

A. Asking about medications taken by the patient.
B. Asking about psychiatric symptoms.
C. Asking about family history.
D. Asking about spirituality.
E. Asking about other medical illness.

The correct response is option D: Asking about spirituality.

The "social" aspect of biopsychosocial refers to the sociological, religious, spiritual, ethnic, and racial issues that may be pertinent to patients (option D). Some of this information may seem like "common knowledge," but exploring specifics will often lead to a discussion of identity, psychology, and culture that can inform an understanding of the patient (Miller et al. 2012; Peteet et al. 2011). Asking routine questions about the patient's medical or psychiatric history is not part of the "social" issues (options A, B, C, E) **(Hales RE, Yudofsky SC, Roberts LW [eds]: APP Textbook of Psychiatry, 6th Edition, Chapter 1, p. 8)**

References

Alegria MJ, Kessler RC, Takeuchi D: National Comorbidity Survey Replication (NCS-R), 2001–2003. Ann Arbor, MI, Inter-university Consortium for Political and Social Research, 2003

American Psychiatric Association: Ethics Primer of the American Psychiatric Association. Washington, DC, American Psychiatric Association, 2001

Centers for Medicare and Medicaid Services: Health Homes for Enrollees with Chronic Conditions (Letter to State Medicaid Directors and State Health Officials, SMDL# 10-024, ACA# 12). Baltimore, MD. Department of Health and Human Services, November 16, 2010. Available at: http://www.cms.gov/smdl/downloads/SMD10024.pdf. Accessed December 2015.

De Hert M, Correll CU, Bobes J, et al: Physical illness in patients with severe mental disorders, I: prevalence, impact of medications and disparities in health care. World Psychiatry 10(1):52–77, 2011 21379357

Elon R, Pawlson LG: The impact of OBRA on medical practice within nursing facilities. J Am Geriatr Soc 40(9):958–963, 1992 1512394

Epstein RS: Psychological characteristics of therapists who commit serious boundary violations, in Keeping Boundaries: Maintaining Safety and Integrity in the Psychotherapeutic Process. Washington, DC, American Psychiatric Press, 1994, pp 239–254

Fry ST: Is health-care delivery by partially trained professionals ever morally justified? J Clin Ethics 2(1):42–44, 1991 11642915

Hoop JG: Hidden ethical dilemmas in psychiatric residency training: the psychiatry resident as dual agent. Acad Psychiatry 28(3):183–189, 2004 15507552

Jones K: Taming the Troublesome Child: American Families, Child Guidance, and the Limits of Psychiatric Authority. Cambridge, MA, Harvard University Press, 1999

Katon WJ: Clinical and health services relationships between major depression, depressive symptoms, and general medical illness. Biol Psychiatry 54(3):216–226, 2003 12893098

Knitzer J: Unclaimed Children: The Failure of Public Responsibility to Children and Adolescents in Need of Mental Health Services. Washington, DC, The Children's Defense Fund, 1982

Lourie IS: A history of community child mental health, in The Handbook of Child and Adolescent Systems of Care: The New Community Psychiatry. Edited by Pumariega AJ, Winters NC. San Francisco, CA, Jossey-Bass, 2003, pp 1–16

Mann C: Re: Integrated Care Models (letter to state Medicaid director) SMDL# 12–001 ICM# 1. Baltimore, MD, Center for Medicaid and CHIP Services, July 10, 2012. Available at: http://www.medicaid.gov/Federal-Policy-Guidance/downloads/SMD-12-001.pdf. Accessed December 6, 2013

Miller L, Wickramaratne P, Gameroff MJ, et al: Religiosity and major depression in adults at high risk: a ten-year prospective study. Am J Psychiatry 169(1):89–94, 2012 21865527

Milne D: Psychologists' disciplinary failure leads to new law in Ohio. Psychiatr News 37:18, 2002

Moussavi S, Chatterji S, Verdes E, et al: Depression, chronic diseases, and decrements in health: results from the World Health Surveys. Lancet 370(9590):851–858, 2007 17826170

Parks J, Singer P, Foti ME, et al: Morbidity and Mortality in People With Serious Mental Illness. Alexandria, VA, National Association of State Mental Health Program Directors Medical Directors Council, 2006

Peteet JR, Lu FG, Narrow WE (eds): Religious and Spiritual Issues in Psychiatric Diagnosis: A Research Agenda for DSM-V. Washington, DC, American Psychiatric Publishing, 2011

Roberts LW: Informed consent and the capacity for voluntarism. Am J Psychiatry 159(5):705–712, 2002 11986120

Roberts LW, Dyer AR: Concise Guide to Ethics in Mental Health Care. Washington, DC, American Psychiatric Publishing, 2004

Vinicky JK, Connors RB Jr, Leader R, Nash JD: Patients as "subjects" or "objects" in residency education? J Clin Ethics 2(1):35–41, discussion 41–44, 1991 1932794

CHAPTER 14

Feeding and Eating Disorders

14.1 Which of the following indicates a major change in the DSM-5 diagnostic criteria for anorexia nervosa in women compared with DSM-IV?

A. The criterion for menorrhagia has been eliminated.
B. The criterion for amenorrhea has been eliminated.
C. The criteria for both amenorrhea and menorrhagia have been eliminated.
D. Body weight is no longer a significant criterion.
E. Developmental stage is no longer a significant issue.

The correct response is option B: The criterion for amenorrhea has been eliminated.

The DSM-IV-TR (American Psychiatric Association 2000) requirement for amenorrhea (option B) (*not* menorrhagia; options A, C) has been eliminated in DSM-5 (American Psychiatric Association 2013). In DSM-5, individuals meeting diagnostic criteria for anorexia nervosa are required to be below a significantly low body weight for their developmental stage (option D). Guidance regarding how to judge whether an individual is at or below a significantly low weight is provided. Criterion B has been expanded to include not only expressed fear of weight gain but also persistent behavior that interferes with weight gain. Developmental stage (option E) has never been a part of the DSM diagnostic criteria for anorexia nervosa. **(Hales RE, Yudofsky SC, Roberts LW [eds]: APP Textbook of Psychiatry, 6th Edition, Chapter 17, pp. 561–563)**

14.2 What is the change in the criteria for bulimia nervosa in DSM-5 compared with DSM-IV?

A. There is an increase in the required numbers of binge-eating episodes and in-appropriate compensatory behaviors per week, from twice to three times weekly.

B. There is an increase in the numbers of episodes of using ipecac or vomiting per week, from three to four.
C. There is a reduction in the required minimum average frequency of binge eating and inappropriate compensatory behavior frequency, from twice to once weekly.
D. There is a requirement for an episode of pica, at least once in the last year.
E. There is a requirement for an electrolyte imbalance to be demonstrated, at least twice in the last 2 years.

The correct response is option C: There is a reduction in the required minimum average frequency of binge eating and inappropriate compensatory behavior frequency, from twice to once weekly.

In DSM-5, the clinical characteristics and course for individuals meeting the diagnostic criteria of bulimia nervosa are similar to DSM-IV criterion. The only change in the criteria for bulimia nervosa from DSM-IV is a reduction (option C) rather than increase (options A, B) in the required minimum average frequency of binge eating and inappropriate compensatory behavior frequency from twice to once weekly for 3 months. The clinical characteristics and outcome of individuals meeting this slightly lower threshold are similar to those meeting the DSM-IV criterion. Pica and electrolyte imbalance (options D, E) have never been part of the DSM diagnostic criteria for bulimia nervosa. **(Hales RE, Yudofsky SC, Roberts LW [eds]: APP Textbook of Psychiatry, 6th Edition, Chapter 17, pp. 571–572)**

14.3   The minimum average frequency of binge eating for a diagnosis of binge-eating disorder in DSM-5 requires which of the following time periods?

A. Once weekly over the last 3 months.
B. Once weekly over the last 4 months.
C. Every other week over the last 3 months.
D. Every other week over the last 4 months.
E. Once a month over the last 3 months.

The correct response is option A: Once weekly over the last 3 months.

Binge eating is reliably associated with obesity and overweight status in individuals who seek treatment. Binge-eating disorder is differentiated from obesity in that most individuals who are obese do not engage in recurrent binge eating. The only significant difference from the preliminary criteria in Appendix B of DSM-IV-TR is that the minimum average frequency of binge eating required to meet the diagnosis is once weekly over the last 3 months, identical to the frequency criterion for bulimia nervosa. **(Hales RE, Yudofsky SC, Roberts LW [eds]: APP Textbook of Psychiatry, 6th Edition, Chapter 17, pp. 577–578)**

14.4 What are the two subtypes of anorexia nervosa?

A. Restricting type and binge-eating/purging type.
B. Energy-sparing type and binge-eating/purging type.
C. Low-calorie/low-carb type and restricting type.
D. Low-carb/low-fat type and restricting type.
E. Restricting type and low-weight type.

The correct response is option A: Restricting type and binge-eating/purging type.

In the restricting type, during the last 3 months, the individual has not engaged in recurrent episodes of binge-eating or purging behavior; in the binge-eating/purging type, during the last 3 months, the individual has engaged in recurrent episodes of binge eating or purging behavior (option A). Options B–E contain distractor specifiers that do not exist. **(Hales RE, Yudofsky SC, Roberts LW [eds]: APP Textbook of Psychiatry, 6th Edition, Chapter 17, pp. 561–562)**

14.5 Which are the three essential diagnostic features of anorexia nervosa in DSM-5?

A. Low self-confidence, low attention, and low motivation.
B. Low libido, disturbance in self-perceived weight or shape, and persistent energy restriction.
C. Low mood, low concentration, and low energy level.
D. Persistent energy restriction, behavior interfering with weight gain or fear of weight gain, and a disturbance in self-perceived weight or shape.
E. Persistent low attention, low motivation, and low mood.

The correct response is option D: Persistent energy restriction, behavior interfering with weight gain or fear of weight gain, and a disturbance in self-perceived weight or shape.

Only option D lists all three essential DSM-5 criteria. Children and adolescents with anorexia nervosa may not make expected weight gain or maintain a normal developmental trajectory, and adolescents and older individuals may maintain a body weight that is below a minimally normal level for age, height, and sex; however, self-confidence (option A), libido (option B), mood (options C, E), and attention and motivation (options A, E), all of which may be affected in anorexia nervosa, are not essential diagnostic features in DSM-5. **(Hales RE, Yudofsky SC, Roberts LW [eds]: APP Textbook of Psychiatry, 6th Edition, Chapter 17, pp. 561–563)**

14.6 What is the most effective treatment for osteopenia and osteoporosis in patients with anorexia nervosa?

A. Calcium.
B. Vitamin D.
C. Bisphosphonates.

D. Weight gain.

E. Hormone replacement therapy.

The correct response is option D: Weight gain.

Osteopenia and osteoporosis are quite common in anorexia nervosa, and available data suggest that many of the treatments that seem most logical for this problem, including vitamin D (option B) and calcium supplementation (option A), as well as the use of bisphosphonates (option C) and hormonal replacement therapy (option E), are generally not very effective; the best available treatment appears to be weight gain (option D). **(Hales RE, Yudofsky SC, Roberts LW [eds]: APP Textbook of Psychiatry, 6th Edition, Chapter 17, p. 565)**

14.7   Which of the following is the most serious complication of weight restoration in patients with anorexia nervosa?

A. Refeeding syndrome.

B. High white blood cell count.

C. Hypocortisolism.

D. Hyperphosphatemia.

E. Hyperkalemia.

The correct response is option A: Refeeding syndrome.

One of the most serious complications of weight restoration is the refeeding syndrome (option A), characterized by marked fluid and electrolyte abnormalities, including low serum phosphate levels (option D). The combination of depletion of total body phosphate stores during catabolic starvation and increased cellular influx of phosphate during anabolic refeeding leads to severe extracellular hypophosphatemia. This well-recognized complication of refeeding, particularly in individuals with very low body weight, can lead to cardiac arrhythmias, delirium, and even sudden death (Solomon and Kirby 1990). Other potential symptoms of the refeeding syndrome include abnormal sodium and fluid balance; alterations in the metabolism of glucose, protein, and fat; thiamine deficiency; hypokalemia (option E); and hypomagnesemia (Mehanna et al. 2008). This syndrome has most often been noted in refeeding with total parenteral nutrition but can be seen with oral and nasogastric refeeding regimens as well (American Psychiatric Association 2006). Cholesterol levels in anorexia nervosa are usually normal or high despite low cholesterol intake. These levels do not result from the de novo synthesis of cholesterol. Rather, abnormal thyroid hormone status, low serum estrogen levels, hypercortisolism (option C), and impaired clearance of cholesterol explain or contribute to hypercholesterolemia in this setting. Weight restoration is typically accompanied by reduction in cholesterol level and apolipoprotein B (Feillet et al. 2000), and no effort should be made to further reduce dietary fat or cholesterol (Rock and Curran-Celentano 1996). Other laboratory abnormalities that characterize starvation and early recovery such as low white blood count (option B) or elevated liver transaminase typically normalize with weight recovery. **(Levenson JL [ed]: The American Psychiatric Publishing Textbook of Psychosomatic Medicine: Psychiatric Care of the Medically Ill, 2nd Edition, Chapter 14, p. 322)**

14.8   Which of the following medical problems is found in patients with anorexia nervosa but not in those with bulimia nervosa?

A. Enlarged parotid glands.
B. Malnutrition.
C. Dental enamel erosion.
D. Constipation.
E. Hematemesis.

The correct response is option B: Malnutrition.

Significantly fewer medical complications are associated with bulimia nervosa than with anorexia nervosa, and the complications themselves are usually less severe. Problems with malnutrition are generally not seen, if present at all, in patients with bulimia nervosa (option B). Enlarged parotid glands (option A), dental enamel erosion (option C), and hematemesis (option E), which in severe rare cases results from gastric dilatation and esophageal rupture, can be seen in both anorexia nervosa and bulimia nervosa. Constipation (option D) and diarrhea, at times alternating, also can occur in both. **(Hales RE, Yudofsky SC, Roberts LW [eds]: APP Textbook of Psychiatry, 6th Edition, Chapter 17, p. 573 and Table 17–1, pp. 564–565)**

14.9   Which of the following compensatory behaviors is most commonly used by patients with bulimia nervosa?

A. Self-induced vomiting.
B. Laxatives.
C. Diuretics.
D. Fasting.
E. Excessive exercise.

The correct response is option A: Self-induced vomiting.

Patients with bulimia engage in inappropriate compensatory behaviors to prevent weight gain, most commonly self-induced vomiting (option A), which occurs in about 90% of patients, as well as using stimulant-type laxatives (option B) as a way of inducing diarrhea and causing a sense of weight loss (40%–60%). Diuretics (option C) are also occasionally used as weight-control techniques. Some patients will fast all day or for several days (option D). Excessive exercise is used by a subgroup of those with bulimia nervosa (option E). **(Hales RE, Yudofsky SC, Roberts LW [eds]: APP Textbook of Psychiatry, 6th Edition, Chapter 17, p. 572)**

14.10 What is the only drug that currently has U.S. Food and Drug Administration (FDA) approval for bulimia nervosa?

A. Imipramine.
B. Sertraline.
C. Fluoxetine.
D. Citalopram.
E. Topiramate.

The correct response is option C: Fluoxetine.

A growing and impressive literature suggests that antidepressant medications can be quite effective in suppressing many of the symptoms of bulimia nervosa. Studies suggest this is true for a variety of agents, including tricyclic antidepressants, monoamine oxidase inhibitors, and—more recently and of particular clinical importance—serotonin reuptake inhibitors. The only drug that is currently approved by the FDA for treatment of bulimia nervosa is fluoxetine. **(Hales RE, Yudofsky SC, Roberts LW [eds]: APP Textbook of Psychiatry, 6th Edition, Chapter 17, p. 575)**

14.11 Which DSM-5 diagnostic criterion differentiates bulimia nervosa from binge-eating disorder?

A. Recurrent episodes of binge eating.
B. Recurrent inappropriate compensatory behavior aimed at preventing weight gain.
C. Binge-eating frequency of at least once a week for 3 months.
D. Eating, in a discrete period of time, an amount of food that is definitely larger than what most individuals would eat in a similar period of time.
E. A sense of loss of control over eating during binge episodes.

The correct response is option B: Recurrent inappropriate compensatory behavior aimed at preventing weight gain.

DSM-5 criteria for both binge-eating disorder and bulimia nervosa include recurrent episodes of binge eating (options A, C) that occur at least once a week for 3 months. In both disorders, the episodes involve eating, in a discrete period of time, an amount of food that is definitely larger than what most individuals would eat in a similar period of time (option D). There is also a sense of lack of control over eating during binge episodes (option E). The criterion that distinguishes the two diagnoses is recurrent inappropriate compensatory behavior in order to prevent weight gain (option B), which is found in bulimia nervosa but not in binge-eating disorder. **(Hales RE, Yudofsky SC, Roberts LW [eds]: APP Textbook of Psychiatry, 6th Edition, Chapter 17, pp. 570–572, 577–578)**

14.12 What is the most commonly abused substance among patients with binge-eating disorder?

    A. Marijuana.
    B. Cocaine.
    C. Alcohol.
    D. Tobacco.
    E. Opiates.

The correct response is option C: Alcohol.

Approximately 20%–25% of individuals with binge-eating disorder also display significant substance use disorder, most typically alcohol use disorder (option C). Abuse of marijuana (option A), cocaine (option B), tobacco (option D), or opiates (option E) may be present in patients with binge-eating disorder but is not as common as alcohol use disorder. **(Hales RE, Yudofsky SC, Roberts LW [eds]: APP Textbook of Psychiatry, 6th Edition, Chapter 17, p. 579)**

14.13 Which of the following statements regarding pica is most accurate?

    A. Ingestion of nonfood, nonnutritive substances must be sustained for at least 1 year.
    B. Pica typically displays an onset in adolescence.
    C. Common substances ingested include paper, soap, and soil.
    D. Psychiatric comorbidities may include bipolar disorder and personality disorders.
    E. Pica does not occur in adults.

The correct response is option C: Common substances ingested include paper, soap, and soil.

Pica is the diagnostic term used to describe the ingestion of nonfood, nonnutritive substances. In DSM-5, this pattern of eating must be sustained for at least 1 month (option A). Pica typically displays an onset in childhood (option B). Common substances ingested might include paper, soap, string, soil, chalk, or paint (option C) (Bryant-Waugh et al. 2010). Psychiatric comorbidities may include autism spectrum disorder and intellectual developmental disorder (option D). When pica occurs in adults, it is most likely to occur in the context of learning disabilities or other mental disorders (option E). **(Hales RE, Yudofsky SC, Roberts LW [eds]: APP Textbook of Psychiatry, 6th Edition, Chapter 17, pp. 557–558)**

14.14 Which of the following best describes the DSM-5 diagnosis of avoidant/restrictive food intake disorder (ARFID)?

    A. ARFID replaces the diagnosis of feeding disorder of infancy or early childhood.
    B. The main diagnostic feature of ARFID is disturbance of body image.

C. Somatic interventions are typically used to treat ARFID.

D. ARFID cannot be diagnosed in the presence of certain medical conditions.

E. ARFID tends to present similarly across different age groups.

The correct response is option A: ARFID replaces the diagnosis of feeding disorder of infancy or early childhood.

The addition of ARFID in DSM-5 addresses an important group of patients who were difficult to classify in DSM-IV-TR and also replaces the diagnosis of feeding disorder of infancy or early childhood (option A), which was rarely utilized. The main diagnostic feature of ARFID is avoidance or restriction of food intake that results in clinically significant reductions in nutritional intake, as evidenced by weight loss, specific nutritional deficiencies, or marked interference with psychosocial functioning (option B). The diagnostic features will to some extent depend on the age of the patient, with presentations ranging from agitation around feeding in infants to more generalized emotional difficulties in older children and adolescents (option E). ARFID can be diagnosed in the presence of other conditions if the eating disturbance requires special clinical attention (option D); examples include individuals with certain medical conditions (e.g., gastrointestinal disorders, food allergies) and individuals with autism spectrum disorder. Currently, there are no recommended somatic treatments (option C), although comorbid conditions may require specific somatic interventions. **(Hales RE, Yudofsky SC, Roberts LW [eds]: APP Textbook of Psychiatry, 6th Edition, Chapter 17, p. 559)**

References

American Psychiatric Association: Diagnostic and Statistical Manual of Mental Disorders, 4th Edition, Text Revision. Washington, DC, American Psychiatric Association, 2000

American Psychiatric Association: Practice guideline for the treatment of patients with eating disorders (revision). Am J Psychiatry 163(suppl):1–54, 2006 16390877

American Psychiatric Association: Diagnostic and Statistical Manual of Mental Disorders, 5th Edition. Arlington, VA, American Psychiatric Association, 2013

Bryant-Waugh R, Markham L, Kreipe RE, Walsh BT: Feeding and eating disorders in childhood. Int J Eat Disord 43(2):98–111, 2010 20063374

Feillet F, Feillet-Coudray C, Bard JM, et al: Plasma cholesterol and endogenous cholesterol synthesis during refeeding in anorexia nervosa. Clin Chim Acta 294(1-2):45–56, 2000 10727672

Mehanna HM, Moledina J, Travis J: Refeeding syndrome: what it is, and how to prevent and treat it. BMJ 336(7659):1495–1498, 2008 18583681

Rock CL, Curran-Celentano J: Nutritional management of eating disorders. Psychiatr Clin North Am 19(4):701–713, 1996 8933603

Solomon SM, Kirby DF: The refeeding syndrome: a review. JPEN J Parenter Enteral Nutr 14(1):90–97, 1990 2109122

CHAPTER 15

Law

15.1   Who decides whether a patient is competent to stand trial?

A. Any licensed physician.
B. A jury.
C. A psychiatrist.
D. A judge.
E. The patient.

The correct response is option D: A judge.

A judge determines the decision of competence (option D); physicians determine issues of capacity (options A, C). A jury or the patient does not determine a patient's competency (options B, E). It is clinically useful to distinguish the terms incompetence and incapacity. *Incompetence* refers to a court adjudication, whereas *incapacity* indicates a functional inability as determined by a clinician (Mishkin 1989). **(Hales RE, Yudofsky SC, Roberts LW [eds]: APP Textbook of Psychiatry, 6th Edition, Chapter 6, pp. 177–178)**

15.2   In addition to communication of choice, understanding of relevant information provided, and appreciation of available options and consequences, what other standard is used to determine competency?

A. Acting in one's own best interest.
B. Deciding in a timely manner.
C. Showing a stable choice over time.
D. Rational decision making.
E. Choosing what is medically indicated.

The correct response is option D: Rational decision making.

A review of case law and scholarly literature reveals four standards for determining competency in decision making. These standards, in order of increasing levels of mental capacity required, are communication of choice, understanding of relevant information provided, appreciation of available options and consequences, and rational decision making (option D). Whether the person is acting in his or her own best interest is generally not for the clinician to decide (option A). The time line of the decision is not a standard measure of competency (option B). Showing a stable choice over time is not a standard criterion; it adds weight to the patient's decision when the choice is reasonable, but could also be evidence for incompetence if the choice is consistently unreasonable (option C). When the patient chooses what is medically indicated, questions of competency rarely come up (option E). If competency is being discussed, typically the patient is choosing contrary to medical recommendations. **(Hales RE, Yudofsky SC, Roberts LW [eds]: APP Textbook of Psychiatry, 6th Edition, Chapter 6, pp. 177–178 and Table 6–1, p. 178)**

15.3   In the landmark case *Rennie v. Klein* (1978), the court recognized the right of psychiatric patients to refuse treatment but concluded that this right could be overridden in which of the following circumstances?

A. The patient is psychotic.
B. The patient denies having a mental illness.
C. The patient is not acting in his or her best interest.
D. The patient is charged with a crime.
E. The patient is a danger to self or others.

The correct response is option E: The patient is a danger to self or others.

In *Rennie v. Klein* (1978), the Third Circuit Court of Appeals recognized a right to refuse treatment in the state of New Jersey. The court concluded, however, that this right could be overridden and antipsychotic drugs administered "whenever, in the exercise of professional judgment, such an action is deemed necessary to prevent the patient from endangering himself or others" (option E). Patients are frequently allowed to refuse treatment despite being psychotic (option A), denying having a mental illness (option B), not acting in their own best interest (option C), or being charged with a crime (option D). **(Hales RE, Yudofsky SC, Roberts LW [eds]: APP Textbook of Psychiatry, 6th Edition, Chapter 6, pp. 181–183)**

15.4   What is the *most common* allegation when patients sue psychiatrists for inappropriate involuntary hospitalization?

A. Abuse of authority.
B. Assault and battery.
C. Malicious prosecution.
D. Intentional infliction of emotional distress.
E. Absence of "good faith" in the psychiatrists' behavior.

The correct response is option E: Absence of "good faith" in the psychiatrists' behavior.

Because psychiatrists are often granted conditional immunity for their good-faith participation in involuntary hospitalization proceedings, it is not surprising that most malpractice claims involving involuntary hospitalization allege an absence of good faith in the psychiatrists' behavior (option E). Often these lawsuits are brought under the theory of false imprisonment. Other areas of liability that may arise from wrongful commitment include abuse of authority (option A), assault and battery (option B), malicious prosecution (option C), and intentional infliction of emotional distress (option D). **(Hales RE, Yudofsky SC, Roberts LW [eds]: APP Textbook of Psychiatry, 6th Edition, Chapter 6, p. 190)**

15.5   Which of the following is seclusion?

A. Informing the patient that he or she must remain in his or her room with the door open and a security guard sitting outside of the room.
B. Hospitalizing the patient involuntarily on a locked unit.
C. Instructing a patient, in the middle of the night, to return to his or her room.
D. Allowing a patient to remain in his or her room with the door closed.
E. Using physical force to limit freedom of movement.

The correct response is option A: Informing the patient that he or she must remain in his or her room with the door open and a security guard sitting outside of the room.

The Center for Medicare Services, the Joint Commission (2006), and most states have developed requirements designed to minimize and avoid the use of seclusion and restraint (Simon and Hales 2006). Where they apply, federal requirements establish a floor but may be superseded by more restrictive state laws. The requirements define seclusion and restraint as follows: *Seclusion* is the involuntary confinement of a person alone in a room where the person is physically prevented from leaving or the separation of the patient from others in a safe, contained, controlled environment (option A). *Restraint* is the direct application of physical force to an individual, with or without the individual's permission, to restrict his or her freedom of movement. Physical force may involve human touch (option E), mechanical devices (e.g., a lock; option B), or a combination thereof. Under the federal rules, the use of these interventions is regarded as presenting an inherent risk to the patient's physical safety and well-being and therefore may be used only when there is "imminent risk" that the patient may inflict harm to self or others. Neither instructing a patient to return to his or her room nor allowing a patient who wishes to stay in the room is a restriction because patients should be in bed in the middle of the night and can elect to stay in their rooms (options C, D). **(Hales RE, Yudofsky SC, Roberts LW [eds]: APP Textbook of Psychiatry, 6th Edition, Chapter 6, p. 192)**

15.6   According to federal law, which of the following is deemed a physical restraint?

A. Verbal commands.
B. Behavior contracts.
C. Medications.
D. Video surveillance cameras.
E. An aide assisting a patient who has difficulty walking.

The correct response is option C: Medications.

Restraint is the direct application of physical force to an individual, with or without the individual's permission, to restrict his or her freedom of movement (options A, B, D, E). Physical force may involve human touch, mechanical devices, or a combination thereof. Under the federal rules, the use of these interventions is regarded as presenting an inherent risk to the patient's physical safety and well-being and therefore may be used only when there is "imminent risk" that the patient may inflict harm to self or others. Like many state laws, federal law includes the use of drugs in the definition of restraint (option C) (Simon and Hales 2006). Federal law permits the use of seclusion and restraint only as a last resort to protect the patient's safety and dignity and never for the convenience of the staff. Specifically, federal requirements permit qualified staff members to initiate seclusion or restraint for the safety and protection of the patient and staff only if they obtain an order from the licensed independent practitioner as soon as possible within 1 hour of initiation. Stringent requirements for face-to-face evaluation of the patient within 1 hour of initiation and for assessment, frequency of reassessment, monitoring, time-limited orders, notification of family members, discontinuation at the earliest possible opportunity, and debriefing with patient and staff members have been carefully defined by the Center for Medicare Services and the Joint Commission (2006). **(Hales RE, Yudofsky SC, Roberts LW [eds]: APP Textbook of Psychiatry, 6th Edition, Chapter 6, p. 192)**

References

Joint Commission: Comprehensive Accreditation Manual for Behavioral Healthcare Restraint and Seclusion Standards for Behavioral Health. Oak Brook Terrace, IL, Joint Commission, 2006
Mishkin B: Determining the capacity for making health care decisions, in Issues in Geriatric Psychiatry (Advances in Psychosomatic Medicine, Vol 19). Edited by Billig N, Rabins PV. Basel, Switzerland, S Karger, 1989, pp 151–166
Rennie v Klein, 462 F.Supp. 1131 (D. N.J. 1978), remanded, 476 F.Supp. 1294 (D.N.J. 1979), aff'd in part, modified in part and remanded, 653 F.2d 836 (3d. Cir. 1980), vacated and remanded, 458 U.S. 1119 (1982), 720 F.2d 266 (3rd Cir. 1983)
Simon RI, Hales RE (eds): The American Psychiatric Publishing Textbook of Suicide Assessment and Management. Washington, DC, American Psychiatric Publishing, 2006

CHAPTER 16

Mental Status

16.1 A psychiatrist observes a sustained muscle contraction in the patient's right forearm, with a flexed wrist and extended fingers. In the write-up, this finding is documented as which of the following?

A. Dystonia.
B. Chorea.
C. Asterixis.
D. Myoclonus.
E. Akathisia.

The correct response is option A: Dystonia.

Dystonia (option A) is characterized by sustained contraction of muscles that can result in abnormal posture, twisting, or repetitive movements (Fahn et al. 1987). *Chorea* (option B) refers to involuntary, irregular, rapid, nonstereotyped, and unpredictable movements that appear to "dance" over the patient's body (Higgins 2001). *Myoclonus* (option D) is characterized by sudden, jerky movements. *Asterixis* (option C) is a repeated momentary loss of postural tone notable for a flapping movement of outstretched hands. Motor restlessness accompanied by an urge to move is referred to as *akathisia* (option E) (Sachdev 1995). **(Yudofsky SC, Hales RE [eds]: APP Textbook of Neuropsychiatry and Behavioral Neuroscience, 5th Edition, Chapter 4, pp. 148–151)**

16.2 A patient's speech is marked by lack of emotional expression. When documenting this type of speech in the mental status examination, which of the following is the correct term?

A. Stuttering.
B. Aprosodia.
C. Echolalia.
D. Palilalia.
E. Dysarthria.

The correct response is option B: Aprosodia.

Aprosodia (option B) is the loss of the production or recognition of affective elements of speech. Classically, aprosodia is associated with lesions in the language areas in the right hemisphere. *Stuttering* (option A) is characterized by a disturbance of the rhythm of speech characterized by repetition, prolongation, or arrest of sounds. In *echolalia* (option C), the patient repeats the speech of another person automatically, without communicative intent or effect (Ford 1989). *Palilalia* (option D) is the patient's automatic repetition of his or her own word or phrase. *Dysarthria* (option E) refers to a disorder of articulation that can have various clinical forms, depending on the etiology. **(Yudofsky SC, Hales RE [eds]: APP Textbook of Neuropsychiatry and Behavioral Neuroscience, 5th Edition, Chapter 4, pp. 144–146)**

16.3   "Misperceptions of actual sensory inputs" describes which of the following?

A. Hallucinations.
B. Derealization.
C. Illusions.
D. Depersonalization.
E. Delusions.

The correct response is option C: Illusions.

Illusions are misperceptions of actual sensory inputs (option C). For example, a delirious patient might misinterpret the shadows on a television screen as crawling bugs. *Hallucinations* (option A) have the clarity and impact of true perceptions but without the pertinent sensory input. *Depersonalization* (option D) refers to a sense of being detached from one's own thoughts, body, or actions, whereas *derealization* (option B) refers to detachment from one's own surroundings. *Delusions* (option E) are unusual, preoccupying, or dangerous ideas and relate to thought content rather than sensory perceptions. **(Hales RE, Yudofsky SC, Roberts LW [eds]: APP Textbook of Psychiatry, 6th Edition, Chapter 1, pp. 23–25)**

16.4   How is attention tested during the mental status examination?

A. By asking patients to name all the animals they can think of in 1 minute.
B. By asking patients where they were born.
C. By asking patients simple logic questions, such as "Does a stone float on water?"
D. By asking patients to subtract 7 from 100, and to keep subtracting 7 from the result for five responses.
E. By asking patients to state their name, the present location, and the date.

The correct response is option D: By asking patients to subtract 7 from 100 and to keep subtracting 7 from the result for five responses.

Attention refers to the ability to sustain interest in a stimulus, whereas *concentration* involves the ability to maintain mental effort. Counting backward by 7s (serial 7s) requires that the patient retain interest in the task, recall the last number, subtract 7, and then continue to the next number (option D). The task also requires competence at math. Spelling *world* backward is a similarly good screening test of attention and concentration, but only for people who are fairly good spellers. For other patients, it is preferable to use a test that is less dependent on education, such as reciting the months backward.

Asking a patient to name all the animals he or she can think of in one minute (option A) is a test of fluency, an aspect of language functioning. Asking a patient where he or she was born (option B) is a test of long-term memory (and can be verified by collateral informants). Asking a patient simple logic questions (option C) tests abstract thinking. Asking patients the date is a measure of orientation (option E). **(Hales RE, Yudofsky SC, Roberts LW [eds]: APP Textbook of Psychiatry, 6th Edition, Chapter 1, pp. 26–27)**

16.5 What is being measured when a clinician asks a patient to recall, after a few minutes, three unrelated objects, such as a penny, an apple, and a chair?

A. Short-term memory.
B. Orientation.
C. Long-term memory.
D. Judgment.
E. Immediate recall.

The correct response is option A: Short-term memory.

A brief mental status examination screens for three types of memory dysfunction. Immediate recall (option E) is essentially an assessment of attention and is most often tested by asking patients to repeat the names of three unrelated objects (e.g., apple, table, penny). Recent or short-term memory (option A) is typically tested by asking the patient to recall after a few minutes the three objects repeated as part of the test for immediate recall. Long-term memory (option C) is generally assessed during the course of the interview through the patient's ability to accurately recall events in recent months and throughout the course of a lifetime.

Orientation (option B) is generally assessed by the patient's accurate recitation of name, location, and date (i.e., orientation to person, place, and time). Judgment (option D) is often extrapolated from recent behavior or by asking such questions as "If you were in a movie theater and smelled smoke, what would you do?" **(Hales RE, Yudofsky SC, Roberts LW [eds]: APP Textbook of Psychiatry, 6th Edition, Chapter 1, pp. 26–27)**

References

Fahn S, Marsden CD, Calne DB: Classification and investigation of dystonia, in Movement Disorders 2. Edited by Marsden CD, Fahn S. London, Butterworths, 1987, pp 332–358
Ford RA: The psychopathology of echophenomena. Psychol Med 19(3):627–635, 1989 2477866
Higgins DS Jr: Chorea and its disorders. Neurol Clin 19(3):707–722, 2001 11532650
Sachdev P: Akathisia and Restless Legs. Cambridge, UK, Cambridge University Press, 1995

CHAPTER 17

Neurocognitive Disorders

17.1 Which of the following laboratory results would be suggestive of Wilson's disease?

A. Low blood ceruloplasmin and low urinary copper.
B. Low blood ceruloplasmin and high urinary copper.
C. High blood ceruloplasmin and low urinary copper.
D. High blood ceruloplasmin and high urinary copper.
E. High blood ceruloplasmin and normal urinary copper.

The correct response is option B: Low blood ceruloplasmin and high urinary copper.

Low blood ceruloplasmin and high urinary copper content aid in the diagnosis of Wilson's disease (option B). **(Hales RE, Yudofsky SC, Roberts LW [eds]: APP Textbook of Psychiatry, 6th Edition, Chapter 24, p. 822)**

17.2 Which of the following is a true statement about delirium?

A. Disorientation to person, place, or time must be present to meet DSM-5 criteria for delirium.
B. The hallmark of delirium is impaired attention.
C. Change in psychomotor activity is an uncommon clinical manifestation of delirium.
D. Delirium has a lower degree of personality disorganization and clouding of consciousness compared with mild or major neurocognitive disorder.
E. Delirium generally takes weeks to months to resolve.

The correct response is option B: The hallmark of delirium is impaired attention.

Delirium is a state of altered consciousness and cognition, usually of acute onset (hours or days) and brief duration (days or weeks; option E). The hallmark of delirium is impaired attention (option B). DSM-5 criteria (American Psychiatric Association 2013) require a disturbance in attention and awareness, as well as an additional disturbance in cognition; however, many persons with delirium remain oriented to person, place, and time (option A) but demonstrate impairment on tests of sustained attention. Reduced or increased psychomotor activity is common (option C). Delirium has a greater degree of personality disorganization and clouding of consciousness than mild or major neurocognitive disorder (option D). **(Hales RE, Yudofsky SC, Roberts LW [eds]: APP Textbook of Psychiatry, 6th Edition, Chapter 24, pp. 825–826)**

17.3   What cerebrospinal fluid (CSF) findings would you expect in Alzheimer's disease?

A. Normal.
B. High β-amyloid 42 and low tau and phosphorylated tau.
C. Low β-amyloid 42 and high tau and phosphorylated tau.
D. High β-amyloid 42 and high tau and phosphorylated tau.
E. Low β-amyloid 42 and low tau and phosphorylated tau.

The correct response is option C: Low β-amyloid 42 and high tau and phosphorylated tau.

The finding of low CSF β-amyloid 42 and high total tau and phosphorylated tau is confirmatory of a suspected diagnosis of major or mild neurocognitive disorder due to Alzheimer's disease (option C). **(Hales RE, Yudofsky SC, Roberts LW [eds]: APP Textbook of Psychiatry, 6th Edition, Chapter 24, p. 831 and Table 24–7, p. 832)**

17.4   Which of the following neurocognitive disorders is associated with rapid eye movement (REM) sleep behavior disorder?

A. Alzheimer's disease.
B. Frontotemporal lobar degeneration.
C. Lewy body disease.
D. Cerebrovascular disease.
E. Neurocognitive disorder associated with traumatic brain injury.

The correct response is option C: Lewy body disease.

A distinctive clinical feature of Lewy body disease is that REM sleep behavior disorder is a frequent concomitant and often precedes cognitive symptoms (option C). Other characteristic clinical features that may aid in the diagnosis include the sudden onset of visual hallucinations, which frequently remit and reoccur. There are marked fluctuations in sensorium, with episodes of confusion lasting days or weeks followed by relative clarity for equal periods of time. Mild parkinsonism occurs early on. Functional brain imaging frequently shows low blood flow or low metabolic activity in the occipital lobes. REM sleep behavior disorder is not associated with Alzheimer's disease (option A), frontotemporal lobar degeneration (option B), cerebrovascular disease (option D), or neurocognitive disorder associated with traumatic brain injury (option E). **(Hales RE, Yudofsky SC, Roberts LW [eds]: APP Textbook of Psychiatry, 6th Edition, Chapter 24, p. 835 and Table 24–7, p. 832;** *Journal of Clinical Sleep Medicine* **3(4):357–362, 2007)**

17.5 Which of the following is a true statement about the diagnosis of language-variant frontotemporal lobar degeneration (FTLD)?

A. Language impairment is the principal cause of the impaired daily functioning.
B. Most often behavioral symptoms, such as disinhibition and hyperorality, are the most prominent clinical manifestations at symptom onset.
C. Language symptoms are directly related to the frequency of word use.
D. The prototypical language variant of FTLD is caused by Pick's disease.
E. FTLD has sudden onset and rapid progression.

The correct response is option A: Language impairment is the principal cause of the impaired daily functioning.

A diagnosis of language-variant FTLD requires that the most prominent feature is difficulty with language, that the language impairment is the principal cause of impaired daily functioning (option A), and that *aphasia* (rather than behavioral symptoms; option B) is the most prominent deficit at symptom onset and for the initial stage of the disease. The language symptoms are unrelated to the frequency of word use (option C). The prototypical behavioral variant of FTLD is caused by Pick's disease (option D) and presents as personality change with progressive impairment of judgment, loss of social graces, disinhibition, stimulus boundedness, and a craving for sweets. FTLD has insidious onset and gradual progression (option E). **(Hales RE, Yudofsky SC, Roberts LW [eds]: APP Textbook of Psychiatry, 6th Edition, Chapter 24, p. 835)**

17.6 Which of the following is a true statement about the categorization of aphasias in neurocognitive disorders?

A. In global aphasia, verbal fluency is impaired but repetition and naming are generally intact.
B. Anomic aphasia is uncommon in Alzheimer's disease.
C. Patients with Broca's aphasia can generally obey commands but have difficulty with repetition.
D. Unlike patients with Broca's aphasia, patients with Wernicke's aphasia have good comprehension.
E. In contrast to the naming difficulty in Wernicke's aphasia, the naming difficulty in Broca's aphasia is usually not helped by prompts.

The correct response is option C: Patients with Broca's aphasia can generally obey commands but have difficulty with repetition.

The categorization of aphasias is based on the language functions they impair. Global aphasia impairs all language functions (option A) and occurs in large left-hemisphere strokes. Anomic aphasia, by contrast, primarily affects word finding, may be related to lesions of the left angular or left posterior middle temporal gyrus, and is common in Alzheimer's disease (option B). Broca's (anterior, nonfluent) aphasia impairs verbal fluency, repetition, and naming and results from lesions of the posterior inferior portion of the left (or dominant) frontal lobe; patients with Broca's aphasia generally understand what is said to them and can obey commands but have difficulty with repetition, reading aloud, and writing (option C). Patients with Wernicke's (posterior, fluent) aphasia have fluent (e.g., good flow of speech), paraphasic, and neologistic speech with poor comprehension, repetition, and naming (option D). Although both Broca's aphasia and Wernicke's aphasia involve difficulty with naming, patients with Broca's aphasia are usually aided by prompting, whereas patients with Wernicke's aphasia are not (option E). **(Hales RE, Yudofsky SC, Roberts LW [eds]: APP Textbook of Psychiatry, 6th Edition, Chapter 24, pp. 839–840)**

17.7 What normal, age-related change in neurotransmitter input to the forebrain increases the likelihood of delirium from anticholinergic drugs?

A. Loss of pigmented cells in the substantia nigra, increasing the sensitivity of dopamine D_2 receptors.
B. Loss of neurons in the nucleus basalis of Meynert and septal nuclei, increasing the cholinergic input to the forebrain.
C. Loss of pigmented cells in the substantia nigra, reducing the sensitivity of D_2 receptors.
D. Loss of neurons in the nucleus basalis of Meynert and septal nuclei, reducing the cholinergic input to the forebrain.
E. Increase in pigmented cells in the substantia nigra, increasing the sensitivity of D_2 receptors.

The correct response is option D: Loss of neurons in the nucleus basalis of Meynert and septal nuclei, reducing the cholinergic input to the forebrain.

Loss of neurons in the nucleus basalis of Meynert and septal nuclei reduces cholinergic input to the forebrain and increases (option D), rather than decreases (option B), the likelihood of delirium from anticholinergic drugs such as bladder or gastrointestinal relaxants. Loss of pigmented substantia nigra cells, another normal, age-related change, increases the sensitivity of D_2 receptors and thus sensitivity to extrapyramidal effects of antipsychotic agents (options A, C, E). **(Hales RE, Yudofsky SC, Roberts LW [eds]: APP Textbook of Psychiatry, 6th Edition, Chapter 24, p. 816)**

17.8 Which of the following clinical features would support a diagnosis of neurocognitive disorder over a diagnosis of depression?

A. Increased psychomotor activity.
B. Mood-congruent auditory hallucinations.

C. Frequent suicidal ideation.

D. Marked change in appetite.

E. Day/night confusion.

The correct response is option E: Day/night confusion.

In contrast to the typical presentation of depression, in neurocognitive disorders psychomotor activity is generally normal (option A), visual hallucinations are more common than auditory (option B), suicidal ideation is uncommon (option C), and appetite is typically normal (option D). Whereas patients with depression tend to report early awakening from sleep, patients with neurocognitive disorder often experience day/night confusion (option E), and many become transiently delirious toward the end of the day, a phenomenon known as *sundowning.* **(Hales RE, Yudofsky SC, Roberts LW [eds]: APP Textbook of Psychiatry, 6th Edition, Chapter 24, pp. 825–826 and Table 24–4, p. 827)**

17.9 Which of the following is a true statement about management of delirium in an inpatient setting?

A. Pharmacological intervention is indicated even in mild delirium that does not cause sleep disturbance or interfere with medical treatment.

B. For delirium lasting longer than 7 days, providers should consider substance withdrawal as the likely cause.

C. Rooms should be kept dimly lit to avoid overstimulating the patient.

D. Mechanical restraints should be used in preference to sitters, because bedside companions often exacerbate confusion.

E. Patients should be frequently reoriented to time, place, and staff members.

The correct response is option E: Patients should be frequently reoriented to time, place, and staff members.

Substance withdrawal delirium should be presumed if symptoms begin 1–3 days after admission (option B), and the patient's substance use should be reviewed with family members when possible. Bedside companions (ideally, a well-liked family member) are preferable to and less dangerous than mechanical restraints (option D). Rooms should be kept well lit to minimize misperceptions (option C); a room with a window can assist with day/night orientation. Patients should be frequently reoriented to their surroundings (option E); for example, clocks and calendars should be provided, and staff members should reintroduce themselves each time they visit. Mild delirium that does not cause sleep loss, interfere with medical treatment, or lead to extreme fear and discomfort does not require treatment (option A). **(Hales RE, Yudofsky SC, Roberts LW [eds]: APP Textbook of Psychiatry, 6th Edition, Chapter 24, p. 827 and Table 24–5, p. 828)**

17.10 Which of the following cognitive abnormalities, if elicited on mental status examination of a patient with depression, would be most suggestive of an underlying comorbid neurocognitive disorder?

A. Impaired episodic memory.
B. Impaired attention.
C. Impaired orientation.
D. Reduced information-processing speed.
E. Impaired working memory.

The correct response is option C: Impaired orientation.

In an evaluation of a person with a cognitive complaint, depression must be considered as the cause or as an aggravating factor. Many depressed persons experience cognitive impairment, although the severity of their impairment does not correlate with the severity of their depressive symptoms. Impaired orientation, on the other hand, is a feature that, if present, would be more suggestive of underlying neurocognitive impairment (option C). Persistent deficits in cognitive function often follow remission of depressive symptoms (Nebes et al. 2003), including deficits in working memory (option E), speed of information processing (option D), episodic memory (option A), and attention (option B). **(Hales RE, Yudofsky SC, Roberts LW [eds]: APP Textbook of Psychiatry, 6th Edition, Chapter 24, pp. 838–839 and Table 24–4, p. 827)**

17.11 Which of the following statements correctly describes an advantage of the Montreal Cognitive Assessment (MoCA) over the Folstein Mini-Mental State Examination (MMSE)?

A. The MoCA takes less time to administer than the MMSE.
B. The MoCA has a larger scoring range than the MMSE.
C. The MoCA takes into account differences in education level.
D. The MoCA has greater sensitivity for detection of mild cognitive impairment.
E. The MoCA is more widely used and therefore more acceptable to the public.

The correct response is option D: The MoCA has greater sensitivity for detection of mild cognitive impairment.

The MMSE (Folstein et al. 1975) is the most widely used brief screening tool for cognitive impairment (option E); it requires 10–15 minutes to administer and has a scoring range of 0–30. Like the MMSE, the MoCA (Nasreddine et al. 2005) requires about 15 minutes to administer and has a scoring range of 0–30 (options A, B). Although the MMSE is confounded by premorbid intelligence and education, the MoCA does not specifically address this problem (option C). An advantage of the MoCA over the MMSE is that the former was designed to detect mild cognitive impairment (option D). **(Hales RE, Yudofsky SC, Roberts LW [eds]: APP Textbook of Psychiatry, 6th Edition, Chapter 24, pp. 840–841)**

17.12 Which of the following is a true statement about cholinesterase inhibitors?

A. They may improve cognitive performance in individuals with neurocognitive disorders, but they do not slow the rate of cognitive decline.
B. Their use is absolutely contraindicated in individuals with bradycardia or bronchopulmonary disease.
C. They are effective only in major neurocognitive disorder due to probable Alzheimer's disease.
D. They are available only in oral formulations.
E. They are used as first-line monotherapy for patients with advanced major neurocognitive disorder.

The correct response is option A: They may improve cognitive performance in individuals with neurocognitive disorders, but they do not slow the rate of cognitive decline.

Cholinesterase inhibitors have been used with some success in patients with Alzheimer's disease, Lewy body disease, and cognitive impairment associated with vascular disease (option C). This class of drugs, which also enhances cognition in persons without brain disease, raises baseline cognitive performance but does not slow the rate of decline (option A). All cholinesterase inhibitors are available in once-a-day preparations. Donepezil and galantamine are administered orally; rivastigmine is characteristically used as a patch (option D). A resting pulse below 50 and severe bronchopulmonary disease are relative contraindications (option B), but the treatment decision should be made on a case-by-case basis.

Cholinesterase inhibitors and memantine have different mechanisms of action; thus, combination therapy could, in theory, confer additional benefits (Tariot et al. 2004). This combination has become the preferred treatment in clinical practice for patients with moderate to severe Alzheimer's disease (option E); however, evidence suggests that the addition of memantine to a cholinesterase inhibitor adds little to therapeutic efficacy (Howard et al. 2012). **(Hales RE, Yudofsky SC, Roberts LW [eds]: APP Textbook of Psychiatry, 6th Edition, Chapter 24, pp. 841–842)**

17.13 An 88-year-old man with major neurocognitive disorder secondary to probable Parkinson's disease begins to develop paranoia and agitation over the course of several months. Behavioral interventions are ineffective, and there is concern about caregiver burnout. Which of the following is a true statement about pharmacological treatment of agitation with psychotic features during the course of a neurocognitive disorder?

A. Numerous antipsychotics have received U.S. Food and Drug Administration (FDA) approval for treatment of behavioral disturbances in persons with neurocognitive disorders.
B. High doses of antipsychotics should be employed initially in order to control the behavior, and then tapered as tolerated with close monitoring for symptom recurrence.
C. Psychotropic medications that are helpful should be continued indefinitely.

D. An antipsychotic would be the first choice for treatment of agitation with psychotic features.
E. FDA warnings have been issued about increased cerebrovascular adverse events and increased mortality with use of typical antipsychotics but not with atypical antipsychotics in older dementia patients.

The correct response is option D: An antipsychotic would be the first choice for treatment of agitation with psychotic features.

No drug treatment has received FDA approval for any of the behavioral and emotional symptoms (except major depression and mania) that may arise during the course of a neurocognitive disorder (option A). Because virtually all drugs used to treat behavioral disturbances in persons with neurocognitive disorders are administered off label, the general guideline for younger adults is to escalate dosage until the behavior is controlled or until untoward side effects occur. The psychopharmacological approach most commonly employed is that of Tariot (1999): Use a drug with known efficacy in the symptom complex that most closely resembles the presenting symptoms. Employ low dosages and escalate slowly, assessing both target symptoms and toxicity (option B). If a psychotropic medication is helpful, attempt to withdraw it at an appropriate time and monitor for recurrence of the problem (option C).

Using Tariot's (1999) approach, antipsychotics would be the first choice for treatment of agitation with psychotic features (option D). However, their therapeutic effects are often small and inconsistent. Their potential side effects (akathisia, parkinsonism, tardive dyskinesia, sedation, neuroleptic malignant syndrome, peripheral and central anticholinergic effects, postural hypotension, cardiac conduction defects, and falls) must be weighed against their potential benefits. There is no overall difference in efficacy between typical and atypical antipsychotic drugs, and little distinguishes them from each other except their side-effect profiles. It is important to note that FDA warnings have been issued about increased cerebrovascular adverse events and increased mortality with both typical and atypical antipsychotics in elderly patients with dementia (option E) (U.S. Food and Drug Administration 2011). **(Hales RE, Yudofsky SC, Roberts LW [eds]: APP Textbook of Psychiatry, 6th Edition, Chapter 24, pp. 843–845)**

17.14 Which of the following is a true statement about the treatment of depression in individuals with neurocognitive disorders?

A. Depression cannot be diagnosed in persons with a neurocognitive disorder, and therefore treatment is not indicated.
B. Serotonin reuptake agents have not been shown to have any benefit in persons with neurocognitive disorders.
C. Methylphenidate may be useful for reducing apathy and depression in Alzheimer's disease.

D. Stimulants are relatively safe agents with few side effects in persons with neurocognitive disorders.

E. Electroconvulsive therapy is the first-line treatment for depression in persons with neurocognitive disorders.

The correct response is option C: Methylphenidate may be useful for reducing apathy and depression in Alzheimer's disease.

No controlled clinical trials of stimulants have been performed in persons with neurocognitive disorders. However, methylphenidate may be useful for reducing apathy and depression in Alzheimer's disease (option C) (Padala et al. 2010). Note that the potential to raise blood pressure and heart rate and to lead to irritability, agitation, and psychosis makes careful patient selection critical. Persons with any neurocognitive disorder may develop superimposed depression that should be treated in the same manner as persons without a neurocognitive disorder (option A). Serotonin reuptake agents can reduce irritability in persons who are and who are not depressed with neurocognitive disorders (Siddique et al. 2009) and may also increase alertness (option B). Stimulants can increase blood pressure and heart rate and lead to irritability, agitation, and psychosis, so caution is advised in using these agents (option D). Although electroconvulsive therapy can be used to treat severe depression in persons with any neurocognitive disorder, it is not first-line treatment, and cognitive side effects are more severe than for cognitively intact persons (option E). **(Hales RE, Yudofsky SC, Roberts LW [eds]: APP Textbook of Psychiatry, 6th Edition, Chapter 24, pp. 843–846)**

17.15 Which of the following is the most problematic limitation of high-dose vitamin E in the treatment of patients with neurocognitive disorders?

A. Association with increased cardiovascular adverse events.
B. Failure to significantly slow functional progression of the disease.
C. Potential to increase irritability, agitation, and psychosis in individuals with neurocognitive disorders.
D. Association with extrapyramidal side effects.
E. Association with postural hypotension and increased falls.

The correct response is option A: Association with increased cardiovascular adverse events.

Vitamin E dosages of 2,000 IU daily have been associated with a small but significant slowing of functional progression of Alzheimer's disease (option B) but no improvement in cognition. This treatment, once in wide use, is now less frequently used because of an association of increased cardiovascular events with the use of high-dose vitamin E (option A). Easy bleeding is a common side effect at this dosage, but this occurs infrequently at daily dosages of 800–1,000 IU. High-dose Vitamin E has not been associated with irritability, agitation, and psychosis (option C); extrapyramidal side effects (option D); or postural hypotension and falls (option E). **(Hales RE, Yudofsky SC, Roberts LW [eds]: APP Textbook of Psychiatry, 6th Edition, Chapter 24, p. 842)**

17.16 Which of the following is a true statement about the drug memantine?

A. Memantine is a reversible inhibitor of the enzyme acetylcholinesterase.
B. Memantine is typically dosed once daily.
C. Memantine is poorly absorbed and has a short half-life of 2.5 hours.
D. Memantine received FDA approval for early Alzheimer's disease.
E. Memantine may cause transient confusion or sedation during the titration phase but generally has few adverse effects.

The correct response is option E: Memantine may cause transient confusion or sedation during the titration phase but generally has few adverse effects.

The principal mechanism of action of memantine is believed to be the blockade of N-methyl-D-aspartate (NMDA)–type glutamate receptors (option A), thereby improving synaptic transmission and/or preventing calcium release that may provide neuroprotection. It is not a cholinesterase inhibitor. Memantine may cause transient confusion or sedation during the titration phase but generally has few adverse effects (option E). Memantine is well absorbed and has a 70-hour or greater half-life (option C) but is typically dosed twice daily (option B) because that was the dosage scheme used in efficacy studies. Memantine has received FDA approval for moderate to severe Alzheimer's disease (option D), and although widely used in patients with early Alzheimer's disease, there are no convincing efficacy data to support this use. **(Hales RE, Yudofsky SC, Roberts LW [eds]: APP Textbook of Psychiatry, 6th Edition, Chapter 24, p. 842)**

17.17 Which of the following is a true statement about the use of antiandrogens in controlling inappropriate sexual behavior?

A. There is no report of successful pharmacotherapy for inappropriate sexual behavior in individuals with cognitive impairment.
B. The antiandrogen medroxyprogesterone is effective in reducing sexual drive and sexually aggressive acts both in men who are cognitively intact and in men with brain injury.
C. The drug medroxyprogesterone is available only in an oral formulation.
D. Women with brain injury who are hypersexual are effectively treated with estrogen patches.
E. Medroxyprogesterone carries the risk of deep vein thrombosis.

The correct response is option B: The antiandrogen medroxyprogesterone is effective in reducing sexual drive and sexually aggressive acts both in men who are cognitively intact and in men with brain injury.

Antiandrogens are used to treat inappropriate sexual behavior or unwanted sexual approaches by persons with cognitive impairment (option A) (Guay 2008).

The antiandrogen medroxyprogesterone is effective in reducing sexual drive and sexually aggressive acts both in men who are cognitively intact and in men with brain injury (option B). The drug can be administered orally or intramuscularly (option C), and side effects are minimal. Other drugs that have been used with some success include selective serotonin reuptake inhibitors, the luteinizing hormone–releasing hormone antagonist leuprolide, and estrogen patches. However, estrogen therapy (not medroxyprogesterone) carries the danger of deep vein thrombosis (option E). There is no report of successful pharmacotherapy for hypersexual women with brain injury (option D). **(Hales RE, Yudofsky SC, Roberts LW [eds]: APP Textbook of Psychiatry, 6th Edition, Chapter 24, p. 846)**

17.18 What is the most preventable cause of neurocognitive disorders in young adults?

A. Substance abuse.
B. Traumatic brain injury due to accidents.
C. HIV infection.
D. Depression.
E. Nutritional deficiency.

The correct response is option B: Traumatic brain injury due to accidents.

The most preventable cause of neurocognitive disorders in young adults is traumatic brain injury. The use of helmets for bicycle and motorcycle riders significantly reduces mortality and morbidity from head injuries, as do helmets in situations in which personnel are exposed to blast injury. Attention is also being paid to head injuries in sports (Khurana and Kaye 2012). **(Hales RE, Yudofsky SC, Roberts LW [eds]: APP Textbook of Psychiatry, 6th Edition, Chapter 24, p. 846)**

17.19 Which of the following is a true statement about the psychopharmacological treatment of insomnia or disturbed sleep in individuals with neurocognitive disorder?

A. Conventional hypnotics are not associated with ataxia.
B. Conventional hypnotics do not cause oversedation.
C. Mood stabilizers should be first-line treatment for insomnia in persons with neurocognitive disorder.
D. The most commonly employed hypnotics for these individuals are diazepam and chlordiazepoxide.
E. The REM sleep behavior disorder that is a frequent concomitant to Lewy body disease often responds to anticholinesterase treatment.

The correct response is option E: The REM sleep behavior disorder that is a frequent concomitant to Lewy body disease often responds to anticholinesterase treatment.

The REM sleep behavior disorder that accompanies Lewy body disease often responds to anticholinesterase treatment (option E). Conventional hypnotics are generally avoided because of their tendency to oversedate and to cause ataxia (options A, B). Mood stabilizers are not indicated for treatment of insomnia (option C). The most commonly prescribed hypnotics are not diazepam and chlordiazepoxide (option D); they are trazodone, mirtazapine, and quetiapine. **(Hales RE, Yudofsky SC, Roberts LW [eds]: APP Textbook of Psychiatry, 6th Edition, Chapter 24, p. 846)**

References

American Psychiatric Association: Diagnostic and Statistical Manual of Mental Disorders, 5th Edition. Arlington, VA, American Psychiatric Association, 2013

Folstein MF, Folstein SE, McHugh PR: "Mini-mental state". A practical method for grading the cognitive state of patients for the clinician. J Psychiatr Res 12(3):189–198, 1975 1202204

Guay DR: Inappropriate sexual behaviors in cognitively impaired older individuals. Am J Geriatr Pharmacother 6(5):269–288, 2008 19161930

Howard R, McShane R, Lindesay J, et al: Donepezil and memantine for moderate-to-severe Alzheimer's disease. N Engl J Med 366(10):893–903, 2012 22397651

Khurana VG, Kaye AH: An overview of concussion in sport. J Clin Neurosci 19(1):1–11, 2012 22153800

Nasreddine ZS, Phillips NA, Bédirian V, et al: The Montreal Cognitive Assessment, MoCA: a brief screening tool for mild cognitive impairment. J Am Geriatr Soc 53(4):695–699, 2005 15817019

Nebes RD, Pollock BG, Houck PR, et al: Persistence of cognitive impairment in geriatric patients following antidepressant treatment: a randomized, double-blind clinical trial with nortriptyline and paroxetine. J Psychiatr Res 37(2):99–108, 2003 12842163

Padala PR, Burke WJ, Shostrom VK, et al: Methylphenidate for apathy and functional status in dementia of the Alzheimer type. Am J Geriatr Psychiatry 18(4):371–374, 2010 20220576

Siddique H, Hynan LS, Weiner MF: Effect of a serotonin reuptake inhibitor on irritability, apathy, and psychotic symptoms in patients with Alzheimer's disease. J Clin Psychiatry 70(6):915–918, 2009 19422762

Tariot PN: Treatment of agitation in dementia. J Clin Psychiatry 60(Suppl 8):11–20, 1999 10335667

Tariot PN, Farlow MR, Grossberg GT, et al; Memantine Study Group: Memantine treatment in patients with moderate to severe Alzheimer disease already receiving donepezil: a randomized controlled trial. JAMA 291(3):317–324, 2004 14734594

U.S. Food and Drug Administration: Information for Healthcare Professionals: Conventional Antipsychotics, 2011. Available at: www.fda.gov/Drugs/DrugSafety/PostmarketDrugSafety InformationforPatientsandProviders/ucm124830.htm. Accessed October 12, 2012.

CHAPTER 18

Neurodevelopmental Disorders

18.1   A 7-year-old boy in second grade displays significant delays in his ability to reason, problem solve, and learn from his experiences. He has been slow to develop reading, writing, and mathematics skills in school. Throughout his development, these skills have lagged behind those of his peers, although he is making slow progress. These deficits significantly impair his ability to play in an age-appropriate manner with peers and to begin to acquire independent skills at home. He requires ongoing assistance with basic skills (dressing, feeding, and bathing himself and doing any type of schoolwork) on a daily basis. Which DSM-5 diagnosis is most appropriate?

A. Global developmental delay.
B. Specific learning disorder.
C. Intellectual disability (intellectual developmental disorder), moderate.
D. Communication disorder.
E. Autism spectrum disorder (ASD).

The correct response is option C: Intellectual disability (intellectual developmental disorder), moderate.

Although IQ testing would be informative (in previous DSM classifications, including DSM-IV and DSM-IV-TR [American Psychiatric Association 1994, 2000], subtypes of mild, moderate, severe, and profound were categories based on IQ scores), DSM-5 (American Psychiatric Association 2013) specifies, "levels of severity are defined on the basis of adaptive functioning, and not IQ scores, because it is adaptive functioning that determines the level of supports required" (DSM-5, p. 33). Thus, the specifiers of "mild," "moderate," "severe," and "profound" relate to adaptive functioning rather than IQ. Adaptive functioning involves adaptive reasoning in three domains: *conceptual*, *social*, and *practical*. The conceptual (academic) domain involves, for example, competence in memory, language, reading, writing, math reasoning, acquisition of practical knowledge,

273

problem solving, and judgment in novel situations. The social domain involves, for example, awareness of others' thoughts, feelings, and experiences; empathy; interpersonal communication skills; friendship abilities; and social judgment. The practical domain involves learning and self-management across life settings, including, for example, personal care, job responsibilities, money management, recreation, managing one's behavior, and organizing school and work tasks. Assessment is based on both clinical assessment and standardized testing. With respect to severity of the intellectual disability for the boy in the question, the "moderate" qualifier reflects skills that have chronically lagged behind peers and the need for assistance in most activities of daily living, as well as the fact that he is slowly developing these skills (which would peak at roughly the elementary school level according to DSM-5) (option C). The diagnosis of global developmental delay (option A) is reserved for children under the age of 5 years, when the severity of the presentation cannot be assessed reliably because of the child's age. These children require reassessment and revision of diagnosis after a period of time. In specific learning disorder (option B) and communication disorders (option D), there is no general intellectual impairment. According to DSM-5, ASD (option E) must include history suggesting "persistent deficits in social communication and social interaction across multiple contexts" that are not accounted for by general developmental delays (Criterion A) or "restricted, repetitive patterns of behavior, interests, or activities" (Criterion B). **(DSM-5, Neurodevelopmental Disorders, pp. 31–58, 66–74; Hales RE, Yudofsky SC, Roberts LW [eds]: APP Textbook of Psychiatry, 6th Edition, Chapter 8, pp. 229–249)**

18.2   Which of the following is a characteristic feature of intellectual disability?

A. Full-scale IQ less than 70.
B. Inability to use money.
C. Inability to make medical decisions.
D. Inability to meet community standards of personal independence.
E. In spite of other deficits, there are adequate communication skills for self-expression.

The correct response is option D: Inability to meet community standards of personal independence.

Deficits in adaptive functioning including age-appropriate independent functioning and social responsibility are characteristic features of intellectual disability (Criterion B; option D). The diagnosis does not require a full-scale IQ of less than 70 (option A), as impairment in adaptive functioning is required. Although inability to use money (option B) and make medical decisions (option C) may be part of the impairment in intellectual disability, an isolated impairment would not in and of itself allow the syndrome to be diagnosed. These individuals lack adequate communication skills for self-expression (option E), and this may lead to aggressive behavior. **(DSM-5, Neurodevelopmental Disorders, pp. 33–40;**

Hales RE, Yudofsky SC, Roberts LW [eds]: APP Textbook of Psychiatry, 6th Edition, Chapter 8, pp. 231–235)

18.3   A 3½-year-old girl with a history of lead exposure and a seizure disorder demonstrates substantial delays across multiple domains of functioning, including communication, learning, attention, and motor development, which limit her ability to interact with same-age peers, and requires substantial support in all activities of daily living at home that are not typical for a child her age. Unfortunately, her mother is an extremely poor historian, and the child has received no formal psychological or learning evaluation to date. She is about to be evaluated by the Committee on Preschool Education. What is her most likely DSM-5 diagnosis?

A. Major neurocognitive disorder.
B. Developmental coordination disorder.
C. Autism spectrum disorder.
D. Global developmental delay.
E. Specific learning disorder.

The correct response is option D: Global developmental delay.

In global development delay, which is a new diagnosis in DSM-5, the deficits may be suggestive of intellectual disability; however, as in this case, there may be a lack of information, such as about the age at onset of the symptoms or standardized testing data. At this point, there is no information to suggest the girl has major neurocognitive disorder (option A), ASD (no evidence of symptoms in the core ASD categories) (option C), a specific disorder relating to coordination (option B), or a specific area of learning weakness (option E) (which generally would not be able to be diagnosed until the elementary years). Therefore, global developmental delay is the appropriate diagnosis (option D). **(Hales RE, Yudofsky SC, Roberts LW [eds]: APP Textbook of Psychiatry, 6th Edition, Chapter 8, pp. 233–249)**

18.4   A 7-year-old boy demonstrates deficits in social-emotional reciprocity, in nonverbal communication, and in developing and maintaining relationships. Symptoms were present in early childhood and caused significant impairment across domains. How many restricted, repetitive patterns of behavior, interests, or activities must he have from Criterion B of the new classification of ASD in DSM-5 to meet criteria for the diagnosis?

A. One symptom.
B. Two symptoms.
C. Three symptoms.
D. Four symptoms.
E. Five symptoms.

The correct response is option B: Two symptoms.

According to the ASD classification scheme in DSM-5, two of the possible symptoms in Criterion B must be present in order to meet criteria for the diagnosis (option B). The list of possible symptoms in Criterion B includes 1) stereotyped or repetitive speech, motor movements, or use of objects; 2) excessive adherence to routines, ritualized patterns of verbal or nonverbal behavior, or excessive resistance to change; 3) highly restricted, fixated interests that are abnormal in intensity or focus; and 4) hyperreactivity or hyporeactivity to sensory input or unusual interest in sensory aspects of environment. In DSM-IV, Criterion A specified that only one example of a restricted repetitive and stereotyped pattern of behavior, interests, and activities needed to be present for the diagnosis (option A), although the sensory input symptom was not present as an option. A child having three (option C) or four (option D) symptoms would also fulfill this criterion, but only two symptoms are required. There are only four symptoms listed in Criterion B, so a choice of five symptoms (option E) is incorrect. **(Hales RE, Yudofsky SC, Roberts LW [eds]: APP Textbook of Psychiatry, 6th Edition, Chapter 8, pp. 243–245)**

18.5   A 5-year-old boy has problems with initiating, sustaining, and having back-and-forth conversation; reading social cues; and sharing his feelings with others. He demonstrates a restricted interest in trains that seems abnormal in intensity and focus, has difficulty making friends, and demonstrates little imaginative or symbolic play. There are no clear deficits in his nonverbal communication; he makes good eye contact, has normal speech intonation, displays facial gestures, and has a range of affect that generally seems appropriate to the situation. His mother attends an autism conference and learns about the new diagnostic criteria for ASD in DSM-5. Which of these DSM-5 criteria does the boy seem to lack?

A. Deficits in social-emotional reciprocity.
B. Deficits in nonverbal communication behaviors used for social interaction.
C. Deficits in developing and maintaining friendships.
D. Two of the specified four categories of restricted, repetitive patterns of behavior, interests, or activities.
E. Symptoms dating to early childhood that cause clinically significant impairment.

The correct response is option B: Deficits in nonverbal communication behaviors used for social interaction.

According to DSM-5, Criterion A for ASD specifies that all three symptom clusters summarized in options A, B, and C must be met for diagnosis. The boy does have two of three symptoms from Criterion A (options A, C), and he meets Criteria C and D (option E). He does not meet Criterion B (option D) because although he has "highly restricted, fixated interests that are abnormal in intensity or focus," he needs to have at least one other symptom from the three remaining categories in Criterion B: stereotyped or repetitive motor movements, use of objects, or speech; insistence on sameness, inflexible adherence to routines, or ritualized patterns of verbal or nonverbal behavior; or hyper- or hyporeactivity to sensory input or unusual interest in sensory aspects of the environment. In addition, he is lacking the deficit in nonverbal communication (Criterion A2; option B) that is required for the diagnosis; DSM-5 requires that "deficits in nonverbal communication behaviors used for social interaction, ranging, for example, from poorly integrated verbal and nonverbal communication; to abnormalities in eye contact and body language or deficits in understanding and use of gestures; to a total lack of facial expressions and nonverbal communication." Because this boy's nonverbal communication is reportedly not impaired (although this should be confirmed using standard instruments such as the Autism Diagnostic Observation Schedule, Second Edition [Lord et al. 2012]), on the basis of the current history he could not be diagnosed with DSM-5 ASD. **(Hales RE, Yudofsky SC, Roberts LW [eds]: APP Textbook of Psychiatry, 6th Edition, Chapter 8, pp. 243–245, 247)**

18.6　A 7-year-old girl presents with a history of normal language skills (vocabulary and grammar intact) but is unable to use language in a socially pragmatic manner to share ideas and feelings. She has never made good eye contact and has difficulty reading social cues. Her difficulty making friends is, in part, due to her obsession with cartoon characters and her tendency to repetitively mimic conversations she hears in the cartoons. She tends to excessively smell objects and has difficulty getting dressed because she insists on wearing the same shirt and shorts every day, regardless of the season. These symptoms have dated from early childhood and cause significant impairment in her functioning. According to DSM-5, what diagnosis would she receive?

A. Asperger's disorder.
B. Autism spectrum disorder (ASD).
C. Pervasive developmental disorder not otherwise specified (PDD NOS).
D. Social (pragmatic) communication disorder.
E. Rett's disorder.

The correct response is option B: Autism spectrum disorder (ASD).

This child might have met DSM-IV criteria for Asperger's disorder (option A) or PDD NOS (option C). ASD in DSM-5 subsumed Asperger's disorder and PDD NOS, so ASD is the correct diagnosis (option B). Although this girl has intact formal language skills, it is the use of language for social communication that is particularly affected in ASD. A specific language delay is not required. She meets all three components of Criterion A (deficits in social-emotional reciprocity, deficits in nonverbal communication behaviors used for social interaction, and deficits in developing and maintaining friendships) and two components of Criterion B (highly restricted, fixated interests that are abnormal in intensity or focus; and hyperreactivity or hyporeactivity to sensory input or unusual interest in sensory aspects of the environment). Children diagnosed with social (pragmatic) communication disorder (option D) must not have symptoms better explained by ASD, intellectual disability (intellectual developmental disorder), global developmental delay, or another mental disorder. In DSM-5, Rett's disorder (option E) is no longer included as a neurodevelopmental disorder because it has a known molecular (biological) basis, which excludes it from being a DSM disorder. **(Hales**

RE, Yudofsky SC, Roberts LW [eds]: APP Textbook of Psychiatry, 6th Edition, Chapter 8, p. 240)

18.7   A 15-year-old boy has a long history of nonverbal communication deficits. As an infant he was unable to follow someone else directing his attention by pointing. As a toddler he was not interested in sharing events, feelings, or games with his parents. From school age into adolescence, his speech was odd in tonality and phrasing, and his body language was awkward. What do these behaviors represent?

    A. Stereotypies.
    B. Restricted range of interests.
    C. Developmental regression.
    D. Prodromal schizophreniform symptoms.
    E. Deficits in nonverbal communication behaviors.

The correct response is option E: Deficits in nonverbal communication behaviors.

This boy's symptoms are examples of deficits listed in Criterion A2 of the DSM-5 ASD criteria (option E). Stereotypies (option A) are repetitive motor movements. Restricted range of interests (option B) is captured in Criterion B but is not described in the case above. There is no evidence that the boy has had developmental regression (option C). Schizophreniform symptoms (option D) must have been present for fewer than 6 months; the symptoms described are not consistent with delusions, hallucinations, disorganized speech or behavior, or negative symptoms. **(Hales RE, Yudofsky SC, Roberts LW [eds]: APP Textbook of Psychiatry, 6th Edition, Chapter 8, p. 284)**

18.8   The parents of a 15-year-old female in tenth grade believe that she should be doing better in high school given that she seems bright and that she received mostly As through eighth grade. She hands in papers late and makes careless mistakes on examinations. Her handwriting has always been messy, and she procrastinates completing written assignments, although there has been some improvement since she started typing her responses. Neuropsychological testing is notable for verbal IQ of 125, Perceptual Reasoning Index of 122, Full Scale IQ of 123, Working Memory Index in the 55th percentile, and Processing Speed Index in the 50th percentile, as well as weaknesses in executive function. In a psychiatric evaluation, she reports a long history of failing to give close attention to details; difficulty sustaining attention while in class or doing homework; failing to finish chores and tasks; and significant difficulties with time management, planning, and organization. She says she is forgetful, often loses things, and is easily distracted. She has no history of restlessness or impulsivity and is well liked by her peers. What is her most likely DSM-5 diagnosis?

    A. Adjustment disorder with anxiety.
    B. Specific learning disorder.
    C. Attention-deficit/hyperactivity disorder (ADHD), predominantly inattentive.
    D. Developmental coordination disorder.
    E. Major depressive disorder.

The correct response is option C: Attention-deficit/hyperactivity disorder (ADHD), predominantly inattentive.

The patient has six symptoms in the inattention cluster of ADHD and meets criteria for this disorder (option C). She has common associated features of ADHD, including weaknesses in working memory and processing speed and problems handing in her work (especially writing) on time. There is no evidence from the testing or history that her writing difficulty is secondary to a primary disorder involving writing or that she has any other specific learning disorder (option B). There is no mention of anxiety or of a recent stressful event (option A), and her description does not fit criteria for major depressive disorder (option E). There is no evidence of coordination difficulties, which must be present in the early developmental period for a diagnosis of developmental coordination disorder (option D). **(Hales RE, Yudofsky SC, Roberts LW [eds]: APP Textbook of Psychiatry, 6th Edition, Chapter 8, pp. 257–258, 260; Chapter 11, pp. 363–365; Chapter 14, pp. 482–483)**

18.9   A 25-year-old man who was raised in the United States, but whose first language was Spanish, presents with avoidance of both leisure and work-related activities that involve reading, which is affecting his ability to function in both settings and is exacerbating feelings of inadequacy and anxiety. He was told that as a young child he was a late speaker of Spanish, and he recalls that he had difficulty learning to read in both languages. He received remediation that helped him, but in middle school he continued to have difficulties due to his slow rate of reading, which was complicated by his need to reread material to understand it. He also experienced difficulty with writing, which continued through high school and college. Currently, he is a poor speller and reads quite slowly. What likely conclusions can be drawn about the developmental course of his problems and treatment?

A. The young man has developed adult ADHD.
B. The source of the problem is that he is bilingual.
C. His anxiety symptoms and feelings of inadequacy are the primary issues.
D. This developmental course is somewhat typical for an individual with a specific learning disorder.
E. Treatment with a selective serotonin reuptake inhibitor (SSRI) will likely resolve his problems.

The correct response is option D: This developmental course is somewhat typical for an individual with a specific learning disorder.

This is a typical developmental course for an individual with a specific learning disorder affecting reading and written expression, with learning problems that accumulate over successive developmental periods (option D). Individuals with specific learning disorders in their primary language will likely have difficulty learning academic skills in another language, but being bilingual is not the cause of the problem (option B). Such difficulties commonly do persist into adulthood. Treating his anxiety (option C) or possible depression with medication may reduce these symptoms (option E) but does not address the underlying etiology for his difficulty, which is related to his reading and writing problem; the emotional symptoms are frequent consequences in individuals with specific learning disorders. ADHD is a common comorbidity of specific learning disorders; however, this young man does not meet diagnostic criteria for ADHD (option A) based on the clinical description above. **(Hales RE, Yudofsky SC, Roberts LW [eds]: APP Textbook of Psychiatry, 6th Edition, Chapter 8, pp. 249–252)**

18.10 An 8-year-old boy comes to your office for his third office visit. He has a 6-month history of excessive eye blinking and intermittent chirping, but now the mother has noticed the development of grunting sounds since starting school this term. What is the most likely DSM-5 diagnosis?

    A. Tourette's disorder.
    B. Provisional tic disorder.
    C. Temporary tic disorder.
    D. Persistent vocal tic disorder.
    E. Transient tic disorder, recurrent.

The correct response is option B: Provisional tic disorder.

According to DSM-5, the presence of single or multiple motor and/or vocal tics for *less* than 1 year meets Criteria A and B for provisional tic disorder (option B). This is in contrast to Tourette's disorder (option A), in which tics must be present for *more* than 1 year. There is no temporary tic disorder (option C). Option D is incorrect because in this case, the boy has *both* motor and vocal tics and they have been present for less than 1 year. Transient tic disorder (option E) has been revised and renamed provisional tic disorder in DSM-5. **(Hales RE, Yudofsky SC, Roberts LW [eds]: APP Textbook of Psychiatry, 6th Edition, Chapter 8, pp. 261–262)**

18.11 When considering the diagnosis of speech sound disorder, it is important to know that the speech of a young child should be fully intelligible by the age of ___, and full mastery of speech sounds of one's native language should occur by the age of ___.

    A. 3 years; 10 years.
    B. 4 years; 8 years.
    C. 2 years; 6 years.
    D. 2 years; 10 years.
    E. 3 years; 7 years.

The correct response is option B: 4 years; 8 years.

Full mastery of the speech sounds of one's native language should occur by age 8 years; however, the speech of a young child should be fully intelligible by age 4 years. **(Hales RE, Yudofsky SC, Roberts LW [eds]: APP Textbook of Psychiatry, 6th Edition, Chapter 8, pp. 237–238)**

18.12 Which of the following dysfluencies involves changing around the order of words spoken?

A. Repetitions.
B. Dyslexia.
C. Circumlocutions.
D. Pauses.
E. Prolongations.

The correct response is option C: Circumlocutions.

In childhood-onset fluency disorder (stuttering), *dysfluencies* (i.e., clinically significant impairment in the production of fluent speech) most often take the form of repetitions of words or parts of words (option A), pauses in the production of connected speech (option D), *circumlocutions* (changing around the order of words or avoiding certain words; option C), or the prolongation of speech sounds (option E). *Dyslexia* (option B) is not dysfluency; rather, it is an alternative term used to refer to a specific learning disorder with impairment in reading that encompasses accurate word recognition but poor decoding and poor spelling abilities. **(Hales RE, Yudofsky SC, Roberts LW [eds]: APP Textbook of Psychiatry, 6th Edition, Chapter 8, pp. 238–239, 257)**

18.13 A 10-year-old girl with a seizure disorder has an IQ of 50, becomes agitated by bright light, and has limited interest in social interaction. What is the most likely diagnosis?

A. Intellectual disability.
B. Asperger's disorder.
C. Childhood disintegrative disorder.
D. Autism spectrum disorder.
E. Major depressive disorder.

The correct response is option D: Autism spectrum disorder.

The combination of social and communication limitations, along with odd or repetitive behaviors, expressed consistently throughout the lifetime, should alert the clinician that ASD (option D) must be part of the differential diagnosis. If additional problems not encompassed by the ASD criteria are present, or if changes from baseline indicate onset of new difficulties, or if the individual is not responding as expected to treatment, comorbidity should be considered (Lainhart 1999). IQ alone is insufficient to diagnose intellectual disability, and the description does not mention deficits in adaptive functioning (option A). Asperger's disorder (option B) and childhood disintegrative disorder (option C), which were diagnoses in DSM-IV, are grouped in DSM-5 under ASD, the diagnosis that replaces several developmental disorders. There is insufficient information to make a diagnosis of major depressive disorder in this case (option E). **(Hales RE, Yudofsky SC, Roberts LW [eds]: APP Textbook of Psychiatry, 6th Edition, Chapter 8, pp. 246–247)**

18.14 A 6-year-old girl is noted to have poor motor coordination for her age. She often bumps into objects and is unable to catch a ball. Although her mother works with her to practice skills, the girl's play is significantly impacted. These symptoms seemed to have started before the girl was age 3 years. What is the most likely diagnosis?

A. Rett's disorder.
B. Childhood disintegrative disorder.
C. Autism spectrum disorder.
D. Developmental coordination disorder.
E. Cerebral palsy.

The correct response is option D: Developmental coordination disorder.

Developmental coordination disorder (option D) is characterized by motor performance below expectations for age and experience, with manifestations including poor coordination, balance problems, clumsiness, or substantial delays in acquiring basic motor skills or meeting developmental milestones. Rett's disorder (option A) is characterized by poor motor coordination, decreased social engagement, and stereotyped hand movements. It is no longer part of DSM because of its known molecular basis; DSM-5 focuses on disorders without molecular or biological markers that must instead be defined behaviorally. Childhood disintegrative disorder (option B) is no longer a DSM diagnosis and is encompassed by ASD, along with the former categories autistic disorder (option C), Asperger's disorder, and pervasive developmental disorder not otherwise specified. Most children with cerebral palsy (option E) are born with the disorder, unlike children with Rett's disorder, who are previously healthy prior to the diagnosis; neither is considered a mental disorder. **(Hales RE, Yudofsky SC, Roberts LW [eds]: APP Textbook of Psychiatry, 6th Edition, Chapter 8, pp. 243, 260)**

18.15 According to DSM-5, by what age must symptoms be present for a child to be diagnosed with ADHD?

A. 5 years.
B. 7 years.
C. 8 years.
D. 10 years.
E. 12 years.

The correct response is option E: 12 years.

A change in DSM-5 relative to DSM-IV is that symptom onset of ADHD no longer needs to have occurred by age 7 years. The new criteria state that several inattentive or hyperactive-impulsive symptoms should be evident by age 12 years (option E). For adults to be diagnosed with ADHD, manifestation of the symptoms should have occurred during childhood rather than representing an acute onset. (**Hales RE, Yudofsky SC, Roberts LW [eds]: APP Textbook of Psychiatry, 6th Edition, Chapter 8, pp. 249–251**)

18.16 Efficacy studies of clonidine in the treatment of pediatric ADHD have demonstrated which of the following?

A. Clonidine is more beneficial than methylphenidate for inattention symptoms.
B. Treatment with clonidine for 2–4 weeks may be necessary before its benefits can be adequately assessed.
C. Children with ADHD and comorbid tics have a more positive response to clonidine than children who have ADHD without tics.
D. Extended-release clonidine is similar to placebo in improvement of inattention and hyperactivity.
E. Clonidine and methylphenidate in combination is superior to either alone in the treatment of children with ADHD.

The correct response is option C: Children with ADHD and comorbid tics have a more positive response to clonidine than children who have ADHD without tics.

Children with ADHD and comorbid tics may have a more positive response to clonidine than children who have ADHD without tics (option C) (Steingard et al. 1993). A randomized controlled trial in children with both ADHD *and a chronic tic disorder* (not simply ADHD [option E]) found significant improvements in all treatment groups (clonidine, methylphenidate, and the combination) (Tourette's Syndrome Study Group 2002). The greatest benefit compared with placebo was seen in the combination medication group. Although clonidine and methylphenidate individually were both noted to be effective for symptoms of ADHD, methylphenidate appeared more beneficial for the inattention symptoms (option A), and clonidine appeared more beneficial for the impulsivity and hyperactivity symptoms.

In a study that examined the addition of either clonidine or placebo to the treatment of children with ADHD and comorbid conduct disorder or oppositional defiant disorder who were already taking a stimulant, after about 5 weeks of treatment clonidine was modestly superior to placebo (Hazell and Stuart 2003). This study suggests that 4–6 weeks of treatment with clonidine may be necessary before its benefits can be adequately assessed (option B).

In a large controlled trial, youth with ADHD combined or hyperactive subtypes who had a partial response to a stimulant were randomly assigned to stimulant plus placebo or extended-release clonidine. Extended-release clonidine was superior to placebo in improvement of inattention and hyperactivity (option D) (Kollins et al. 2011). Common adverse effects were somnolence, headache, and fatigue. (**Hales RE, Yudofsky SC, Roberts LW [eds]: APP Textbook of Psychiatry, 6th Edition, Chapter 34, pp. 1200–1201**)

References

American Psychiatric Association: Diagnostic and Statistical Manual of Mental Disorders, 4th Edition. Washington, DC, American Psychiatric Association, 1994

American Psychiatric Association: Diagnostic and Statistical Manual of Mental Disorders, 4th Edition, Text Revision. Washington, DC, American Psychiatric Association, 2000

American Psychiatric Association: Diagnostic and Statistical Manual of Mental Disorders, 5th Edition. Arlington, VA, American Psychiatric Association, 2013

Hazell PL, Stuart JE: A randomized controlled trial of clonidine added to psychostimulant medication for hyperactive and aggressive children. J Am Acad Child Adolesc Psychiatry 42(8):886–894, 2003 12874489

Kollins SH, Jain R, Brams M, et al: Clonidine extended-release tablets as add-on therapy to psychostimulants in children and adolescents with ADHD. Pediatrics 127(6):e1406–e1413, 2011 21555501

Lainhart JE: Psychiatric problems in individuals with autism, their parents, and siblings. Int J Psychiatry 11:278–298, 1999

Lord C, Rutter M, DiLavore PC, et al: Autism Diagnostic Observation Schedule, Second Edition (ADOS-2) Manual. Torrance, CA, Western Psychological Services, 2012

Steingard R, Biederman J, Spencer T, et al: Comparison of clonidine response in the treatment of attention-deficit hyperactivity disorder with and without comorbid tic disorders. J Am Acad Child Adolesc Psychiatry 32(2):350–353, 1993 8444764

Tourette's Syndrome Study Group: Treatment of ADHD in children with tics: a randomized controlled trial. Neurology 58(4):527–536, 2002 11865128

CHAPTER 19

Nonpharmacological Somatic Treatments

19.1   How do the antidepressant effects and safety of daily left prefrontal transcranial magnetic stimulation (TMS) for 3–6 weeks compare with those of psychopharmacological treatments for depression?

A. TMS has a substantially greater risk of seizures.
B. Effect sizes are consistently smaller for TMS.
C. TMS results were not clinically meaningful.
D. TMS has been shown to be effective in "real-world" patients with treatment-resistant depression.
E. High rates of patient discontinuation of TMS limit its applicability in real-world populations.

The correct response is option D: TMS has been shown to be effective in "real-world" patients with treatment-resistant depression.

Studies of TMS in real-world clinical practice settings have highlighted its effectiveness in patients with treatment-resistant depression (option D) (Carpenter et al. 2012). In addition, industry-independent clinical studies (George et al. 2010; Mantovani et al. 2012; McDonald et al. 2011) have demonstrated that left prefrontal TMS daily for 3–6 weeks has antidepressant effects that are significantly greater than sham and that these effects are clinically meaningful (option C) (30% remission rate). Even more important, the outcomes are at least as robust as those for the next-best choice of antidepressant medication; the procedure was found to be safe and well tolerated, with a low incidence of treatment discontinuation (option E); and the therapeutic effects, once obtained, are reasonably durable.

Effect sizes for left prefrontal TMS are of similar or greater magnitude compared with those observed with the majority of currently approved antidepressant medication treatments (option B) (Demitrack and Thase 2009; O'Reardon et al. 2007). The estimated risk of seizure associated with TMS under ordinary clinical use is approximately 1 in 30,000 treatments (0.003% of treatments) or 1 in

1,000 patients (0.1% of patients). This risk is less than or comparable to the risk of seizure associated with antidepressant medications (option A). **(Hales RE, Yudofsky SC, Roberts LW [eds]: APP Textbook of Psychiatry, 6th Edition, Chapter 28, pp. 1011, 1014–1016)**

19.2   A typical initial course of electroconvulsive therapy (ECT) involves administration ___ times per week for a total of ___ treatments?

A. Two times per week for a total of 9–12 treatments.
B. Three times per week for a total of 12–16 treatments.
C. Two to three times per week for a total of 8–12 treatments.
D. Two to three times per week for a total of 16–18 treatments.
E. Four to five times per week for a total of 16–18 treatments.

The correct response is option C: Two to three times per week for a total of 8–12 treatments.

For a typical series or a course of ECT, treatments are usually given two to three times per week for 8–12 treatments. This course may then be followed by maintenance treatment in the form of medication, additional ECT given at less frequent intervals, or both. **(Hales RE, Yudofsky SC, Roberts LW [eds]: APP Textbook of Psychiatry, 6th Edition, Chapter 28, p. 1008)**

19.3   Approximately how strong a magnetic field is typically used in TMS?

A. 0.5 tesla.
B. 1.5 teslas.
C. 4 teslas.
D. 7 teslas.
E. 10 teslas.

The correct response is option B: 1.5 teslas.

The electricity flowing in an electromagnetic coil on the scalp creates an extremely potent (near 1.5-teslas) but brief (microseconds) magnetic field. **(Hales RE, Yudofsky SC, Roberts LW [eds]: APP Textbook of Psychiatry, 6th Edition, Chapter 28, p. 1010)**

19.4   Which of the following aspects of TMS has been useful for researchers studying the brain?

A. Repetitive TMS over a brain region can cause a temporary augmentation of a brain function controlled by that region.
B. Paired-pulse TMS can demonstrate the behavior of local interneurons in the motor cortex and indirectly measure serotonin activity.
C. Brain circuit excitation caused by TMS reverts to baseline when stimulation ends.

D. There is no evidence that TMS can induce neurogenesis, which can confound the collection of functional data.

E. TMS can be conducted in a magnetic resonance imaging (MRI) machine.

The correct response is option E: TMS can be conducted in a magnetic resonance imaging (MRI) machine.

TMS can be performed within an MRI scanner, which is itself a huge magnet and is constantly on (option E) (Bohning 2000; Bohning et al. 1998).

One of the more interesting repetitive TMS (rTMS) effects is that for brief periods of time, during stimulation, rTMS can block or inhibit a brain function (option A). That is, rTMS over the motor area that controls speech can *temporarily* leave the patient speechless (motor aphasia), but only while the device is firing (option C). Additionally, two pulses of TMS in quick succession can provide information about the underlying excitability of a region of cortex. This diagnostic technique, called paired-pulse TMS, can demonstrate the behavior of local interneurons in the motor cortex and serve as an indirect measure of γ-aminobutyric acid (GABA) or glutamate (option B) (Heide et al. 2006). Single nerve cells form themselves into functioning circuits over time through repeated discharges. Externally stimulating a single nerve cell with low-frequency electrical stimulation can cause long-term depression, where the efficiency of links between cells diminishes. High-frequency stimulation over time can cause the opposite effect, called long-term potentiation. These behaviors are thought to be involved in learning, memory, and dynamic brain changes associated with networks. Many TMS studies have now shown inhibition or excitation lasting for up to several hours beyond the time of stimulation (Di Lazzaro et al. 2005). Animal studies have found that TMS can induce neurogenesis (option D) (Post and Keck 2001). **(Hales RE, Yudofsky SC, Roberts LW [eds]: APP Textbook of Psychiatry, 6th Edition, Chapter 28, pp. 1011–1014)**

19.5 Which of the following statements best describes the relationship between TMS and seizures?

A. The site of stimulation is not significant in terms of the risk of a seizure.

B. Concurrent use of medications plays no role in seizure risk.

C. TMS intensity and frequency have no impact on the risk of a seizure.

D. The estimated risk of a seizure in ordinary clinical use is approximately 10%.

E. All TMS seizures have occurred during stimulation rather than later.

The correct response is option E: All TMS seizures have occurred during stimulation rather than later.

TMS pulses applied in rhythmic succession are referred to as repetitive TMS. rTMS can create behaviors that do not occur with single pulses, including the potential risk of causing an unintended seizure, particularly if the stimulation is conducted near the motor cortex (option A). Over 20 seizures have occurred in the history of TMS use, out of an unclear total number of people stimulated but easily over 100,000 sessions (Rossi et al. 2009). Since market introduction of the Neuro-Star TMS Therapy system in October 2008, seven seizures have been reported with Neuro-Star TMS Therapy, over a usage of more than 250,000 treatment sessions and over 8,000 patients. In five of the seven seizures, patients had concurrent use of medications that may have altered the seizure threshold (option B). The estimated risk of seizure under ordinary clinical use is approximately 1 in 30,000 treatments (0.003% of treatments) (option D) or 1 in 1,000 patients (0.1% of patients) (M. Demitrack, Neuronetics, personal communication, November 12, 2012). This risk is less than or comparable to the risk of seizure associated with antidepressant medications. All TMS seizures have occurred during stimulation, rather than later, and have been self-limited with no sequelae (option E). rTMS seizures are more likely to occur with certain combinations of TMS intensity, frequency, duration, and interstimulus interval (option C) (Wassermann 1997). **(Hales RE, Yudofsky SC, Roberts LW [eds]: APP Textbook of Psychiatry, 6th Edition, Chapter 28, p. 1011)**

19.6 Which of the following brain stimulation treatments has been approved by the U.S. Food and Drug Administration (FDA) for the treatment of depression?

A. Focal electrically administered seizure therapy (FEAST).
B. Transcutaneous electrical nerve stimulation (TENS).
C. Magnetic seizure therapy (MST).
D. Repetitive transcranial magnetic stimulation (rTMS).
E. Deep brain stimulation (DBS).

The correct response is option D: Repetitive transcranial magnetic stimulation (rTMS).

The FDA has approved one device for administering rTMS for the treatment of depression in adult patients who have failed to achieve satisfactory improvement from one previous antidepressant medication (option D). FEAST is an experimental form of ECT that uses direct current to initiate a focal seizure (option A). TENS, which uses electrical stimulation of peripheral nerves to block pain signals, was grandfathered in by the FDA for treatment of pain conditions, but it has not been rigorously tested for the treatment of depression (option B). MST uses magnetic fields to initiate seizures. Although MST is promising in terms of causing fewer acute cognitive side effects than traditional ECT, it does not yet have adequate clinical data and remains an experimental treatment for depression (option C). DBS has a humanitarian device exemption for use in conjunction with medications for the treatment of treatment-resistant obsessive-compulsive disorder. Despite promising preliminary data in patients with treatment-resistant depression, DBS does not have FDA approval for this condition (option E). **(Hales RE, Yudofsky SC, Roberts LW [eds]: APP Textbook of Psychiatry, 6th Edition, Chapter 28, pp. 1005–1010, 1028 and Table 28–1, p. 1007)**

19.7 How do functional brain changes seen in depressed patients after ECT compare with changes seen in depressed patients after TMS?

A. ECT increases global activity following the seizure.
B. TMS increases limbic activity.
C. Both TMS and ECT decrease limbic activity.
D. ECT increases prefrontal activity following the seizure.
E. No changes in brain activity are seen after TMS stimulation.

The correct response is option B: TMS increases limbic activity.

TMS at different frequencies appears to have divergent effects on brain activity (option E). In contrast to imaging studies with ECT that have found that ECT shuts off global and regional activity following the seizure (options A, C, D) (Nobler et al. 2001), most studies using serial scans in depressed patients undergoing TMS have found increased activity in the cingulate and other limbic regions (option B) (Teneback et al. 1999). **(Hales RE, Yudofsky SC, Roberts LW [eds]: APP Textbook of Psychiatry, 6th Edition, Chapter 28, pp. 1012–1013)**

19.8 Which of the following is a true statement about transcranial direct current stimulation (tDCS)?

A. The costs and inconvenience of tDCS are major obstacles to its wider use.
B. The most promising effects of tDCS have been observed in depression studies.
C. tDCS affects neuronal excitability by causing neurons to fire at particular frequencies.
D. tDCS is a relatively safe treatment that can be administered in a patient's home.
E. tDCS dosing is based on motor threshold, similar to TMS.

The correct response is option D: tDCS is a relatively safe treatment that can be administered in a patient's home.

tDCS is a brain stimulation technique achieved through application of constant weak (typically ≤1 mA) electrical current through scalp electrodes. Unlike TMS, tDCS does not elicit action potentials in cortical neurons. Instead, the constant direct current of tDCS induces subthreshold changes in membrane potential that increase or decrease the ease with which an action potential may be triggered (option C) (Leung et al. 2009).

There are currently no FDA-approved therapeutic uses for tDCS. Nevertheless, tDCS remains an active area of research because of the ease with which it can be applied and the flexibility derived from its various potential electrode placements. A small current source and damp sponges (electrodes) are all that is required for tDCS administration. This portable, safe, inexpensive setup (option A) is particularly alluring because it may enable tDCS to be used in nontraditional ways, including in a patient's home (option D) or during therapeutic interventions such as cognitive-behavioral therapy or rehabilitation exercises. Thus far, the most promising effects of tDCS have been found in rehabilitation studies (option B). Although more research is needed, there is emerging evidence that tDCS may enhance poststroke aphasia rehabilitation therapies. Appropriate dosing of tDCS remains an unresolved issue. Unlike TMS, which can be titrated based on motor threshold, tDCS is not typically tailored for each individual patient (option E). **(Hales RE, Yudofsky SC, Roberts LW [eds]: APP Textbook of Psychiatry, 6th Edition, Chapter 28, pp. 1026–1027)**

19.9　How is vagus nerve stimulation (VNS) thought to impact neuropsychiatric disorders?

　　A. By blocking efferent motor and autonomic signals.
　　B. By modulating afferent fibers.
　　C. By directly increasing sympathetic tone.
　　D. By initiating seizures.
　　E. By modulating abdominal vagus tone.

The correct response is option B: By modulating afferent fibers.

Traditionally, the vagus nerve has been considered a parasympathetic efferent nerve (option C) (controlling and regulating autonomic functions such as heart rate and gastric tone). The afferent role of the vagus has been underemphasized in the traditional literature. The vagus nerve is composed of about 80% afferent sensory fibers carrying information *to the brain* from the head, neck, thorax, and abdomen (Foley and Dubois 1937). The brain region stimulated always follows the same initial route: the vagus nerve in the neck (option E). VNS offers the potential for modulating and modifying function in many brain regions, through transsynaptic connections (option A) (George et al. 2000). The incoming sensory (afferent) connections of the vagus nerve provide direct projections to many of the brain regions implicated in neuropsychiatric disorders. These connections provide a basis for understanding how VNS might be a portal to the brain stem and connected limbic and cortical regions. These pathways likely account for the neuropsychiatric effects of VNS (option B). VNS has been most extensively studied as a treatment for epilepsy. Two double-blind studies have been conducted in patients with epilepsy, with a total of 313 treatment-resistant completers (Ben-Menachem et al. 1994; Handforth et al. 1998). In this difficult-to-treat group, the average decline in seizure frequency was about 25%–30% compared with baseline (option D). **(Hales RE, Yudofsky SC, Roberts LW [eds]: APP Textbook of Psychiatry, 6th Edition, Chapter 28, pp. 1019–1021)**

19.10　Which of the following is a true statement about relapse after symptom remission in response to ECT?

　　A. Most patients who experience symptom remission in response to ECT will relapse after 6 months.
　　B. Remission is typically maintained for at least 12 months.
　　C. Medication does not affect the relapse rate after symptom remission with ECT.

D. A robust body of evidence shows that maintenance ECT prevents relapse.

E. ECT is the most effective treatment for both acute and chronic depression.

The correct response is option A: Most patients who experience symptom remission in response to ECT will relapse after 6 months.

Although ECT is the most effective acute treatment for depression (option E), it is disappointing that at 6 months many ECT patients who have responded or remitted will relapse (option A, not option B). For example, one study randomly assigned ECT remitters to placebo, nortriptyline, or nortriptyline plus lithium after patients had remitted (Sackeim et al. 2001). At 6 months, the relapse rate was 84% with placebo, 60% with nortriptyline, and 39% with nortriptyline plus lithium (option C). Some psychiatrists administer maintenance ECT treatments every 3–5 weeks to prevent relapse, although few formal studies with maintenance ECT have been reported (option D). **(Hales RE, Yudofsky SC, Roberts LW [eds]: APP Textbook of Psychiatry, 6th Edition, Chapter 28, p. 1009)**

19.11 The FDA has approved VNS for treatment of which of the following conditions?

A. Treatment-resistant depression.

B. Obsessive-compulsive disorder.

C. Parkinson's disease.

D. Acute depression.

E. Chronic pain.

The correct response is option A: Treatment-resistant depression.

VNS has been approved since 2005 for use in patients with treatment-resistant depression (option A), but it is not used for acute episodes of depression (option D). It is currently being studied for the treatment of anxiety, obesity, and pain (not options B, C, E). **(Hales RE, Yudofsky SC, Roberts LW [eds]: APP Textbook of Psychiatry, 6th Edition, Chapter 28, pp. 1019, 1023)**

19.12 DBS has FDA approval for which of the following conditions?

A. Epilepsy.

B. Obsessive-compulsive disorder.

C. Parkinson's disease.

D. Depression.

E. Chronic pain.

The correct response is option C: Parkinson's disease.

DBS has FDA approval for the treatment of Parkinson's disease (option C). A humanitarian device exemption was granted by the FDA for using DBS in patients with treatment-resistant obsessive-compulsive disorder (option B). DBS is also being studied in depression, Tourette's disorder, substance abuse, addictions, obesity, and schizophrenia (not options A, E). DBS for depression is not FDA approved and should be performed only in well-controlled research studies (option D). **(Hales RE, Yudofsky SC, Roberts LW [eds]: APP Textbook of Psychiatry, 6th Edition, Chapter 28, pp. 1024–1026 and Table 28–1, p. 1007)**

19.13 What is the preferred electrical stimulation in current ECT treatment?

A. Long pulse widths.
B. Ultrabrief pulse widths.
C. Delivery through bilateral electrode placement.
D. Delivery through left electrode placement.
E. Application of the pulse after the neuron has depolarized.

The correct response is option B: Ultrabrief pulse widths.

Data suggest that shorter pulse (option A) widths have fewer side effects than the fatter pulse widths used in traditional ECT (Sackeim et al. 2001). Applying electricity after the neuron has depolarized is not needed and is perhaps cognitively harmful (option E). Sackeim et al. (2008) determined that the most efficient pulse width for an ECT pulse was about 0.25 milliseconds; they label this as "ultrabrief pulse width" and have shown that right unilateral ultrabrief pulse (not options C, D) width ECT applied at a dose 6 times that needed to produce a seizure (the seizure threshold) is as effective as older forms of ECT (option B), with markedly fewer cognitive side effects. It is not just the seizure that is needed for the antidepressant response; electrode placement and optimal stimulation parameters, such as pulse width and suprathreshold dose, enhance clinical profiles. **(Hales RE, Yudofsky SC, Roberts LW [eds]: APP Textbook of Psychiatry, 6th Edition, Chapter 28, pp. 1008–1009)**

19.14 Which of the following brain stimulation treatments targets the subcortical regions of the brain?

A. Electroconvulsive therapy (ECT).
B. Deep brain stimulation (DBS).
C. Transcranial magnetic stimulation (TMS).
D. Vagus nerve stimulation (VNS).
E. Transcutaneous electrical nerve stimulation (TENS).

The correct response is option B: Deep brain stimulation (DBS).

In DBS, an electrode is implanted deep within the brain, allowing electrical current to be delivered to subcortical locations (option B). ECT and TMS target cortical circuits (options A, C). VNS stimulates a cranial nerve (option D). TENS works on peripheral nerves (option E). **(Hales RE, Yudofsky SC, Roberts LW [eds]: APP Textbook of Psychiatry, 6th Edition, Chapter 28, pp. 1011, 1019, 1027–1028 and Table 28–1, p. 1007)**

19.15 Which of the following disorders has the *least* evidence supporting the use of ECT?

A. Catatonia associated with an underlying medical condition.
B. Depression in bipolar disorder.
C. Parkinson's disease.
D. Negative symptoms of schizophrenia.
E. Nonmelancholic symptoms of depression.

The correct response is option D: Negative symptoms of schizophrenia.

There is no evidence to indicate that ECT has efficacy for the negative symptoms of schizophrenia (option D). The strongest evidence base is for the use of ECT in major depression, including the subtypes of depression (option E) as well as bipolar depression (option B). Catatonia—associated with underlying psychiatric or medical conditions—is highly responsive to ECT (option A). Evidence suggests that ECT can be useful in the treatment of Parkinson's disease (option C). **(Steffens DC, Blazer DG, Thakur ME [eds]: APP Textbook of Geriatric Psychiatry, 5th Edition, Chapter 21, pp. 590–591)**

19.16 Which of the following is a true statement about the relationship between ECT and cognitive side effects?

A. Cumulative deterioration of cognitive functions should be expected.
B. Association between the magnitude of cognitive effects and ECT treatment parameters increases as time from ECT progresses.
C. During and shortly after a course of ECT, retrograde amnesia is greater for personal information than for impersonal or public events.
D. Cognitive side effects are the major factor limiting the use of ECT.
E. Patients' scores on intelligence tests will typically worsen shortly after ECT compared with scores obtained in the pretreatment depressed state.

The correct response is option D: Cognitive side effects are the major factor limiting the use of ECT.

Although ECT is a highly effective treatment for a number of psychiatric disorders, its cognitive side effects are the major factor limiting its use (option D). With alterations in ECT technique, cumulative deterioration of cognitive functions need not occur, and improvements may even be seen (option A) (Sackeim 1992). Associations between the magnitude of cognitive effects and ECT treatment parameters decrease as time from ECT increases (option B). The retrograde amnesia seen during and shortly after a course of ECT is worse for impersonal or public events than for autobiographical information (option C). Depressed patients can achieve improved scores on intelligence testing after ECT (option E). **(Yudofsky SC, Hales RE [eds]: APP Textbook of Neuropsychiatry and Behavioral Neuroscience, 5th Edition, Chapter 14, pp. 584–585)**

19.17 Which of the following accurately describes the relationship between ECT treatment parameters and memory?

A. Unilateral placement of stimulus electrodes increases the risk of amnesia.
B. Lower stimulus intensity decreases the risk of amnesia.
C. Lower number of ECT treatments increases the risk of amnesia.
D. Higher doses of barbiturate anesthetic decrease the risk of amnesia.
E. More time between treatments increases the risk of amnesia.

The correct response is option B: Lower stimulus intensity decreases the risk of amnesia.

Technical factors can affect objective memory side effects in ECT. Compared with higher stimulus intensity, lower intensity decreases the risk of amnesia (option B). Greater risk of amnesia is associated with bilateral electrode placement (option A), a higher number of treatments (option C), higher doses of barbiturate anesthetic (option D), and less time between treatments (option E). **(Steffens DC, Blazer DG, Thakur ME [eds]: APP Textbook of Geriatric Psychiatry, 5th Edition, Chapter 21, p. 594)**

19.18 What is the overall mortality rate for ECT?

A. 0.02 deaths per 100,000 treatments.
B. 0.2 deaths per 100,000 treatments.
C. 2 deaths per 100,000 treatments.
D. 20 deaths per 100,000 treatments.
E. 200 deaths per 100,000 treatments.

The correct response is option C: 2 deaths per 100,000 treatments.

Although it is difficult to establish an accurate mortality rate for any medical procedure, the overall mortality rate for ECT is estimated to be 2 deaths per 100,000 treatments (Shiwach et al. 2001). **(Steffens DC, Blazer DG, Thakur ME [eds]: APP Textbook of Geriatric Psychiatry, 5th Edition, Chapter 21, p. 593)**

19.19 Which of the following is *not* considered to be a routine component of a pre-ECT evaluation?

A. Obtaining a thorough psychiatric history.
B. Obtaining a medical history and physical examination.
C. Obtaining a dental history and examination of teeth.
D. Eliciting a history of personal experiences with anesthesia.
E. Obtaining a neuropsychological assessment.

The correct response is option E: Obtaining a neuropsychological assessment.

The pre-ECT evaluation should be performed by the ECT provider in conjunction with an anesthesia provider. The evaluation should include a thorough psychiatric history and examination including prior response to ECT and other treatments (option A), a medical history and physical examination (option B), a dental history and examination (option C), and a history of personal and family experiences with anesthesia (option D). The decision about whether to pursue testing of cerebral function such as neuropsychological testing or imaging should be made on an individual basis (option E). **(Steffens DC, Blazer DG, Thakur ME [eds]: APP Textbook of Geriatric Psychiatry, 5th Edition, Chapter 21, p. 599)**

19.20 For which of the following patients would bright light therapy be a first-line treatment option?

A. Elderly moderately depressed patient.
B. Psychotically depressed patient.
C. Mildly depressed pregnant patient.
D. Bipolar I patient in a depressed phase.
E. Severely depressed pregnant patient.

The correct response is option C: Mildly depressed pregnant patient.

Because the use of antidepressants during pregnancy is not without some risk, these medications should be withheld if possible. Bright light therapy is a noninvasive treatment option for antenatal depression (option C). Patients described in options A, B, D, and E would be treated with other therapeutic modalities as a first-line option. **(Hales RE, Yudofsky SC, Roberts LW [eds]: APP Textbook of Psychiatry, 6th Edition, Chapter 38, p. 1325)**

19.21 A 55-year-old woman with a history of major depressive disorder, gastroesophageal reflux disease (GERD), coronary artery disease, and asthma is admitted for ECT. Which of her currently prescribed medications should be discontinued prior to starting an index ECT course?

A. Metoprolol.
B. Lithium.
C. Ranitidine.
D. Albuterol.
E. Sertraline.

The correct response is option B: Lithium.

There are considerable differences of opinion and great variations in practice regarding the use of psychotropic medications during the ECT course. The following psychotropic medications are among those best avoided or maintained at the lowest possible levels: 1) lithium (option B), which increases the risks for delirium or prolonged seizures; and 2) benzodiazepines, whose anticonvulsant properties may decrease efficacy (but can be reversed with flumazenil at the time of ECT) (Krystal et al. 1998). Individuals with coronary artery disease are at risk for ischemia during both the periods of relative parasympathetic tone and the periods of increased sympathetic system tone (Christopher 2003; Weiner et al. 2000). β-Adrenergic blockers, such as metoprolol (option A), can be used to decrease cardiac workload. For patients with GERD, complications of aspiration may be diminished with the use of a pretreatment histamine type 2 antagonist the night before and the morning of treatment (Weiner et al. 2000); therefore, continuing ranitidine (option C) is prudent. Patients with asthma or chronic obstructive pulmonary disease have an increased risk of posttreatment bronchospasm, which should be mitigated by the use of bronchodilators such as albuterol (option D). The literature regarding the benefits of an antidepressant medication such as sertraline (option E) as a means to augment the ECT response is unclear, although it does not appear that such a combination is associated with significantly increased risk; hence, it may be continued. **(Steffens DC, Blazer DG, Thakur ME [eds]: APP Textbook of Geriatric Psychiatry, 5th Edition, Chapter 21, pp. 596–598, 601)**

19.22 In a _____ patient receiving ECT, prolonged paralysis and associated apnea induced by _____ may occur.

A. Hyperkalemic; succinylcholine.
B. Hypokalemic; succinylcholine.
C. Hyperkalemic; rocuronium.
D. Hyponatremic; succinylcholine.
E. Hypercalcemic; rocuronium.

The correct response is option A: Hyperkalemic; succinylcholine.

Hyperkalemia is a concern in patients receiving ECT, because of the risk of cardiac arrhythmia and because of the transient rise in serum potassium caused by succinylcholine and the muscle activity that may occur during the induced seizures (Christopher 2003; Weiner et al. 2000). In individuals with hyperkalemia, prolonged paralysis and associated apnea induced by succinylcholine may be seen (option A). In cases where correction of hyperkalemia is not possible, the use of paralytic agents other than succinylcholine should be considered. These include nondepolarizing muscle relaxants such as rocuronium (options C, E). Hypokalemia and hyponatremia (options B, D) do not have the same risks as hyperkalemia. **(Steffens DC, Blazer DG, Thakur ME [eds]: APP Textbook of Geriatric Psychiatry, 5th Edition, Chapter 21, p. 597)**

19.23 Biofeedback from electromyography (EMG) is used as a treatment for which of the following?

A. Migraine headaches.
B. Phantom limb pain.
C. Fibromyalgia.

D. Cancer pain.

E. Chronic regional pain syndrome.

The correct response is option C: Fibromyalgia.

Biofeedback refers to a procedure in which physical parameters (e.g., muscle tension) are continuously monitored and fed back to the patient, who then attempts to alter the physiological parameter. Biofeedback from EMG assists the patient in learning to reduce muscle tension; the levels of measured muscle tension are signaled back to the patient for modification. This technique is useful in tension headaches, temporomandibular joint disorders, fibromyalgia (option C), and other myofascial pain disorders. *Thermal* biofeedback monitors skin temperature to give the patient an indication of the degree of peripheral vasodilation. The cooler the skin, the greater the vascular constriction; this reflects the amount of prevailing sympathetic activity. By increasing the skin temperature, one is able to suppress the extent of sympathetic activity. This approach has been used in the treatment of migraine (option A) and sympathetically mediated pain (chronic regional pain syndrome; option E). Phantom limb pain (option B) and cancer pain (option D) are not pain syndromes classically mediated by muscle tension. **(Leo RJ: Clinical Manual of Pain Management in Psychiatry, Chapter 6, pp. 151–152)**

19.24 Which of the following are the three key components of hypnosis?

A. Distraction, dissociation, reattribution.

B. Distraction, emotional processing, suggestibility.

C. Absorption, emotional processing, reattribution.

D. Absorption, dissociation, suggestibility.

E. Distraction, dissociation, mentalization.

The correct response is option D: Absorption, dissociation, suggestibility.

Hypnosis has three main components: absorption, dissociation, and suggestibility (option D). *Absorption* is the tendency to become fully involved in a perceptual, imaginative, or ideational experience. Individuals prone to this type of cognition are more highly hypnotizable than are those who never fully engage in such experience. *Dissociation* is the mental separation of components of experience that would ordinarily be processed together. This may involve discontinuities in the sensations in one part of the body compared with another or a sense of involuntariness in motor functions (e.g., in the movement of one arm compared with the other). *Suggestibility* is heightened responsiveness to social cues, leading to an enhanced tendency to comply with hypnotic instructions. This represents not a loss of will but rather a suspension of critical judgment because of the intense absorption of the hypnotic state. Hypnotic instructions are acted upon automatically and often are mistakenly perceived as internally generated. *Distraction* (options A, B, E) is a technique used in dialectical behavioral therapy to help individuals with distress tolerance. *Reattribution* (options A, C) is used in cognitive-behavioral therapy to help test automatic thoughts and assumptions. *Emotional processing* (options B, C) is part of cognitive processing therapy, to help individuals with posttraumatic stress disorder. *Mentalization* (option E) is the natural human imaginative capacity to perceive and interpret behavior in self and others as conjoined with intentional mental states, such as desires, motives, feelings, and beliefs. **(*Journal of Neuropsychiatry and Clinical Neurosciences* 3(4):440–445, 1991; Spiegel H, Spiegel D: Trance and Treatment: Clinical Uses of Hypnosis, 2nd Edition, Chapter 2, p. 19)**

References

Ben-Menachem E, Mañon-Espaillat R, Ristanovic R, et al; First International Vagus Nerve Stimulation Study Group: Vagus nerve stimulation for treatment of partial seizures: 1. A controlled study of effect on seizures. Epilepsia 35(3):616–626, 1994 8026408

Bohning DE: Introduction and overview of TMS physics, in Transcranial Magnetic Stimulation in Neuropsychiatry. Edited by George MS, Belmaker RH. Washington, DC, American Psychiatric Press, 2000, pp 13–44

Bohning DE, Shastri A, Nahas Z, et al: Echoplanar BOLD fMRI of brain activation induced by concurrent transcranial magnetic stimulation. Invest Radiol 33(6):336–340, 1998 9647445

Carpenter LL, Janicak PG, Aaronson ST, et al: Transcranial magnetic stimulation (TMS) for major depression: a multisite, naturalistic, observational study of acute treatment outcomes in clinical practice. Depress Anxiety 29(7):587–596, 2012 22689344

Christopher EJ: Electroconvulsive therapy in the medically ill. Curr Psychiatry Rep 5(3):225–230, 2003 12773277

Demitrack MA, Thase ME: Clinical significance of transcranial magnetic stimulation (TMS) in the treatment of pharmacoresistant depression: synthesis of recent data. Psychopharmacol Bull 42(2):5–38, 2009 19629020

Di Lazzaro V, Pilato F, Saturno E, et al: Theta-burst repetitive transcranial magnetic stimulation suppresses specific excitatory circuits in the human motor cortex. J Physiol 565(Pt 3):945–950, 2005 15845575

Foley JO, Dubois F: Quantitative studies of the vagus nerve in the cat, I: the ratio of sensory and motor studies. J Comp Neurol 67:49–67, 1937

George MS, Sackeim HA, Rush AJ, et al: Vagus nerve stimulation: a new tool for brain research and therapy. Biol Psychiatry 47(4):287–295, 2000 10686263

George MS, Lisanby SH, Avery D, et al: Daily left prefrontal transcranial magnetic stimulation therapy for major depressive disorder: a sham-controlled randomized trial. Arch Gen Psychiatry 67(5):507–516, 2010 20439832

Handforth A, DeGiorgio CM, Schachter SC, et al: Vagus nerve stimulation therapy for partial-onset seizures: a randomized active-control trial. Neurology 51(1):48–55, 1998 9674777

Heide G, Witte OW, Ziemann U: Physiology of modulation of motor cortex excitability by low-frequency suprathreshold repetitive transcranial magnetic stimulation. Exp Brain Res 171(1):26–34, 2006 16307247

Krystal AD, Watts BV, Weiner RD, et al: The use of flumazenil in the anxious and benzodiazepine-dependent ECT patient. J ECT 14(1):5–14, 1998 9661088

Leung A, Donohue M, Xu R, et al: rTMS for suppressing neuropathic pain: a meta-analysis. J Pain 10(12):1205–1216, 2009 19464959

Mantovani A, Pavlicova M, Avery D, et al: Long-term efficacy of repeated daily prefrontal transcranial magnetic stimulation (TMS) in treatment-resistant depression. Depress Anxiety 29(10):883–890, 2012 22689290

McDonald WM, Durkalski V, Ball ER, et al: Improving the antidepressant efficacy of transcranial magnetic stimulation: maximizing the number of stimulations and treatment location in treatment-resistant depression. Depress Anxiety 28(11):973–980, 2011 21898711

Nobler MS, Oquendo MA, Kegeles LS, et al: Decreased regional brain metabolism after ECT. Am J Psychiatry 158(2):305–308, 2001 11156816

O'Reardon JP, Solvason HB, Janicak PG, et al: Efficacy and safety of transcranial magnetic stimulation in the acute treatment of major depression: a multisite randomized controlled trial. Biol Psychiatry 62(11):1208–1216, 2007 17573044

Post A, Keck ME: Transcranial magnetic stimulation as a therapeutic tool in psychiatry: what do we know about the neurobiological mechanisms? J Psychiatr Res 35(4):193–215, 2001 11578638

Rossi S, Hallett M, Rossini PM, Pascual-Leone A; Safety of TMS Consensus Group: Safety, ethical considerations, and application guidelines for the use of transcranial magnetic stimulation in clinical practice and research. Clin Neurophysiol 120(12):2008–2039, 2009 19833552

Sackeim HA: The cognitive effects of electroconvulsive therapy, in Cognitive Disorders: Pathophysiology and Treatment. Edited by Moos WH, Gamzu ER, Thal LJ. New York, Marcel Dekker, 1992, pp 183–228

Sackeim HA, Haskett RF, Mulsant BH, et al: Continuation pharmacotherapy in the prevention of relapse following electroconvulsive therapy: a randomized controlled trial. JAMA 285(10):1299–1307, 2001 11255384

Sackeim HA, Prudic J, Nobler MS, et al: Effects of pulse width and electrode placement on the efficacy and cognitive effects of electroconvulsive therapy. Brain Stimulat 1(2):71–83, 2008 19756236

Shiwach RS, Reid WH, Carmody TJ: An analysis of reported deaths following electroconvulsive therapy in Texas, 1993-1998. Psychiatr Serv 52(8):1095–1097, 2001 11474057

Teneback CC, Nahas Z, Speer AM, et al: Changes in prefrontal cortex and paralimbic activity in depression following two weeks of daily left prefrontal TMS. J Neuropsychiatry Clin Neurosci 11(4):426–435, 1999 10570754

Wassermann EM: Report on risk and safety of repetitive transcranial magnetic stimulation (rTMS): suggested guidelines from the International Workshop on Risk and Safety of rTMS (June 1996). Electroencephalogr Clin Neurol 108:1–16, 1997

Weiner RD, Coffey CE, Krystal AD: Electroconvulsive therapy in the medical and neurologic patient, in Psychiatric Care of the Medical Patient, 2nd Edition. Edited by Stoudemire A, Fogel BS, Greenberg D. New York, Oxford University Press, 2000, pp 419–428

CHAPTER 20

Obsessive-Compulsive and Related Disorders

20.1 Which of the following is a compulsion commonly seen in obsessive-compulsive disorder (OCD)?

A. Purging.
B. Fear of contamination.
C. Intrusive sexual thoughts.
D. Checking.
E. Skin picking.

The correct response is option D: Checking.

Compulsions are repetitive behaviors or mental acts that an individual feels driven to perform in response to an obsession or according to rules that must be applied rigidly. Common compulsive behaviors include excessive cleaning (e.g., hand washing), checking (option D), ordering, rearranging, counting, repeating, and mental rituals. Fear of contamination (option B) and intrusive sexual thoughts (option C) are common *obsessions* in OCD. Purging and skin picking (options A, E) are features of other disorders. **(Hales RE, Yudofsky SC, Roberts LW [eds]: APP Textbook of Psychiatry, 6th Edition, Chapter 13, pp. 431–432 and Table 13–1, p. 433)**

20.2 Among individuals with OCD, what is the most common comorbid psychiatric diagnosis?

A. Obsessive-compulsive personality disorder.
B. Major depressive disorder.
C. Substance use disorder.
D. Generalized anxiety disorder.
E. Schizophrenia.

The correct response is option B: Major depressive disorder.

Psychiatric comorbidity is common in OCD, with the Epidemiologic Catchment Area study finding that two-thirds of patients with OCD met criteria for at least one other psychiatric illness during their lifetime (Karno et al. 1988). The most common comorbid psychiatric diagnosis is major depressive disorder (option B). Approximately one-third of individuals with OCD are currently experiencing a major depressive episode, and two-thirds will have a major depressive episode during their lifetime. Other commonly comorbid psychiatric illnesses include anxiety disorders (option D), eating disorders, and substance use disorders (option C). The differential diagnosis of OCD includes the ruminations of depression, the delusions of psychosis (option E), anxiety symptoms associated with other anxiety disorders, and severe obsessive-compulsive personality disorder (OCPD; option A). OCPD is defined as a rigid, perfectionistic personality type. A general rule of thumb is that whereas OCPD tends to be experienced as ego-syntonic, the obsessions and compulsions of OCD are experienced as ego-dystonic. Despite the similarity of their names, OCPD is clearly a separate disorder from OCD and does not respond to the treatments used for OCD. **(Hales RE, Yudofsky SC, Roberts LW [eds]: APP Textbook of Psychiatry, 6th Edition, Chapter 13, pp. 433–434)**

20.3   What are the concordance rates of OCD in monozygotic twins?

A. 5%–12%.
B. 10%–17%.
C. 24%–31%.
D. 80%–87%.
E. 93%–100%.

The correct response is option D: 80%–87%.

A review of twin studies found that there is a strong heritable component to OCD, with concordance rates of 80%–87% in monozygotic twins compared with rates of 47%–50% in dizygotic twins (van Grootheest et al. 2005). OCD also tends to run in families, with a study of 1,209 first-degree relatives of OCD probands indicating an increased risk of OCD among relatives of probands (8.2%) compared with control subjects (2.0%) (Hettema et al. 2001). Candidate gene studies have found a number of genes that may be associated with OCD, including many associated with serotonin, dopamine, and glutamate. Larger-scale studies are needed to confirm these initial findings. **(Hales RE, Yudofsky SC, Roberts LW [eds]: APP Textbook of Psychiatry, 6th Edition, Chapter 13, p. 434)**

20.4   A patient presents with obsessive ruminations about a defect in the appearance of his genitalia that prevents him from sexual interaction with any partner. What is the most likely diagnosis?

A. Body dysmorphic disorder.
B. Major depressive disorder.
C. Anorexia nervosa.

D. Obsessive-compulsive disorder (OCD).

E. Schizophrenia presenting with somatic delusions.

The correct response is option A: Body dysmorphic disorder.

The diagnosis of body dysmorphic disorder (BDD) requires a preoccupation with one or more perceived defects or flaws in physical appearance that are not observable by or appear very mild to others. Patients believe they look ugly, unattractive, abnormal, or deformed (option A). The perceived defects can involve any area of the body. As opposed to the generally good insight seen in patients with OCD (option D), most patients with BDD have poor insight into their illness. They tend to firmly believe that the perceived defect is present and not imagined. BDD patients often suffer from delusions of reference and believe that others are laughing at them or mocking them because of the perceived appearance flaw. Perhaps the most important factor to consider in the differential diagnosis of BDD is the possibility of normal appearance concerns or actual clearly noticeable physical defects. Concerns with bodily defects that are clearly noticeable (i.e., not slight) are not diagnosed as BDD. Weight concerns occurring in the context of an eating disorder such as anorexia nervosa (option C) preclude the diagnosis of BDD. Finally, the feelings of low self-worth associated with major depression (option B) may manifest physically, and delusions associated with psychosis (option E) may focus on physical appearance. **(Hales RE, Yudofsky SC, Roberts LW [eds]: APP Textbook of Psychiatry, 6th Edition, Chapter 13, p. 438)**

20.5   Findings from studies examining psychiatric comorbidity in individuals with body dysmorphic disorder (BDD) show that approximately what percentage will experience OCD at some point in life?

A. 5%.

B. 10%.

C. 25%.

D. 33%.

E. 60%.

The correct response is option D: 33%.

Psychiatric comorbidity is common in BDD; major depressive disorder, with a lifetime prevalence of 75%, is the most common comorbid diagnosis. Approximately one-third of patients with BDD experience comorbid OCD during their lifetime, and almost 40% have comorbid social anxiety disorder at some point. Comorbid substance use disorders are also common. **(Hales RE, Yudofsky SC, Roberts LW [eds]: APP Textbook of Psychiatry, 6th Edition, Chapter 13, p. 438)**

20.6   Which of the following is a true statement about treatment of hoarding disorder?

A. Patients with hoarding disorder are usually fairly agreeable to treatment.
B. Serotonin reuptake inhibitors (SRIs) are considered the first-line treatment for hoarding disorder.
C. Behavioral therapy is considered the first-line treatment for hoarding disorder.
D. Rates of response to behavioral therapy for hoarding disorder are similar to those for OCD.
E. There is no role for motivational interviewing in the treatment of hoarding disorder.

The correct response is option C: Behavioral therapy is considered the first-line treatment for hoarding disorder.

One of the most difficult aspects of treating individuals with hoarding disorder is getting them to accept treatment (option A). Although their hoarding behavior often causes great distress to those around them, individuals with hoarding disorder may not find these behaviors distressing. The first-line treatment of hoarding disorder is behavioral therapy (option C) that focuses on removing hoarded items from the environment (increasing outflow) and providing skills to decrease future hoarding (decreasing inflow) (Frost and Tolin 2008). Some data suggest that cognitive-behavioral therapy (CBT) (e.g., addition of motivational interviewing) may be a more effective approach to treating hoarding behavior (option E) (Steketee et al. 2010). There are few to no data regarding pharmacotherapy specifically for hoarding disorder, as hoarding has been considered a subtype of OCD. Overall, in pharmacological trials for OCD, hoarding appears to exhibit a lesser response to SRIs than other OCD spectrum disorders (option B) (e.g., Mataix-Cols et al. 1999). Most studies have found hoarding symptoms to be chronic and unchanging. Individuals with hoarding disorder who participate in behavioral therapy have lower response rates than individuals with OCD (option D) (Abramowitz et al. 2003; Mataix-Cols et al. 2002). This may be partly due to poor motivation to engage in treatment and higher dropout rates. Some data suggest that CBT may be more effective than behavioral therapy alone for hoarding symptoms. Because hoarding has been considered a subtype of OCD rather than a distinct disorder until DSM-5 (American Psychiatric Association 2013), there is little prognostic data regarding pharmacotherapy for hoarding behavior. **(Hales RE, Yudofsky SC, Roberts LW [eds]: APP Textbook of Psychiatry, 6th Edition, Chapter 13, p. 442)**

20.7   What is the DSM-5 definition of obsessions?

A. Chronic impulses that occur within a person's life but do not cause the patient internal distress.
B. Pursuits that give people pleasure, such as attending sporting events or shopping.
C. Recurrent delusions that are intrusive, causing a patient distress.

D. Behaviors meant to suppress thoughts through avoidance or suppression.

E. Recurrent thoughts that are experienced as intrusive and unwanted and that cause anxiety to the patient.

The correct response is option E: Recurrent thoughts that are experienced as intrusive and unwanted and that cause anxiety to the patient.

Per DSM-5, *obsessions* are recurrent and persistent thoughts, urges, or images that are experienced, at some time during the disturbance, as intrusive and unwanted, and that in most individuals cause marked anxiety or distress (option E). The individual attempts to ignore or suppress such thoughts, urges, or images, or to neutralize them with some other thought or action (i.e., by performing a compulsion; option D). Obsessions must be time-consuming or cause significant distress or impairment in social, occupational, or other important areas of functioning (options A, B). *Delusions* are fixed false beliefs (option C). Patients with obsessions generally have insight into their persistent thoughts and find them to be distressing. **(Hales RE, Yudofsky SC, Roberts LW [eds]: APP Textbook of Psychiatry, 6th Edition, Chapter 13, pp. 431–433)**

20.8 Which of the following is a true statement about hair-pulling disorder (trichotillomania)?

A. Trichotillomania occurs exclusively in times of elevated distress.

B. Trichotillomania is time limited in presentation and does not become chronic in the majority of patients.

C. Trichotillomania occurs more frequently in women than in men.

D. Trichotillomania does not respond to pharmacotherapy with antipsychotics.

E. Trichotillomania has a consistently high incidence of response to SRIs.

The correct response is option C: Trichotillomania occurs more frequently in women than in men.

Most studies of trichotillomania have found that females are much more commonly affected than males (option C), with some studies estimating that 93% of individuals with hair-pulling disorder are female (Christenson et al. 1991). Whereas some patients report pulling hair when distressed, others report hair pulling during states of relaxation (option A); most report pulling during both conditions. Some studies have found that with early childhood onset, the duration of hair pulling may be brief and not require treatment. However, if the hair-pulling symptoms are of longer duration, the usual course is chronic with some waxing and waning of symptoms (option B) (Keuthen et al. 2001).

Pharmacotherapy studies have shown mixed results with SRIs, with a meta-analysis failing to show any evidence of improvement with SRIs compared with placebo (option E) (Bloch et al. 2007). Encouraging initial results with antipsychotic medications (both as SRI augmentation and as monotherapy) have been reported (option D). Finally, one controlled trial each for naltrexone (Christenson et al. 1994) and *N*-acetylcysteine (Grant et al. 2009) demonstrated efficacy superior to placebo. **(Hales RE, Yudofsky SC, Roberts LW [eds]: APP Textbook of Psychiatry, 6th Edition, Chapter 13, pp. 442–445)**

References

Abramowitz JS, Franklin ME, Schwartz SA, Furr JM: Symptom presentation and outcome of cognitive-behavioral therapy for obsessive-compulsive disorder. J Consult Clin Psychol 71(6):1049–1057, 2003 14622080

American Psychiatric Association: Diagnostic and Statistical Manual of Mental Disorders, 5th Edition. Arlington, VA, American Psychiatric Association, 2013

Bloch MH, Landeros-Weisenberger A, Dombrowski P, et al: Systematic review: pharmacological and behavioral treatment for trichotillomania. Biol Psychiatry 62(8):839–846, 2007 17727824

Christenson GA, Mackenzie TB, Mitchell JE: Characteristics of 60 adult chronic hair pullers. Am J Psychiatry 148(3):365–370, 1991 1992841

Christenson GA, Crow SJ, MacKenzie TB, et al: A placebo controlled double-blind study of naltrexone for trichotillomania (NR 597), in 1994 New Research Program and Abstracts, American Psychiatric Association 147th Annual Meeting, Philadelphia, PA, May 21–26, 1994. Washington, DC, American Psychiatric Association, 1994, p 212

Frost RO, Tolin DF: Compulsive hoarding, in Clinical Handbook of Obsessive-Compulsive Disorder and Related Problems. Edited by Abramowitz JS, Taylor S, McKay D. Baltimore, MD, Johns Hopkins University Press, 2008, pp 76–94

Grant JE, Odlaug BL, Kim SW: N-acetylcysteine, a glutamate modulator, in the treatment of trichotillomania: a double-blind, placebo-controlled study. Gen Psychiatry 66(7):756–763, 2009 19581567

Hettema JM, Neale MC, Kendler KS: A review and meta-analysis of the genetic epidemiology of anxiety disorders. Am J Psychiatry 158(10):1568–1578, 2001 11578982

Karno M, Golding JM, Sorenson SB, Burnam MA: The epidemiology of obsessive-compulsive disorder in five US communities. Arch Gen Psychiatry 45(12):1094–1099, 1988 3264144

Keuthen NJ, Fraim C, Deckersbach T, et al: Longitudinal follow-up of naturalistic treatment outcome in patients with trichotillomania. J Clin Psychiatry 62(2):101–107, 2001 11247093

Mataix-Cols D, Rauch SL, Manzo PA, et al: Use of factor-analyzed symptom dimensions to predict outcome with serotonin reuptake inhibitors and placebo in the treatment of obsessive-compulsive disorder. Am J Psychiatry 156(9):1409–1416, 1999 10484953

Mataix-Cols D, Marks IM, Greist JH, et al: Obsessive-compulsive symptom dimensions as predictors of compliance with and response to behaviour therapy: results from a controlled trial. Psychother Psychosom 71(5):255–262, 2002 12207105

Steketee G, Frost RO, Tolin DF, et al: Waitlist-controlled trial of cognitive behavior therapy for hoarding disorder. Depress Anxiety 27(5):476–484, 2010 20336804

van Grootheest DS, Cath DC, Beekman AT, Boomsma DI: Twin studies on obsessive-compulsive disorder: a review. Twin Res Hum Genet 8(5):450–458, 2005 16212834

CHAPTER 21

Paraphilic Disorders

21.1 Which of the following paraphilic disorders can be diagnosed only if a patient reports experiencing distress or psychosocial role impairment from the urges or behaviors?

A. Exhibitionistic disorder.
B. Fetishistic disorder.
C. Frotteuristic disorder.
D. Pedophilic disorder.
E. Sexual sadism disorder.

The correct response is option B: Fetishistic disorder.

Fetishistic disorder is sexual arousal that often involves the use of nonliving objects, such as women's underpants, bras, stockings, shoes, boots, or other apparel, but it may also include a highly specific focus on nongenital body parts (Kafka 2010). The inclusion of nongenital body parts is new in DSM-5 (American Psychiatric Association 2013). One of the most important features of the diagnosis is that the individual must experience clinically significant distress or impairment (option B). If an individual has strong fantasies, urges, and behaviors involving the use of nonliving objects but experiences no distress or psychosocial role impairment, then a diagnosis would not be appropriate. Therefore, the diagnosis of fetishistic disorder cannot be made in a nonadmitter using objective evidence alone. This is in contrast to exhibitionistic disorder (option A), frotteuristic disorder (option C), pedophilic disorder (option D), and sexual sadism disorder (option E), all of which can be diagnosed in a nonadmitter provided that substantial objective evidence is present. **(Hales RE, Yudofsky SC, Roberts LW [eds]: APP Textbook of Psychiatry, 6th Edition, Chapter 26, pp. 902–903)**

21.2 To qualify for a diagnosis of pedophilia, an individual must have been at least how old at the onset of symptoms and be at least how many years older than the child?

A. At least 16 years of age and at least 5 years older than the child.
B. At least 16 years of age and at least 7 years older than the child.
C. At least 18 years of age and at least 5 years older than the child.
D. At least 18 years of age and at least 7 years older than the child.
E. At least 18 years of age and at least 10 years older than the child.

The correct response is option A: At least 16 years of age and at least 5 years older than the child.

Pedophilic disorder is defined as intense, recurrent, sexually arousing fantasies, urges, or behaviors involving a prepubescent child or children over a period of at least 6 months. A diagnosis is suggested if an individual has acted on these urges or if the urges or fantasies caused marked distress. To receive a diagnosis of pedophilia, an individual must have been at least age 16 years and at least 5 years older than the child. **(Hales RE, Yudofsky SC, Roberts LW [eds]: APP Textbook of Psychiatry, 6th Edition, Chapter 26, p. 901)**

21.3 Which of the following is a true statement about exhibitionistic disorder?

A. It is generally thought to be a disorder of women.
B. It is directed primarily at men.
C. Its onset is almost invariably between ages 18 and 22 years.
D. Seventy percent of the victims are adolescents.
E. It is typically found in individuals who have high levels of sexual behavior in general.

The correct response is option E: It is typically found in individuals who have high levels of sexual behavior in general.

Exhibitionistic disorder, known in DSM-IV-TR (American Psychiatric Association 2000) as exhibitionism, is identified as either the exposure of one's genitals to an unsuspecting person or the manifestation of urges to do so in the form of fantasy. When the behavior does occur, it may involve masturbation during the exposure, and in some cases the individual tries to surprise or shock the observer. The exhibitionistic individual may hope or desire that the observer will become sexually aroused or join in sexual activity. Exhibitionistic disorder is generally thought to be a disorder of males (option A), sometimes has an early onset (before age 18 years; option C), and is directed primarily at females (option B) (Murphy and Page 2008). Victims can be adults, children, or adolescents (option D) (Gittleson et al. 1978; MacDonald and Rickles 1973; Riordan 1999). The DSM-5 criteria provide specifications for exposing to prepubertal or early pubertal children, to physically mature individuals, or to both. As with many types of paraphilic disorders, there are no good personality profiles for those with exhibitionistic disorder (Blair and

Lanyon 1981). Långström and Seto (2006) found that individuals who admitted to having engaged in exhibitionistic behavior also tended to have higher levels of sexual activity in general (option E), replicating results from Långström and Hanson (2006). **(Hales RE, Yudofsky SC, Roberts LW [eds]: APP Textbook of Psychiatry, 6th Edition, Chapter 26, pp. 897–898)**

21.4   What is the minimum time frame that symptoms must be present in order to meet diagnostic criteria for a paraphilic disorder?

A. 1 month.
B. 3 months.
C. 6 months.
D. 1 year.
E. 2 years.

The correct response is option C: 6 months.

The paraphilic disorders are characterized by experiencing, over a period of at least 6 months, recurrent, intense sexually arousing fantasies, sexual urges, or behaviors generally involving nonhuman objects or nonconsenting partners. In diagnosing any of the paraphilic disorders, the clinician should also consider whether the person has acted on the urges or is markedly distressed by them. **(Hales RE, Yudofsky SC, Roberts LW [eds]: APP Textbook of Psychiatry, 6th Edition, Chapter 26, p. 895)**

21.5   A 25-year-old woman presents to your office and says that for the past year she has been into "rough sex," and has fantasies of being dominated or humiliated by a sexual partner. What other necessary piece of information do you need prior to diagnosing her with sexual masochism disorder?

A. Whether she has acted on these urges.
B. Whether she has these fantasies about men, women, or both.
C. What age these fantasies began.
D. Whether she is significantly distressed by these fantasies.
E. Whether she has a diagnosis of personality disorder.

The correct response is option D: Whether she is significantly distressed by these fantasies.

The DSM-5 diagnostic criteria for sexual masochism disorder require intense sexually arousing fantasies, urges, or behaviors involving the act of being humiliated, beaten, bound, or otherwise made to suffer. It is important to recall in the context of these paraphilic disorders, which do not necessarily involve nonconsenting partners, that an individual can meet criteria for a diagnosis only if he or she indicates distress or impairment (option D). The arousal must occur over a period of at least 6 months, but diagnosis is not contingent on age that arousal began (option C). Behaviors associated with sexual masochism disorder are typically practiced in a consenting, nondistressing, nonpathological way and are not specific to behaviors with the same or opposite sex partners (options A, B) (Baumeister and Butler 1997). Though a comorbid personality disorder may be present, it does not preclude diagnosis of sexual masochism disorder (option E). **(Hales RE, Yudofsky SC, Roberts LW [eds]: APP Textbook of Psychiatry, 6th Edition, Chapter 26, p. 899)**

References

American Psychiatric Association: Diagnostic and Statistical Manual of Mental Disorders, 4th Edition, Text Revision. Washington, DC, American Psychiatric Association, 2000

American Psychiatric Association: Diagnostic and Statistical Manual of Mental Disorders, 5th Edition. Arlington, VA, American Psychiatric Association, 2013

Baumeister R, Butler JL: Sexual masochism: deviance without pathology, in Sexual Deviance: Theory, Assessment, and Treatment. Edited by Laws DR, O'Donohue W. New York, Guilford, 1997, pp 225–239

Blair CD, Lanyon RI: Exhibitionism: etiology and treatment. Psychol Bull 89(3):439–463, 1981 7255626

Gittleson N, Eacott S, Mehta B: Victims of indecent exposure. Br J Psychiatry 132:61–66, 1978

Kafka MP: The DSM diagnostic criteria for fetishism. Arch Sex Behav 39(2):357–362, 2010 19795202

Långström N, Hanson RK: High rates of sexual behavior in the general population: correlates and predictors. Arch Sex Behav 35(1):37–52, 2006 16502152

Långström N, Seto MC: Exhibitionistic and voyeuristic behavior in a Swedish national population survey. Arch Sex Behav 35(4):427–435, 2006 16900414

MacDonald JM, Rickles NK: Indecent Exposure. Springfield, IL, Charles C Thomas, 1973

Murphy WD, Page IJ: Exhibitionism: psychopathology and theory, in Sexual Deviance: Theory, Assessment, and Treatment, 2nd Edition. Edited by Laws DR, O'Donohue WT. New York, Guilford, 2008, pp 61–75

Riordan S: Indecent exposure: the impact upon the victim's fear of sexual crime. J Forensic Psychiatry 10:309–316, 1999

CHAPTER 22

Personality Disorders

22.1 What percentage of patients with borderline personality disorder (BPD) commit suicide?

A. 1%.
B. 10%.
C. 20%.
D. 30%.
E. 40%.

The correct response is option B: 10%.

About 10% of patients with BPD commit suicide (Oldham 2006). Overall, the longer-term course of BPD may be more benign than previously thought (Gunderson et al. 2011; Zanarini et al. 2012) and may be predicted from historical, clinical, functional, and personality features (Zanarini et al. 2006). Roughly half of patients with BPD have significant remissions of their overt psychopathology within 2 years. Social dysfunction, severe childhood trauma, and persistence of substance abuse are predictive of a worse prognosis (Gunderson et al. 2006). **(Hales RE, Yudofsky SC, Roberts LW [eds]: APP Textbook of Psychiatry, 6th Edition, Chapter 25, pp. 878–879)**

22.2 Which of the following personality disorders (PDs) is characterized by an excessive need to be cared for by others, leading to submissive and clinging behavior and excessive fears of separation?

A. Narcissistic PD.
B. Antisocial PD.
C. Borderline PD.
D. Dependent PD.
E. Schizotypal PD.

The correct response is option D: Dependent PD.

Although individuals with dependent PD are able to care for themselves, they doubt their abilities and judgment, and they view others as much stronger and more capable than they are. Dependent PD (option D) is characterized by an excessive need to be cared for by others, which leads to submissive and clinging behavior and excessive fears of separation.

Dependent PD would be diagnosed as PD–trait specified (PD-TS) according to the alternate model of PDs in Section III of the DSM-5 manual (American Psychiatric Association 2013). Typical impairments in personality functioning are at the moderate level, and pathological traits include submissiveness, separation insecurity, and anxiousness. These traits that characterize dependent PD are not found in narcissistic PD (option A), antisocial PD (option B), or schizotypal PD (option E). BPD (option C) is characterized by fears of abandonment, which may lead to clinging behaviors. However, unlike in dependent PD, close relationships in BPD are often viewed in extremes of idealization and devaluation and alternating between overinvolvement and withdrawal. **(Hales RE, Yudofsky SC, Roberts LW [eds]: APP Textbook of Psychiatry, 6th Edition, Chapter 25, p. 886 and Tables 25–5 and 25–7, pp. 870–871, 880–881)**

22.3   Which of the following is a key element in Linehan's concept of BPD?

A. In contrast to psychodynamic theories, it is silent on the importance of the development of a stable sense of self.
B. It downplays the importance of physiological responses to emotional arousal.
C. It defines a major problem in BPD as a difficulty in inhibiting inappropriate behavior related to intense affect.
D. It considers refocusing of attention as a maladaptive defense mechanism.
E. It downplays the importance of developing interpersonal strategies when setting interpersonal goals.

The correct response is option C: It defines a major problem in BPD as a difficulty in inhibiting inappropriate behavior related to intense affect.

The key characteristics of emotional dysregulation in Linehan's (1993) theory of BPD include difficulty 1) inhibiting inappropriate behavior related to intense affect (option C), 2) organizing oneself to meet behavioral goals (option E), 3) regulating physiological arousal associated with intense emotional arousal (option B), and 4) refocusing attention when emotionally stimulated (option D). Deficits in emotion regulation lead to other problems, such as difficulties with interpersonal functioning and the development of a stable sense of self (option A). **(Oldham JM, Skodol AE, Bender DS [eds]: APP Textbook of Personality Disorders, 2nd Edition, Chapter 2, p. 18)**

22.4   In a randomized controlled trial of transference-focused psychotherapy, dialectical behavior therapy, and supportive therapy, which treatment modality achieved an increased number of patients classified as secure after treatment?

A. Treatment results were inconclusive.
B. Transference-focused psychotherapy.
C. Dialectical behavior therapy.
D. Supportive therapy.
E. Treatment has no effect on attachment

The correct response is option B: Transference-focused psychotherapy.

Some studies have shown changes in patients' attachment resulting from treatment (options A, E). Transference-focused psychotherapy achieved an increased number of patients classified as secure after treatment (option B). Neither of the other study conditions (options C, D) exhibited this outcome (Levy et al. 2006). **(Oldham JM, Skodol AE, Bender DS [eds]: APP Textbook of Personality Disorders, 2nd Edition, Chapter 4, p. 72)**

22.5   Criterion A of the general criteria for the diagnosis of PD in the alternative DSM-5 model of PD requires moderate or greater impairment in which of the following personality functioning?

A. Conscientiousness.
B. Emotional stability.
C. Extraversion.
D. Lucidity.
E. Self/interpersonal relatedness.

The correct response is option E: Self/interpersonal relatedness.

The general diagnostic criteria for a PD in Section II of DSM-5 indicate that a pattern of inner experience and behavior is manifest by characteristic patterns of 1) cognition (i.e., ways of perceiving and interpreting self, other people, and events); 2) affectivity (i.e., the range, intensity, lability, and appropriateness of emotional response); 3) interpersonal functioning; and 4) impulse control. Persons with PDs are expected to have manifestations in at least two of these areas. In contrast, the Section III general criteria focus on impairment in personality functioning and the presence of pathological personality traits. Personality functioning consists of sense of self (identity and self-direction) and interpersonal relatedness (empathy and intimacy) (option E), capturing aspects of all four Section II areas.

Options A–D are considered to be personality trait domains whose polar opposites are considered to be pathological personality trait domains: conscientiousness (vs. disinhibition), emotional stability (vs. negative affectivity), extraversion (vs. detachment), and lucidity (vs. psychoticism). **(DSM-5, Personality Disorders, pp. 646–647; Alternative DSM-5 Model for Personality Disorders, pp. 761–762, 770)**

22.6 Why were PDs initially placed on a separate axis (Axis II) of the multiaxial system in DSM-III?

A. Assessment for presence of additional disorders is often overlooked in the presence of an Axis I disorder.
B. The diagnostic construct of PD did not evolve over time.
C. To enhance recognition of the instability of both Axis I and Axis II PDs.
D. To encourage clinicians to focus on a specific disorder.
E. To enhance recognition of the pattern of instability of personality traits.

The correct response is option A: Assessment for presence of additional disorders is often overlooked in the presence of an Axis I disorder.

In DSM-III (American Psychiatric Association 1980), the assignment of PDs to Axis II was intended, in part, to encourage clinicians to assess for additional disorders that might be overlooked when focusing on Axis I psychiatric disorders (option A), broadening rather than narrowing the focus (option D). Conceptually, this reflected, in part, the putative stability of PDs relative to the episodically unstable course of so-called Axis I psychiatric disorders (options C, E) (Grilo et al. 1998; Shea and Yen 2003; Skodol 1997; Skodol et al. 2002). The diagnostic construct of PD has evolved considerably over the past few decades, and substantial changes have occurred over time in the number and types of specific PD diagnoses and their criteria (option B). **(Oldham JM, Skodol AE, Bender DS [eds]: APP Textbook of Personality Disorders, 2nd Edition, Chapter 8, pp. 165–166)**

22.7 A patient describes excessive anxiety in social situations and in intimate relationships. Although she would like to have more friends, she avoids others because of fears of being ridiculed, criticized, rejected, or humiliated. What is the most likely PD diagnosis for this patient?

A. Paranoid PD.
B. Avoidant PD.
C. Schizoid PD.
D. Schizotypal PD.
E. Dependent PD.

The correct response is option B: Avoidant PD.

Persons with avoidant PD experience excessive and pervasive anxiety and discomfort in social situations and in intimate relationships. Although strongly desiring relationships, they avoid them because they fear being ridiculed, criticized, rejected, or humiliated (option B). Individuals with paranoid PD (option A), schizoid PD (option C), or schizotypal PD (option D) are often isolated with few friends; however, they also frequently lack a desire for close relationships. Patients with dependent PD (option E) have an excessive need to be cared for by others, leading to submissive and clinging behavior and excessive fears of separation. **(Hales RE, Yudofsky SC, Roberts LW [eds]: APP Textbook of Psychiatry, 6th Edition, Chapter 25, pp. 885–886)**

References

American Psychiatric Association: Diagnostic and Statistical Manual of Mental Disorders, 3rd Edition. Washington, DC, American Psychiatric Association, 1980

American Psychiatric Association: Diagnostic and Statistical Manual of Mental Disorders, 5th Edition. Arlington, VA, American Psychiatric Association, 2013

Grilo CM, McGlashan TH, Oldham JM: Course and stability of personality disorders. J Pract Psychiatry Behav Health 4:61–75, 1998

Gunderson JG, Daversa MT, Grilo CM, et al: Predictors of 2-year outcome for patients with borderline personality disorder. Am J Psychiatry 163(5):822–826, 2006 16648322

Gunderson JG, Stout RL, McGlashan TH, et al: Ten-year course of borderline personality disorder: psychopathology and function from the Collaborative Longitudinal Personality Disorders study. Arch Gen Psychiatry 68(8):827–837, 2011 21464343

Levy KN, Meehan KB, Kelly KM, et al: Change in attachment patterns and reflective function in a randomized control trial of transference-focused psychotherapy for borderline personality disorder. J Consult Clin Psychol 74(6):1027–1040, 2006 17154733

Linehan M: Cognitive-Behavioral Treatment of Borderline Personality Disorder. New York, Guilford, 1993

Oldham JM: Borderline personality disorder and suicidality. Am J Psychiatry 163(1):20–26, 2006 16390884

Shea MT, Yen S: Stability as a distinction between Axis I and Axis II disorders. J Pers Disord 17(5):373–386, 2003 14632373

Skodol AE: Classification, assessment, and differential diagnosis of personality disorders. J Pract Psychiatry Behav Health 3:261–274, 1997

Skodol AE, Siever LJ, Livesley WJ, et al: The borderline diagnosis II: biology, genetics, and clinical course. Biol Psychiatry 51(12):951–963, 2002 12062878

Zanarini MC, Frankenburg FR, Hennen J, et al: Prediction of the 10-year course of borderline personality disorder. Am J Psychiatry 163(5):827–832, 2006 16648323

Zanarini MC, Frankenburg FR, Reich DB, Fitzmaurice G: Attainment and stability of sustained symptomatic remission and recovery among patients with borderline personality disorder and axis II comparison subjects: a 16-year prospective follow-up study. Am J Psychiatry 169(5):476–483, 2012 22737693

CHAPTER 23

Principles of Psychopharmacology

23.1   Which second-generation antipsychotic is most likely to cause hyperprolactinemia?

A. Quetiapine.
B. Ziprasidone.
C. Risperidone.
D. Aripiprazole.
E. Olanzapine.

The correct response is option C: Risperidone.

Hyperprolactinemia may cause impotence, menstrual dysregulation, infertility, and sexual dysfunction (Bostwick et al. 2009). Risk factors for drug-induced hyperprolactinemia include increased potency of dopamine D_2 blockade, female sex, and increased age (Kinon et al. 2003). Additionally, an increased risk is identified in individuals with the cytochrome P450 (CYP450) 2D6*10 allele (Ozdemir et al. 2007). Hyperprolactinemia is most likely to occur with risperidone (option C) and high-potency first-generation antipsychotics and least likely to occur with aripiprazole (option D). Quetiapine, ziprasidone, and olanzapine are all less likely to cause hyperprolactinemia than risperidone (options A, B, E). Current American Psychiatric Association guidelines recommend routine monitoring of prolactin serum levels only in symptomatic patients (Lehman et al. 2004). Treatment strategies include 1) decreasing the dosage of the offending agent, 2) changing medication to an agent less likely to affect prolactin, 3) using a dopamine partial agonist such as aripiprazole (Mir et al. 2008), and 4) preventing long-term complications such as bone demineralization. **(Hales RE, Yudofsky SC, Roberts LW [eds]: APP Textbook of Psychiatry, 6th Edition, Chapter 27, p. 950 and Table 27–3, pp. 937–942)**

23.2   Which of the following describes a *pharmacodynamic* interaction?

A. Two medications with similar or opposing effects are combined.
B. One medication blocks the absorption of another medication.
C. One medication enhances the distribution of another medication.
D. One medication induces the metabolism of another medication.
E. One medication inhibits the excretion of another medication.

The correct response is option A: Two medications with similar or opposing effects are combined.

A drug interaction is the alteration of the pharmacological effect of one drug by another concurrently administered drug or substance. A *pharmacodynamic* interaction occurs when drugs with similar or opposing effects are combined (option A). These interactions alter the body's responses to a drug by altering drug binding to a receptor site or indirectly through other mechanisms. A *pharmacokinetic* interaction occurs when an interacting substance alters a drug's concentration because of a change in its absorption (option B), distribution (option C), metabolism (option D), or excretion (option E). These interactions are most likely to be clinically meaningful when the drug involved has a low therapeutic index or active metabolites. **(Hales RE, Yudofsky SC, Roberts LW [eds]: APP Textbook of Psychiatry, 6th Edition, Chapter 27, pp. 930–931)**

23.3   What is the proposed mechanism for the parkinsonian side effects seen with antipsychotic medications?

A. Nigrostriatal dopamine receptor blockade.
B. Muscarinic cholinergic receptor blockade.
C. Tuberoinfundibular dopamine receptor blockade.
D. Hypothalamic histaminergic H_1 receptor blockade.
E. α_1-Adrenergic receptor antagonism.

The correct response is option A: Nigrostriatal dopamine receptor blockade.

Many side effects of antipsychotic drugs can be understood in terms of the drugs' receptor-blocking properties. When antipsychotics reduce dopamine activity in the nigrostriatal pathway (via dopamine receptor blockade), extrapyramidal signs and symptoms (e.g., cogwheel rigidity, masked facies, bradykinesia, pill-rolling tremor) similar to those of Parkinson's disease result (option A). Blockade of dopamine in the tuberoinfundibular pathway can cause an increase in blood prolactin levels resulting in hyperprolactinemia (option C). Muscarinic cholinergic receptor blockade is responsible for anticholinergic side effects such as dry mouth, blurred vision, constipation, and urinary retention (option B). Hypothalamic histaminergic H_1 receptor blockade results in increased appetite and sedation (option D). α_1-Adrenergic receptor antagonism can cause orthostatic hypotension (option E). **(Hales RE, Yudofsky SC, Roberts LW [eds]: APP Textbook of Psychiatry, 6th Edition, Chapter 27, Table 27–4, pp. 945–947)**

23.4   A 34-year-old woman with comorbid attention-deficit/hyperactivity disorder and depression is treated with selegiline 45 mg/day for 6 months. Although her depressive symptoms resolve, she continues to experience difficulty with attention. Her psychiatrist suggests treatment with dextroamphetamine. How long should the psychiatrist wait after discontinuing selegiline before starting the stimulant?

A. 0 days.
B. At least 3 days.
C. At least 7 days.
D. At least 14 days.
E. At least 28 days.

The correct response is option D: At least 14 days.

All stimulants may interact with sympathomimetics and monoamine oxidase inhibitors (MAOIs) (including selegiline), resulting in headache, arrhythmias, hypertensive crisis, and hyperpyrexia. Stimulants should not be administered with MAOIs or within 14 days of MAOI discontinuation. Methylphenidate may interact pharmacodynamically with tricyclic antidepressants (TCAs) to cause increased anxiety, irritability, agitation, and aggression. Higher doses of stimulants may also reduce the therapeutic effectiveness of antihypertensive medications. When stimulants are used concurrently with β-blockers, the excessive α-adrenergic activity may cause hypertension, reflex bradycardia, and possible heart block. **(Hales RE, Yudofsky SC, Roberts LW [eds]: APP Textbook of Psychiatry, 6th Edition, Chapter 27, p. 985)**

23.5   Concomitant use of which of the following medications might be responsible for an increase in plasma clozapine levels in an adherent patient?

A. Carbamazepine.
B. Clonazepam.
C. Fluvoxamine.
D. Propranolol.
E. Temazepam.

The correct response is option C: Fluvoxamine.

Fluvoxamine inhibits CYP450 enzymes that metabolize clozapine (CYP2D6, CYP3A4, and CYP1A2), thus increasing clozapine levels (option C). This may result in clozapine toxicity. Carbamazepine is a CYP450 cytochrome inducer (option A). β-Blockers, such as propranolol, are substrates of CYP2D6 (option D). Benzodiazepines, except lorazepam, oxazepam, and temazepam, are substrates at CYP3A4. Therefore, carbamazepine, clonazepam, propranolol, and temazepam do not increase clozapine levels (options B, E). **(Hales RE, Yudofsky SC, Roberts**

LW [eds]: APP Textbook of Psychiatry, 6th Edition, Chapter 27, pp. 931–932 and Table 27–2, pp. 933–934)

23.6   Which of the following is a common side effect of MAOIs?

A. Anxiety.
B. Leukopenia.
C. Hypertensive crisis.
D. Orthostatic hypotension.
E. Urinary retention.

The correct response is option D: Orthostatic hypotension.

Irreversible inhibitors of monoamine oxidase A (MAO-A) and monoamine oxidase B (MAO-B) are used as third-line pharmacotherapy in the treatment of major depressive disorder or atypical depression. Common adverse effects of MAOIs include orthostatic hypotension (option D), dizziness, headache, sedation, insomnia or hypersomnia, tremor, and hyperreflexia. Hypertensive crisis can occur in patients taking MAOIs who ingest sympathomimetic drugs, including over-the-counter decongestants, other agents (e.g., meperidine), or foods containing tyramine (option C). These serious drug-drug and drug-food interactions are not common. Anxiety (option A), leukopenia (option B), and urinary retention (option E) are not typical side effects of MAOIs. Anxiety can be a common key side effect of bupropion or vilazodone. Leukopenia or agranulocytosis is a key side effect of mirtazapine. Urinary retention is commonly observed with TCAs. **(Hales RE, Yudofsky SC, Roberts LW [eds]: APP Textbook of Psychiatry, 6th Edition, Chapter 27, pp. 976–977 and Table 27–12, p. 970)**

23.7   Discontinuation of which of the following selective serotonin reuptake inhibitor (SSRI) medications would be most likely to result in withdrawal symptoms?

A. Citalopram.
B. Escitalopram.
C. Fluoxetine.
D. Sertraline.
E. Paroxetine.

The correct response is option E: Paroxetine.

Antidepressants, like all psychoactive medications, should be gradually withdrawn when possible. Discontinuation symptoms can cause misdiagnosis and inappropriate treatment, particularly in a patient with an active medical illness, as well as erode future compliance. Abrupt discontinuation of SSRIs or serotonin-norepinephrine reuptake inhibitors (SNRIs), especially those with short half-lives (e.g., fluvoxamine, paroxetine, venlafaxine), may give rise to a discontinuation syndrome characterized by a wide variety of symptoms, including psychiatric, neurological, and flulike symptoms (nausea, vomiting, sweats); sleep disturbances; and headache, usually resolving within 3 weeks (Schatzberg et al. 1997). Some patients experience the symptoms even with very gradual withdrawal over months. Paroxetine (option E) has the shortest half-life of the medications listed (20 hours), making cessation most likely to result in discontinuation or withdrawal symptoms. Citalopram (option A) has a half-life of 35 hours, escitalopram (option B) has a half-life of 27–32 hours, fluoxetine (option C) has the longest half-life at 72 hours (216 hours for active metabolites), and sertraline (option D) has a half-life of 26 hours (66 hours for active metabolites). **(Hales RE, Yudofsky SC, Roberts LW [eds]: APP Textbook of Psychiatry, 6th Edition, Chapter 27, pp. 965–966, 975 and Table 27–11, pp. 967–969)**

23.8 Which of the following is *not* considered a common side effect of SSRIs?

A. Acne.
B. Dry mouth.
C. Sexual dysfunction.
D. Impaired sleep.
E. Sweating.

The correct response is option A: Acne.

Dry mouth (option B), sexual dysfunction (option C), impaired sleep (option D), and sweating (option E) are known side effects of SSRIs. Acne (option A) is the only condition that is not a common side effect of SSRIs. **(Hales RE, Yudofsky SC, Roberts LW [eds]: APP Textbook of Psychiatry, 6th Edition, Chapter 27, p. 971)**

23.9 A 47-year-old man presents to the emergency department after being found wandering aimlessly in the street. Upon examination, he is disoriented, his skin is hot and dry, he has dilated pupils, and he has absent bowel sounds. An electrocardiogram reveals a supraventricular arrhythmia. The patient most likely overdosed on which of the following medications?

A. Amitriptyline.
B. Bupropion.
C. Fluoxetine.
D. Sertraline.
E. Venlafaxine.

The correct response is option A: Amitriptyline.

Amitriptyline is a TCA. Complications of TCA, including amitriptyline, overdose may include neuropsychiatric impairment, hypotension, cardiac arrhythmias, and seizures. Anticholinergic delirium may occur, as well as other complications of anticholinergic overdose, including agitation, supraventricular arrhythmias, hallucinations, severe hypertension, and seizures. Patients with anticholinergic delirium may also have hot dry skin, tachycardia, dilated pupils, dry mucous membranes, and absent bowel sounds.

TCA overdose carries a risk of death from cardiac conduction abnormalities that result in malignant ventricular arrhythmias. Initial symptoms of overdose involve central nervous system (CNS) stimulation, in part due to anticholinergic effects, and include hyperpyrexia, delirium, hypertension, hallucinations, seizure, agitation, hyperreflexia, and parkinsonian symptoms. The initial stimulation phase is typically followed by CNS depression with drowsiness, areflexia, hypothermia, respiratory depression, severe hypotension, and coma. Risk of cardiotoxicity is high if the QRS interval is 100 msec or more or if the total TCA plasma concentration is greater than 1,000 ng/mL; concentrations greater than 2,500 ng/mL are often fatal. SSRIs (options C, D) in overdose or in combination with other serotonergic agents can contribute to serotonin syndrome, which presents with confusion, hemodynamic changes (hypertension, hypotension, tachycardia), diaphoresis, tremor, and myoclonus. Venlafaxine (option E) could also contribute to serotonin syndrome, and causes sedation in overdose, but does not have a well-established withdrawal syndrome. Bupropion (option B) can cause tachycardia, arrhythmia, mental status changes, and seizures in overdose. None of these other options would fully explain the entire constellation of symptoms described in this question, which are classic signs of TCA overdose (option A). **(Hales RE, Yudofsky SC, Roberts LW [eds]: APP Textbook of Psychiatry, 6th Edition, Chapter 27, pp. 971–972, 976 and Tables 27–13, 27–14, p. 973)**

23.10 What are the main mechanisms of action of mirtazapine?

A. Inhibition of serotonin and norepinephrine reuptake transporters.
B. Increases norepinephrine and serotonin via blockade of inhibitory receptors.
C. Antagonism of norepinephrine type $\alpha 1$, muscarinic, and histamine receptors.
D. Partial agonism at serotonin type 1A ($5\text{-}HT_{1A}$) receptors.
E. Norepinephrine and dopamine modulation.

The correct response is option B: Increases norepinephrine and serotonin via blockade of inhibitory receptors.

Antidepressants are classified according to their activity at monoamine receptors. Mirtazapine increases norepinephrine and serotonin concentrations by blocking inhibitory receptors (option B). It is a novel tetracyclic antidepressant. Serotonin-norepinephrine reuptake inhibition (option A) refers to the mechanism of action of both venlafaxine and duloxetine. Antagonism of norepinephrine type $\alpha 1$, muscarinic, and histamine receptors (option C), along with inhibition of norepinephrine and serotonin reuptake transporters describes the mechanism of action of TCAs. Partial agonism at $5\text{-}HT_{1A}$ receptors (option D) is the mechanism of action of buspirone, and inhibition of norepinephrine and dopamine reuptake transporters (option E) is the mechanism of action of bupropion. **(Hales RE, Yudofsky SC, Roberts LW [eds]: APP Textbook of Psychiatry, 6th Edition, Chapter 27, p. 979; Levenson JL [ed]: APP Textbook of Psychosomatic Medicine: Psychiatric Care of the Medically Ill, 2nd Edition, Chapter 8, pp. 186–188)**

23.11 A 30-year-old woman with no medical problems and a history of two major depressive episodes is evaluated for medication consultation. She has a history of involuntary inpatient hospitalization for suicidal ideation 1 year ago. Six months ago her maintenance dose of fluoxetine 40 mg/day was reduced to 10 mg/day under psychiatric supervision. She subsequently suffered a severe depression relapse. Fluoxetine was then increased to 40 mg/day, and the patient has been euthymic since then. She just discovered that she is pregnant. How should she be advised about the risks of fluoxetine during her pregnancy?

A. Recommend continuing fluoxetine because exposure to fluoxetine has no significant adverse fetal effects.
B. Recommend discontinuing fluoxetine because the risks of fluoxetine are greater than the risks of maternal depression.
C. Recommend continuing fluoxetine because maternal depression carries a significant risk of adverse fetal effects.
D. Recommend discontinuing fluoxetine because the risk of depression relapse is decreased during pregnancy.
E. Recommend continuing fluoxetine because fluoxetine has independently been found to improve neonatal outcomes.

The correct response is option C: Recommend continuing fluoxetine because maternal depression carries a significant risk of adverse fetal effects.

Pregnancy is not a time of improved emotional stability (option D). SSRIs have been shown in humans to be associated with poor neonatal adaptability, persistent pulmonary hypertension of the newborn, shorter gestation, and small-for-gestational age neonates, but the data are conflicting, most studies use nondepressed mothers as the comparison group, and the absolute risk is very small. However, some potential for risk and no direct benefit have been shown (options A, E). Untreated maternal depression has been shown to be associated with low birth weight, preeclampsia, placental abnormalities, preterm labor, fetal distress, and lower cognitive and language achievements in exposed children (option B). The risk of depression relapse in pregnancy is high—about 26% for women staying on their antidepressants and almost 70% for those who choose to stop antidepressants for the pregnancy (Cohen et al. 2006). Overall, in cases of women who have had severe symptoms, particularly those who have relapsed when medication was withdrawn, severe maternal depression is considered to have higher fetal risks than in utero exposure to SSRIs (option C). **(Hales RE, Yudofsky SC, Roberts LW [eds]: APP Textbook of Psychiatry, 6th Edition, Chapter 38, pp. 1323–1330 and Table 38–3, p. 1324; Levenson JL [ed]: APP Textbook of Psychosomatic Medicine: Psychiatric Care of the Medically Ill, 2nd Edition, Chapter 33, pp. 807, 812–813)**

23.12 What are the adverse effects frequently observed with clozapine?

A. Dry mouth and impaired thermoregulation.
B. Activation and hyperprolactinemia.
C. Akathisia and diabetic ketoacidosis.

D. Tardive dyskinesia and sedation.
E. Seizures and hypotension.

The correct response is option E: Seizures and hypotension.

Clozapine is the first and a uniquely important second-generation antipsychotic. Clozapine has been shown in multiple clinical trials, including the Clinical Antipsychotic Treatment Effectiveness (CATIE) trial, to be efficacious for treatment-resistant schizophrenia. Clozapine rarely causes extrapyramidal symptoms and does not produce tardive dyskinesia (options C, D). Clozapine is a desirable agent for patients with tardive dyskinesia who need an antipsychotic medication (Lieberman et al. 1991; van Harten and Tenback 2011). This clinical profile is thought to be due to clozapine's selective blockade of mesolimbic dopamine pathways, with minimal effects on the tuberoinfundibular and nigrostriatal dopamine tracts. It is important to monitor for orthostatic hypotension (option E) and sedation. Hyperprolactinemia (option B) is most likely to occur with risperidone and high-potency first-generation antipsychotics and least likely to occur with aripiprazole. Impaired thermoregulation stems from hypothalamic histaminergic H_1 receptor blockade. Excessive salivation is a commonly observed side effect of clozapine therapy (option A). Agranulocytosis was previously estimated to occur in 0.8% of the patients receiving clozapine during the first year of treatment, with a peak incidence at 3 months. A system of hematological monitoring, the Clozaril National Registry (www.clozapineregistry.com), has reduced agranulocytosis-related fatalities to less than half of previous levels. Clozapine is associated with a dose-dependent risk of seizures, most often tonic-clonic (option E). Dosages less than 300 mg/day are associated with a 1%–3% risk of seizures; dosages of 300–600 mg/day carry a 2.7% risk; and dosages greater than 600 mg/day are associated with a 4.4% risk (Devinsky et al. 1991). **(Hales RE, Yudofsky SC, Roberts LW [eds]: APP Textbook of Psychiatry, 6th Edition, Chapter 27, pp. 944–949, 953–954)**

23.13 What is the initial standard of treatment for neuroleptic malignant syndrome (NMS)?

A. Dantrolene started immediately for all cases of suspected NMS.
B. Expectant management on the psychiatric unit because this is a self-limited illness.
C. Rapid cessation of antipsychotics, lithium, and antiemetics.
D. Initiation of benzodiazepines until vital signs stabilized then taper.
E. Switch to a less potent dopamine D_2 blocking agent until symptoms resolve.

The correct response is option C: Rapid cessation of antipsychotics, lithium, and antiemetics.

The incidence of NMS is about 0.02% among patients treated with antipsychotic drugs (Caroff 2003; Strawn et al. 2007). Classic signs are hyperthermia, generalized

rigidity with tremors, altered consciousness with catatonia, and autonomic instability. Several lines of evidence implicate drug-induced dopamine blockade as the
primary triggering mechanism in the pathogenesis of NMS. Once all dopamine-
blocking drugs are withheld (option C), two-thirds of NMS cases resolve within
1–2 weeks, with an average duration of 7–10 days (Caroff 2003). NMS is potentially fatal in some cases due to renal failure, cardiorespiratory arrest, dissemi-
nated intravascular coagulation, pulmonary emboli, or aspiration pneumonia
(option B). Treatment consists of early diagnosis, discontinuing dopamine antagonists (option E), and supportive medical care. Benzodiazepines (option D), dopamine agonists, dantrolene (option A), and electroconvulsive therapy have been
advocated in clinical reports, but randomized controlled trials comparing these
treatments with supportive care have not been done. These treatments may be
considered empirically in individual cases, based on symptoms, severity, and duration of the episode (Strawn et al. 2007). **(Hales RE, Yudofsky SC, Roberts LW
[eds]: APP Textbook of Psychiatry, 6th Edition, Chapter 27, p. 949)**

23.14 Which benzodiazepine would be an appropriate choice for the inpatient treatment of mild to moderate acute alcohol withdrawal in an elderly man with
known liver cirrhosis?

A. Midazolam.
B. Diazepam.
C. Triazolam.
D. Oxazepam.
E. Alprazolam.

The correct response is option D: Oxazepam.

Benzodiazepine choice is based primarily on pharmacokinetic properties, including half-life, rapidity of onset, metabolism, and potency. In general, longer-acting
agents possess active metabolites and tend to produce a steady serum drug concentration and few rebound effects between doses, whereas shorter-acting agents
are prone to emergence of symptoms between doses. All benzodiazepines are metabolized by the liver, increasing the risk of sedation, confusion, and frank hepatic
encephalopathy in patients with hepatic failure. In patients with liver failure, lorazepam, temazepam, and oxazepam (option D) may be preferred because they
undergo hepatic conjugation and renal excretion and have no active metabolites,
whereas other benzodiazepines (options A, B, C, E) undergo hepatic microsomal
metabolism and may have long-acting active metabolites. **(Hales RE, Yudofsky
SC, Roberts LW [eds]: APP Textbook of Psychiatry, 6th Edition, Chapter 27, p. 979)**

23.15 A 37-year-old woman with schizophrenia is brought to the clinic by her mother. She has a history of five hospitalizations in the last 7 years for severe psychotic symptoms in the setting of nonadherence to oral medications. You consider using risperidone long-acting injectable (LAI) and propose a treatment plan to the team. The patient has not used risperidone in the past. What is your plan for initiation of this medication?

A. Initial injection of risperidone LAI 25 mg intramuscularly today without oral medication.
B. Initial treatment with risperidone oral for 2 weeks and then switch to LAI.
C. Initial treatment with risperidone oral until tolerability is established and continued for 3 weeks after LAI is administered.
D. Initial treatment with risperidone oral and LAI today for 2 weeks, then LAI monotherapy.
E. Initial treatment with risperidone LAI today with plan to titrate LAI dose weekly to desired efficacy.

The correct response is option C: Initial treatment with risperidone oral until tolerability is established and continued for 3 weeks after LAI is administered.

For patients with chronic psychotic symptoms who are not compliant with antipsychotic medication, an LAI or depot preparation should be considered after stabilization with oral medication. Risperdal Consta is a long-acting injectable form of risperidone; the recommended starting dosage is 25 mg every 2 weeks. It takes about 3 weeks (not 2 weeks; options B, D) for Risperdal Consta to build up adequate blood levels, thus oral risperidone or another antipsychotic medication must be continued for 3 weeks after the first dose of Risperdal Consta is given (option C) in order to prevent worsening of symptoms. Injections are given every 2 weeks, and steady-state plasma concentrations are achieved after four injections. Dose adjustments should not be made more often than once a month (option E); the maximum dose is 50 mg every 2 weeks. If a patient has not taken risperidone before, a trial of oral risperidone is recommended to determine whether the patient has a hypersensitivity reaction to the medication (option A) **(Chew RH, Hales RE, Yudofsky SC: What Your Patients Need to Know About Psychiatric Medications, 2nd Edition, p. 296; Hales RE, Yudofsky SC, Roberts LW [eds]: APP Textbook of Psychiatry, 6th Edition, Chapter 10, pp. 340, 342–343)**

23.16 You are evaluating a patient who has developed acute symptoms suggestive of either serotonin syndrome or NMS. The patient was recently started on fluoxetine, olanzapine, trazodone, and as-needed intramuscular haloperidol. Which of the following signs or symptoms is more indicative of serotonin syndrome than of NMS?

A. Spontaneous or inducible clonus.
B. Tachycardia.
C. Elevated body temperature.
D. Elevated creatine phosphokinase.
E. Diaphoresis.

The correct response is option A: Spontaneous or inducible clonus.

Tachycardia (option B), elevated body temperature (option C), elevated creatine phosphokinase (option D), and diaphoresis (option E) are symptoms of both serotonin syndrome and NMS. Spontaneous or inducible clonus is indicative of serotonin syndrome (option A). **(Levenson JL [ed]: APP Textbook of Psychosomatic Medicine: Psychiatric Care of the Medically Ill, 2nd Edition, Chapter 38, pp. 961, 969–970, 976–977 and Tables 38–5, 38–6, 38–7, pp. 971, 977, 978)**

23.17 A 46-year-old man with bipolar I disorder and a co-occurring seizure disorder is maintained on valproate extended release for mood stabilization and seizure prophylaxis. His neurologist has suggested adding lamotrigine for adjunctive seizure prophylaxis given a recent increase in number of partial seizures. What is the appropriate recommendation?

A. Decrease the maintenance dose of valproate.
B. Increase the maintenance dose of valproate.
C. Start the patient on a lower than usual dose of lamotrigine.
D. Start the patient on a higher than usual dose of lamotrigine.
E. No change in doses of either medication.

The correct response is option C: Start the patient on a lower than usual dose of lamotrigine.

The maintenance valproate dose will not require a change based on addition of lamotrigine (options A, B). Valproate can inhibit several enzymes, resulting in increased levels of other medications, particularly lamotrigine, resulting in increased risk of rash. The incidence of adverse effects increases with anticonvulsant multitherapy (option D). Current lamotrigine product labeling provides specific lamotrigine dosing guidelines for patients who are taking valproate. For patients who are taking valproate or other medications that decrease the clearance of lamotrigine, the dosing schedule and target dose are halved (option C, not option E). Valproate may also increase concentrations of phenobarbital, ethosuximide, and the active 10,11 epoxide metabolite of carbamazepine, increasing the risk of toxicity. Valproate metabolism may be induced by other anticonvulsants, including carbamazepine, phenytoin, primidone, and phenobarbital, resulting in an increased total clearance of valproate and perhaps decreased efficacy when taken in combination with those above-named CYP450 inducers. **(Hales RE, Yudofsky SC, Roberts LW [eds]: APP Textbook of Psychiatry, 6th Edition, Chapter 27, pp. 962–965)**

23.18 A 28-year-old man with schizophrenia with poor medication adherence presents to the emergency department with severe agitation. He receives haloperidol 20 mg and lorazepam 4 mg intramuscularly over the next 12 hours. On examination, his neck is flexed to the left and he is unable to turn it to the right. He is able to breathe, and his vital signs are normal. Which medication is first-line treatment for this patient's motor condition?

A. Amantadine.
B. Benztropine.
C. Clozapine.
D. Dantrolene.
E. Propranolol.

The correct response is option B: Benztropine.

Extrapyramidal side effects include acute dystonic reactions, parkinsonian symptoms, akathisia, tardive dyskinesia, and NMS. Acute dystonic reactions are perhaps the most disturbing extrapyramidal side effects for patients and may be life threatening in the case of laryngeal dystonias. Amantadine (option A) is a dopaminergic agent indicated for parkinsonian syndrome. Benztropine (option B) and diphenhydramine are anticholinergic agents indicated for dystonia, parkinsonian syndrome, and acute dystonia. Clozapine (option C) is an antipsychotic with efficacy in the management of treatment-resistant schizophrenia or in the presence of tardive dyskinesias. Dantrolene (option D) is a medication sometimes used in the management of NMS. Propranolol (option E) is a β-blocking agent with a psychiatric indication for treatment of akathisia. **(Hales RE, Yudofsky SC, Roberts LW [eds]: APP Textbook of Psychiatry, 6th Edition, Chapter 27, p. 944 and Tables 27–4, 27–5, pp. 945, 948)**

23.19 A 45-year-old man has a history of diabetes, hyperlipidemia, chronic low back pain, and recurrent major depressive disorder. He has a history of medication nonadherence with paroxetine and fluoxetine, due to complaints of sedation and sexual side effects. He is requesting treatment for symptoms consistent with a recurrent episode of major depression. What regimen will you recommend considering his prior medication nonadherence?

A. Restart paroxetine daily in the morning.
B. Start duloxetine in twice-daily dosing.
C. Start fluvoxamine daily.
D. Restart fluoxetine daily at night.
E. Start bupropion daily in the morning.

The correct response is option E: Start bupropion daily in the morning.

In general, all drugs indicated for the treatment of a particular psychiatric disorder have similar therapeutic efficacy. However, each patient may respond better to or tolerate one agent over another because of differences in each drug's pharmacokinetics, spectrum of secondary pharmacological effects, or drug interactions. A patient's personal or family history of response and tolerance can guide future drug selection. Strategies to maximize medical adherence can be clustered into the following four categories: patient education, convenient dosing schedule, minimizing adverse effects, and checking for patient compliance. Once-daily dosing of bupropion in the morning (option E) may be a more acceptable regimen for this patient with a history of nonadherence and a history of sedation and sexual side effects with other agents. Compliance is maximized with once-daily dosing (option B). Selecting drugs with minimum pharmacokinetic interactions where possible can minimize adverse effects (option C). It is important to select drugs with an adverse effect profile that the patient can best tolerate (option D) and schedule the dose so that the side effects are less bothersome. If possible, prescribe activating drugs in the morning and sedating drugs at night (option A). **(Hales RE, Yudofsky SC, Roberts LW [eds]: APP Textbook of Psychiatry, 6th Edition, Chapter 27, General Principles/Choice of Medication, pp. 930–931 and Table 27–1, p. 931)**

23.20 A 72-year-old woman living with her daughter has a history of depression. She was fully independent in activities of daily living at her last follow-up appointment 1 month ago but needed assistance with shopping and bill paying. She has been maintained on a stable dose of amitriptyline for the last 25 years without symptoms of depression. She also takes cyclobenzaprine as needed for muscle relaxation in the evening. At the evaluation today, her daughter tells you that the patient has experienced mild confusion during the day and difficulty urinating in the last 2 weeks. On examination, she is oriented to place and season only, and demonstrates mild impairment in attention and memory. On review of her medication list, you learn that her primary care physician started meclizine daily for dizziness. What is your treatment recommendation?

A. Discontinue meclizine and call the primary care physician.
B. Direct hospital admission for stroke evaluation.
C. Increase amitriptyline for depression leading to pseudodementia.
D. Initiate donepezil treatment for dementia.
E. Refer patient to memory disorders clinic for likely Alzheimer's dementia.

The correct response is option A: Discontinue meclizine and call the primary care physician.

Pharmacodynamic interactions occur when drugs with similar or opposing effects are combined. Generally, pharmacodynamic interactions are most apparent in individuals with compromised physiological functions such as those with cardiovascular disease or the elderly. Drugs with anticholinergic activity (e.g., TCAs, antihistamines, and antispasmodics, among many others) can cause a degree of cognitive impairment, an effect exacerbated when several are combined. Unfortunately, anticholinergic activity is an often unrecognized property of many common drugs. This additive interaction is most disruptive in cognitively compromised patients, such as the elderly or those with Alzheimer's disease, and forms the basis for many cases of delirium. In the vignette, the patient was previously stable on two medications that have anticholinergic activity and developed acute cognitive impairment with urinary retention only when a third drug with anticholinergic activity was started. There is no indication that she has experienced an acute stroke (option B) or that she has worsening depressive symptoms (option C). The time course of the development of cognitive impairment is too rapid for dementia of Alzheimer's type (option E). The most appropriate recommendation would be to address polypharmacy, discontinue the offending medications, and coordinate care with the other physician (option A). Adding additional medications would not be useful or appropriate in this case of polypharmacy and anticholinergic overactivity (option D). **(Hales RE, Yudofsky SC, Roberts LW [eds]: APP Textbook of Psychiatry, 6th Edition, Chapter 27, p. 935 and Table 27–19, p. 990)**

23.21 What is the function of the CYP450 enzymes?

A. Phase I oxidative metabolism.
B. Phase II glucuronidation.
C. P-glycoprotein efflux transportation.
D. Renal elimination.
E. Regulation of protein binding.

The correct response is option A: Phase I oxidative metabolism.

A pharmacokinetic interaction occurs when an interacting substance alters a drug's concentration due to a change in its absorption, distribution, metabolism, or excretion. The majority of drugs are substrates for Phase I oxidative metabolism by one or more CYP450 enzymes (option A). Phase II hepatic metabolism refers to conjugation reactions including glucuronidation (option B). The P-glycoprotein efflux transporter system forms a barrier to absorption in the gut wall (option C). CYP450 enzymes are not part of renal elimination of drugs (option D). Changes in protein binding, either disease induced or the result of protein-binding drug interactions, can lead to toxic effects through an increase in concentrations of free drug (option E). **(Hales RE, Yudofsky SC, Roberts LW [eds]: APP Textbook of Psychiatry, 6th Edition, Chapter 27, pp. 930–934; Levenson JL [ed]: APP Textbook of Psychosomatic Medicine: Psychiatric Care of the Medically Ill, 2nd Edition, Chapter 38, pp. 958–960)**

23.22 What is an anticipated protein-binding interaction?

A. Drugs competing to bind at a receptor, leading to an additive effect at that receptor.
B. Drugs competing to bind with a plasma protein, leading to an increase in the level of circulating free drug of the first medication.
C. Drugs competing to bind with a plasma protein, leading to a decrease in the level of circulating free drug of the first medication.

D. Drugs competing to bind with a plasma protein, leading to negligible changes in the level of circulating free drug of the first medication.

E. Drugs competing to be metabolized by a CYP450 enzyme, leading to increased enzyme inhibition.

The correct response is option B: Drugs competing to bind with a plasma protein, leading to an increase in the level of circulating free drug of the first medication.

Protein-bound interactions occur when two medications that both bind to plasma proteins compete for available binding sites. The fraction of either medication that is protein bound is inactive and the free fraction, or portion of circulating drug, is active; therefore administering multiple medications that are protein bound is likely to increase the activity of both medications, which can be very important for medications with a narrow therapeutic window (option B). Most psychiatric medications, with the notable exception of lithium, are protein bound. In general, acidic drugs (e.g., valproate, barbiturates) bind to albumin, and basic medications (e.g., phenothiazines, TCAs, amphetamines, benzodiazepines) bind mostly to globulins. One of the concerns for medication dosing in pregnant patients or patients with multiple medical comorbidities is that the albumin binding is often decreased.

Drugs competing to bind at a receptor, leading to an additive effect at that receptor (option A), describes a pharmacodynamic interaction not a pharmacokinetic interaction. Adding a protein-binding medication will increase, not decrease, the unbound fraction of the first (option C). Protein-binding interactions usually result in significant changes in levels of circulating or free drug even if the amount of protein-bound medication displaced was small (option D). Option E describes a CYP450 interaction. **(Hales RE, Yudofsky SC, Roberts LW [eds]: APP Textbook of Psychiatry, 6th Edition, Chapter 27, pp. 930–935; Levenson JL [ed]: APP Textbook of Psychosomatic Medicine: Psychiatric Care of the Medically Ill, 2nd Edition, Chapter 38, pp. 957–958)**

23.23 What is a critical substrate drug?

A. A drug with a wide therapeutic window and a single CYP enzyme mediating its metabolism.

B. A drug with a wide therapeutic window and multiple CYP enzymes mediating its metabolism.

C. A drug with a narrow therapeutic window and a single CYP enzyme mediating its metabolism.

D. A drug with a narrow therapeutic window and multiple CYP enzymes mediating its metabolism.

E. A drug with a narrow therapeutic window metabolized outside the CYP450 system.

The correct response is option C: A drug with a narrow therapeutic window and a single CYP enzyme mediating its metabolism.

A critical substrate drug is a medication that is likely to have a clinically relevant alteration in concentration and activity based on CYP450 pharmacokinetic interactions (option E). Medications with narrow therapeutic windows and a single (or primary) metabolic pathway are most susceptible to these interactions because inhibition or induction of the single metabolizing CYP450 enzyme can result in clinically significant supratherapeutic or subtherapeutic medication levels (option C). A wide therapeutic window means that changes in drug metabolism are less likely to translate into clinically significant effects (options A, B). Medications that are metabolized by multiple enzymes are less likely to be affected by the induction or inhibition of a single CYP enzyme (option D). This concept is most clinically relevant in cases of polypharmacy in which critical substrates and strong inducers or inhibitors are best avoided (Cozza et al. 2003). **(Levenson JL [ed]: APP Textbook of Psychosomatic Medicine: Psychiatric Care of the Medically Ill, 2nd Edition, Chapter 38, pp. 960–961)**

23.24 A 25-year-old woman presents to you for treatment of her first episode of moderate depression. She has never taken antidepressants. After deciding that she can be treated as an outpatient, you prescribe fluoxetine 20 mg/day. Six weeks later, she reports no side effects but still has significant symptoms of depression without notable improvement. What do you recommend next?

A. Wait an additional 4 weeks before considering a dose change.
B. Discontinue fluoxetine and initiate sertraline.
C. Augment fluoxetine by initiating bupropion.
D. Increase fluoxetine dose to 80 mg/day and reassess in 4 weeks.
E. Increase fluoxetine dose to 40 mg/day and reassess in 4 weeks.

The correct response is option E: Increase fluoxetine dose to 40 mg and reassess in 4 weeks.

In patients with depression, there is evidence that all classes of antidepressants are effective. The starting dose of fluoxetine is 20 mg/day, and the usual daily dose goal is 20–60 mg/day. Antidepressants do work better at higher doses within the standard range, and therefore, considering the lack of side effects, increasing the dose (option E) instead of changing (option B) or augmenting (option C) the medication is the appropriate next step. Because higher doses have not yet been subject to trial, it is also too soon to consider a dose greater than the standard dose (option D). It takes approximately 4–6 weeks for a given dose of an SSRI to achieve full effect, and there is not sufficient evidence that waiting longer will result in clinically significant therapeutic effects (option A). **(Hales RE, Yudofsky SC, Roberts LW [eds]: APP Textbook of Psychiatry, 6th Edition, pp. 965–971 and Table 27–11, pp. 967–969)**

23.25 How do generic medications compare with brand-name medications?

    A. Generic and brand-name medications are equivalent biochemically and therapeutically.

    B. Generic and brand-name medications are bioequivalent but may have different clinical effects.

    C. Generic medications often have 20%–30% differences in potency.

    D. Generic and brand-name medications have identical active ingredients, but the bioavailability can vary.

    E. Generic and brand-name medications may have different chemical structure but must be similar therapeutically.

The correct response is option B: Generic and brand-name medications are bioequivalent but may have different clinical effects.

Generic drugs are less expensive alternatives to brand-name formulations, which can benefit patients from the cost savings. The U.S. Food and Drug Administration requires generic medications to be bioequivalent to the brand-name formulations; however, varying clinical effects can occur (option B). Bioequivalents have no significant difference in the active ingredient, the rate of absorption, or the bioavailability of the medication (options D, E). The difference in bioavailability has been found to be approximately 3.5% (option C), which is the same as the variability between brand-name medications (Kesselheim et al. 2008). However, generic formulations are not exactly the same because the coating and inactive ingredients can vary. Therefore, it is possible for someone to have an allergic reaction to the dye or coating materials in one generic brand but not the brand-name medication (option A). If a patient tells you that they responded differently to a generic medication, the concern should be taken seriously. **(Hales RE, Yudofsky SC, Gabbard GO [eds]: APP Textbook of Psychiatry, 5th Edition, Chapter 26, p. 1054)**

References

Bostwick JR, Guthrie SK, Ellingrod VL: Antipsychotic-induced hyperprolactinemia. Pharmacotherapy 29(1):64–73, 2009 19113797

Caroff SN: Neuroleptic malignant syndrome, in Neuroleptic Malignant Syndrome and Related Conditions, 2nd Edition. Edited by Mann SC, Caroff SN, Keck PE Jr, et al. Washington, DC, American Psychiatric Publishing, 2003, pp 1–44

Cohen LS, Altshuler LL, Harlow BL, et al: Relapse of major depression during pregnancy in women who maintain or discontinue antidepressant treatment. JAMA1 295(5):499–507, 2006 16449615

Cozza K, Armstrong S, Oesterheld J: Concise Guide to the Cytochrome P450 System: Drug Interaction Principles for Medical Practice. Washington, DC, American Psychiatric Publishing, 2003

Devinsky O, Honigfeld G, Patin J: Clozapine-related seizures. Neurology 41(3):369–371, 1991 2006003

Kesselheim AS, Misono AS, Lee JL, et al: Clinical equivalence of generic and brand-name drugs used in cardiovascular disease: a systematic review and meta-analysis. JAMA 300(21):2514–2526, 2008 19050195

Kinon BJ, Gilmore JA, Liu H, Halbreich UM: Prevalence of hyperprolactinemia in schizophrenic patients treated with conventional antipsychotic medications or risperidone. Psychoneuroendocrinology 28(Suppl 2):55–68, 2003 12650681

Lehman AF, Lieberman JA, Dixon LB, et al: Practice guideline for the treatment of patients with schizophrenia, second edition. American Psychiatric Association Steering Committee on Practice Guidelines. Am J Psychiatry 161 (2 suppl):1–56, 2004

Lieberman JA, Saltz BL, Johns CA, et al: The effects of clozapine on tardive dyskinesia. Br J Psychiatry 158:503–510, 1991 1675900

Mir A, Shivakumar K, Williamson RJ, et al: Change in sexual dysfunction with aripiprazole: a switching or add-on study. J Psychopharmacol 22(3):244–253, 2008 18308789

Ozdemir V, Bertilsson L, Miura J, et al: CYP2D6 genotype in relation to perphenazine concentration and pituitary pharmacodynamic tissue sensitivity in Asians: CYP2D6-serotonin-dopamine crosstalk revisited. Pharmacogenet Genomics 17(5):339–347, 2007 17429316

Schatzberg AF, Haddad P, Kaplan EM, et al; Discontinuation Consensus Panel: Serotonin reuptake inhibitor discontinuation syndrome: a hypothetical definition. Discontinuation Consensus panel. J Clin Psychiatry 58(Suppl 7):5–10, 1997 9219487

Strawn JR, Keck PE Jr, Caroff SN: Neuroleptic malignant syndrome. Am J Psychiatry 164(6):870–876, 2007 17541044

van Harten PN, Tenback DE: Tardive dyskinesia: clinical presentation and treatment. Int Rev Neurobiol 98:187–210, 2011 21907088

CHAPTER 24

Professionalism

24.1 Intrinsic consequences of boundary violations may include which of the following?

A. Ethics complaint to the professional society.
B. Civil lawsuit.
C. Board of registration complaint.
D. Criminal lawsuit.
E. Patient suicide.

The correct response is option E: Patient suicide.

The consequences of boundary problems may be divided into those intrinsic to the therapy and those extrinsic to the therapy. A serious and exploitative boundary violation may doom the therapy and cause the patient to feel (accurately) betrayed and used. The clinical consequences of boundary violations, including sexual misconduct, may encompass the entire spectrum of emotional harms from mild and transient distress to suicide (option E). The *extrinsic* harms fall into three major categories: civil lawsuits (in some jurisdictions, criminal charges for overtly sexual activity) (options B, D); complaints to the board of registration, the licensing agency (option C); and ethics complaints to the professional society (such as the district branch of the American Psychiatric Association), usually directed to the ethics committee of the relevant organization (option A). **(Oldham JM, Skodol AE, Bender DS [eds]: APP Textbook of Personality Disorders, 2nd Edition, Chapter 17, p. 372)**

24.2 When a boundary crossing occurs in therapy, it is essential to first do which of the following?

A. Discuss with the patient at the next available occasion.
B. Apologize to the patient at the next session.
C. Only discuss it if the patient brings it up at the next session.
D. Transfer the patient to another therapist.
E. Emphasize to the patient that this is considered a normal part of therapy.

The correct response is option A: Discuss with the patient at the next available occasion.

When a boundary crossing occurs, the therapist should review the matter with the patient on the next available occasion (option A) and fully document the rationale, the discussion with the patient, and the description of the patient's response. This advice may be summarized as the "3 Ds": demeanor (remaining professional at all times), debriefing (with the patient at the next session), and documentation (of both the crossing event and its rationale). Under some circumstances, a tactful apology to the patient for misreading a situation may be in order when there is a potential boundary violation (option B), but the subject should first be discussed. It is not recommended that discussion be dependent on the patient bringing up the subject (option C) or that the patient be transferred (option D) or told that boundary crossings are "normal" (option E). **(Oldham JM, Skodol AE, Bender DS [eds]: APP Textbook of Personality Disorders, 2nd Edition, Chapter 17, pp. 371, 380)**

24.3   Which of the following is defined as the "red flag" that should alert a therapist of an impending boundary violation with a patient who has borderline personality disorder (BPD)?

A. The therapist's realization that an exception to his or her usual practice is about to be made.
B. The patient's sense of entitlement and of being "special."
C. A history of early sexual trauma in the patient.
D. The therapist's recognition of the patient's unconscious manipulation.
E. Recognition of "borderline rage" in a patient.

The correct response is option A: The therapist's realization that an exception to his or her usual practice is about to be made.

The patient's sense of entitlement and of being "special" may infect the therapist with the same view of the patient's specialness, such that the clinician is tempted to make inappropriate exceptions to usual practice. However, just noting the sense of entitlement (option B) or "borderline rage" (option E) or a history of sexual trauma (option C) does not indicate an imminent boundary violation because these are common in many, if not most, patients with BPD. The surprising power of the manipulation to slip under the clinician's radar, as it were, is one of the more striking findings in the boundary realm: "I sensed that I was doing something that was outside my usual practice and, in fact, outside the pale," the therapist will lament to the consultant, "but somehow I just found myself making an exception with this patient and doing it anyway." Gutheil (1989) described his experience with therapists seeking consultation who would begin their narratives with "I don't ordinarily do this with my patients, but in this case I [insert a broad spectrum of inappropriate behaviors here]." Recognizing the patient's unconscious manipulation does not indicate a potential boundary violation (option D).

However, a therapist who realizes that an exception to usual practice is about to be made should view this impulse as a red flag signaling the need for reflection and consultation (option A). **(Oldham JM, Skodol AE, Bender DS [eds]: APP Textbook of Personality Disorders, 2nd Edition, Chapter 17, p. 376)**

24.4 Which of the following is the definition of *integrity*?

A. The virtue of truthfulness.
B. The virtue of fully regarding and according intrinsic value to someone or something.
C. The virtue of promise keeping.
D. The virtue of acting for the good of another person rather than for oneself.
E. The virtue of coherence and adherence to professionalism in intention and action.

The correct response is option E: The virtue of coherence and adherence to professionalism in intention and action.

Honesty is the virtue of truthfulness (option A), *respect* is the virtue of fully regarding and according intrinsic value to someone or something (option B), *fidelity* is the virtue of promise keeping (option C), and *altruism* is the virtue of acting for the good of another person rather than for oneself (option D). *Integrity* is the virtue of coherence and adherence to professionalism in intention and action (option E). **(Hales RE, Yudofsky SC, Roberts LW [eds]: APP Textbook of Psychiatry, 6th Edition, Chapter 7, Table 7–2, p. 208)**

24.5 Posting a photograph of someone identified as a patient on Facebook is acceptable under which of these circumstances?

A. If it is a former patient.
B. Under no circumstances.
C. If the patient is not identified.
D. If the patient is a Facebook "friend."
E. If appropriate privacy settings are used.

The correct response is option B: Under no circumstances.

An emerging area of ethical significance for psychiatrists is the maintenance of ethics and professionalism in the digital age. The Internet, e-mail, blogs, social networking, and other online media pose a number of new ethical challenges (Mostaghimi and Crotty 2011). There are obvious hazards in posting online content about oneself or others that may affect individual patients' as well as societal perceptions of the professionalism of psychiatrists. Both intentional and unintentional online disclosures of patient information (including photographs) have been documented in studies (Lagu et al. 2008). By acting carefully and proactively, psychiatrists can maintain appropriate boundaries, ethics, and professionalism online. Recommended guidelines for dealing with online media require adherence to basic standards of trust, privacy, professional conduct, and awareness of potential implications of all digital content and interactions (Gabbard et al. 2011). Respect for the privacy of patients' personal information has been an established ethical duty of physicians for millennia. From the standpoint of United States law, doctor-patient confidentiality is a legal privilege granted to patients. The privilege requires physicians to keep patient information private unless the doctor is legally compelled to make a disclosure or the patient waives the privilege.

Information about former patients remains confidential (option A). Even in circumstances where the patient is not identified, it is not permissible to identify someone as a psychiatric patient; this would be a breach of privacy and trust (option C). Having a patient as a Facebook "friend" or utilizing privacy settings do not alter the fact that revealing someone is your patient in a public forum is a breach of privacy and confidentiality (options D, E). Therefore, patient information or photographs indicating someone is your patient should never be posted on social media (option B). Patients should be reasonably able to expect that the information they tell their psychiatrist or other mental health professional will be kept confidential and that disclosure will not occur without their consent. Unfortunately, several studies have shown that many patients are not informed about specific safeguards for their confidentiality and do not seek treatment out of fear about lack of confidentiality (Roberts and Dyer 2004). **(Hales RE, Yudofsky SC, Roberts LW [eds]: APP Textbook of Psychiatry, 6th Edition, Chapter 7, pp. 211–212, 215–216)**

24.6 Which of the following scenarios exemplifies a "dual agency" conflict?

A. While moonlighting in an emergency room, a psychiatrist evaluates a patient she has treated in another mental health facility.
B. A military psychiatrist lives on a military base near his patients who are currently enlisted for active duty.
C. A psychiatrist works in a correctional facility treating prisoners for mental health issues.
D. A psychiatrist is asked to complete disability forms for someone who is his patient.
E. A psychiatrist is asked to evaluate a police officer's fitness for duty after the officer completed a drug rehabilitation program.

The correct response is option E: A psychiatrist is asked to evaluate a police officer's fitness for duty after the officer completed a drug rehabilitation program.

A psychiatrist evaluating a police officer's fitness for duty after drug rehabilitation must place the safety and welfare of the community above the interests of the officer being evaluated (option E). "Dual agency" situations are ones in which a psychiatrist is given additional professional duties to fulfill that may not be fully congruent with the role of physician. An extreme example is the forensic psychiatrist who may be asked to evaluate a death-row inmate to determine whether he or she is "sane enough" to be executed (Gutheil 2009). In this instance, the forensic psychiatrist's first duty is to veracity—telling the truth—in the service of society above all other interests, including those of the individual who is being evaluated. Options A, B, C, and D represent situations in which the professional duties are congruent with the role of physician, although other types of conflict might be present. **(Hales RE, Yudofsky SC, Roberts LW [eds]: APP Textbook of Psychiatry, 6th Edition, Chapter 7, p. 218)**

References

Gabbard GO, Kassaw KA, Perez-Garcia G: Professional boundaries in the era of the Internet. Acad Psychiatry 35(3):168–174, 2011 21602438

Gutheil TG: Borderline personality disorder, boundary violations, and patient-therapist sex: medicolegal pitfalls. Am J Psychiatry 146(5):597–602, 1989 2653055

Gutheil TG: Ethics and forensic psychiatry, in Psychiatric Ethics, 4th Edition. Edited by Bloch S, Chodoff P, Green SA. New York, Oxford University Press, 2009, pp 435–452

Lagu T, Kaufman EJ, Asch DA, Armstrong K: Content of weblogs written by health professionals. J Gen Intern Med 23(10):1642–1646, 2008 18649110

Mostaghimi A, Crotty BH: Professionalism in the digital age. Ann Intern Med 154(8):560–562, 2011 21502653

Roberts LW, Dyer AR: Concise Guide to Ethics in Mental Health Care. Washington, DC, American Psychiatric Publishing, 2004

CHAPTER 25

Psychiatric Consultation

25.1 A surgeon requests a capacity consultation for a patient with colon cancer. The patient is refusing surgery that has a high probability of a cure. In assessing this patient's capacity, you elect to follow the four-pronged approach developed by P. S. Appelbaum and T. Grisso. Which of the following is *not* one of the four factors requiring consideration in this model?

A. Rational manipulation of information.
B. Absence of a serious mental disorder.
C. Preference.
D. Appreciation of the facts presented.
E. Factual understanding of the procedure.

The correct response is option B: Absence of a serious mental disorder.

Assessing the rationality of a patient's decision-making process, rather than the presence or absence of a mental disorder itself (option B), is the key element in determining whether patients with serious mental illness have sufficient capacity for specific medical decisions. A patient's decisional capacity depends on an understanding of the underlying illness, proposed interventions, prognosis, and consequences of treatment and nontreatment. The most established method of capacity determination for medical decision making is a four-pronged analysis developed by Appelbaum and Grisso (Appelbaum 2007; Appelbaum and Grisso 1988). Under this model, the four factors for consideration in determining decisional capacity are preference (option C), factual understanding (option E), appreciation of the facts presented (i.e., how they relate to the specific individual; option D), and rational manipulation of information (option A). All four elements must be met in order for the individual to demonstrate decisional capacity. In practice, a patient's decisional capacity is rarely questioned when the patient is in agreement with the proposed medical interventions. **(Levenson JL [ed]: APP Textbook of Psychosomatic Medicine: Psychiatric Care of the Medically Ill, 2nd Edition, Chapter 2, p. 24)**

25.2   In recent years, the clinical and ethical appropriateness of the use of physical re-
        straints in the medical setting has come under increasing scrutiny, leading to an
        evolution in medical and nursing practice regarding the use of restraints. In re-
        gard to the ethics of restraint use for an acutely agitated and confused medical pa-
        tient, which of the following statements is true?

        A. Agitated and confused patients should never be restrained.
        B. Agitated and confused patients may be restrained only after a formal determi-
           nation of decision-making capacity.
        C. Immediate safety concerns transcend ethics discussions and allow for restraint
           as the unequivocal standard of care in acute agitation and confusion.
        D. Restraints may be legally permissible but are always unethical.
        E. Refusal of care by an agitated and confused patient should be treated no dif-
           ferently from refusal of care by a competent and informed patient.

        **The correct response is option C: Immediate safety concerns transcend ethics
        discussions and allow for restraint as the unequivocal standard of care in acute
        agitation and confusion.**

        Physical restraint of patients should be used only when no less restrictive method
        is available to protect them and staff from harm (option C). The Centers for Medi-
        care and Medicaid Services (U.S. Department of Health and Human Services
        2006) and the Joint Commission (2009) require that hospitals have policies on
        physical restraint and seclusion. Most physicians and nurses are comfortable de-
        ciding whether and when a patient's behavior warrants physical restraints. In
        cases of extreme agitation (option A) and violence, nuanced mental status exam-
        inations are unnecessary (option B). It is both ethical and legal to physically re-
        strain patients when safety of both patients and staff is concerned (option D).
            Evaluating the necessity of clinical tests for a confused patient necessitates
        clinical judgment about the necessity of the diagnostic test, its associated risks,
        and the degree to which the patient's condition is deemed to threaten life or risk
        permanent serious injury. For minimally invasive testing judged to be urgent and
        of critical importance, physicians have an obligation to act in the best medical in-
        terests of their patients, even if this entails the use of force. The critical distinction
        to be made to justify the use of force or restraint is between competent, informed
        refusal of care that warrants respect versus refusal due to compromised decision-
        making capacity (option E). **(Levenson JL [ed]: APP Textbook of Psychosomatic
        Medicine: Psychiatric Care of the Medically Ill, 2nd Edition, Chapter 3, pp. 37–38)**

25.3   Which of the following clinical scenarios would *not* routinely prompt early use of
        neuroimaging for evaluation?

        A. Acute onset of psychotic illness, without delirium, in a previously healthy pa-
           tient.
        B. First presentation of apparent dementia.
        C. Pretreatment workup for electroconvulsive therapy (ECT) in a patient with
           psychotic depression.

D. Mental status changes associated with lateralizing neurological signs.

E. Delirium following documented overdose with anticholinergic medication with normal motor examination.

The correct response is option E: Delirium following documented overdose with anticholinergic medication with normal motor examination.

Dougherty and Rauch (2004) suggest that the following conditions and situations merit consideration of neuroimaging: new-onset psychosis (option A), new-onset dementia (option B), delirium of unknown cause, testing prior to an initial course of ECT (option C), and an acute mental status change with an abnormal neurological examination in a patient with either a history of head trauma or an age of 50 years or older (option D). Neuroimaging is not indicated for patients who have overdosed with anticholinergic medications (option E). **(Levenson JL [ed]: APP Textbook of Psychosomatic Medicine: Psychiatric Care of the Medically Ill, 2nd Edition, Chapter 1, p. 10)**

25.4 Treatment of anxiety disorders in terminally ill patients may require modification of usual psychopharmacological practices. For example, many terminally ill patients can no longer reliably take oral medications. Which of the following benzodiazepines can be administered rectally?

A. Oxazepam.
B. Clonazepam.
C. Lorazepam.
D. Diazepam.
E. Temazepam.

The correct response is option D: Diazepam.

For patients who feel persistently anxious, the first-line antianxiety drugs are the benzodiazepines. Dying patients can be administered diazepam rectally when no other route is available, with dosages equivalent to those used in oral regimens. Rectal diazepam (Twycross and Lack 1984) has been used widely in palliative care to control anxiety, restlessness, and agitation associated with the final days of life (option D). For patients with severely compromised hepatic function, the use of shorter-acting benzodiazepines such as oxazepam, lorazepam, and temazepam (options A, C, E) is preferred, because these drugs are metabolized by conjugation with glucuronic acid and have no active metabolites (Roth and Massie 2009). Clonazepam is available in an orally disintegrating formulation for patients with swallowing difficulties (option B). **(Levenson JL [ed]: APP Textbook of Psychosomatic Medicine: Psychiatric Care of the Medically Ill, 2nd Edition, Chapter 41, p. 1059)**

25.5   Suicide accounts for a very low number of deaths in cancer patients. Which of the following risk factors has been reported?

A. The risk of suicide in cancer patients was five times that in the general population.
B. Female cancer patients had a higher suicide rate than male patients.
C. Caucasians had a lower rate of suicide than other racial groups.
D. Young age at cancer diagnosis predicted suicide risk.
E. Head and neck cancers were associated with a notably high suicide risk.

The correct response is option E: Head and neck cancers were associated with a notably high suicide risk.

In the United States, a large retrospective cohort study comparing cancer patients with the general population reported that patients with cancer had nearly twice the incidence of suicide (option A) (Misono et al. 2008). Higher suicide rates were associated with male gender, white race, and older age at diagnosis (options B–D). The highest suicide rates were observed in cancers of the respiratory system, stomach, and head and neck (option E). **(Levenson JL [ed]: APP Textbook of Psychosomatic Medicine: Psychiatric Care of the Medically Ill, 2nd Edition, Chapter 23, p. 528)**

25.6   A patient you treat in the HIV/AIDS clinic exhibits a change in his level of alertness, confusion, headache, fever, and focal neurological signs. The brain computed tomography (CT) scan shows multiple bilateral, ring-enhancing lesions in the basal ganglia. What is the *most likely* medical diagnosis for this patient?

A. Cytomegalovirus.
B. Cryptococcal meningitis.
C. Progressive multifocal leukoencephalopathy.
D. Toxoplasmosis.
E. Central nervous system (CNS) lymphoma.

The correct response is option D: Toxoplasmosis.

Infection with *Toxoplasma gondii* (option D) generally occurs in 30% of patients with fewer than 100 CD4 cells/mm^3 (Kaplan et al. 2009). In AIDS patients, toxoplasmosis is the most common reason for intracranial masses, affecting between 2% and 4% of the AIDS population. Symptoms of CNS infection are fever, change in level of alertness, headache, confusion, focal neurological signs (approximately 80% of cases), and partial or generalized seizures (approximately 30% of cases). CT scanning usually shows multiple bilateral, ring-enhancing lesions in the basal ganglia or at the gray/white matter junction.

Cytomegalovirus (CMV) infection (option A) is found at autopsy in about 30%–50% of brains from HIV-infected patients (Jellinger et al. 2000). Short-term memory is especially impaired in CMV encephalitis in HIV-infected patients, mimicking Korsakoff's syndrome (Pirskanen-Matell et al. 2009).

Although meningitis caused by *Cryptococcus neoformans* (option B) is rare in immunocompetent persons, it is a devastating illness that has occurred in approximately 8%–10% of AIDS patients in the United States and in up to 30% of AIDS patients in other parts of the world (Powderly 2000). Patients generally present with fever and delirium. Meningeal signs are not universally seen. Seizures and focal neurological deficits occur in about 10% of patients, and intracranial pressure is elevated in about 50% of patients.

Progressive multifocal leukoencephalopathy (option C) is a demyelinating disease of white matter in immunocompromised patients. The clinical syndrome consists of multiple focal neurological deficits, such as monoparetic or hemiparetic limb weakness, dysarthria, gait disturbances, sensory deficits, and progressive dementia, with eventual coma and death. Occasionally, seizures or visual losses may occur.

Lymphoma (option E) is the most common neoplasm seen in AIDS patients, affecting between 0.6% and 3% of these patients. The patient is generally afebrile; may develop a single lesion with focal neurological signs or small, multifocal lesions; and most commonly presents with mental status change. Seizures occur in about 15% of these patients. CNS lymphoma presents late in the course of HIV infection and is associated with a very poor prognosis. CNS lymphoma is at times misdiagnosed as toxoplasmosis, HIV dementia, or other encephalopathy. CT scan of the brain may be normal or show one or multiple hypodense or patchy, nodular enhancing lesions. Magnetic resonance imaging generally shows enhanced lesions that may be difficult to differentiate from CNS toxoplasmosis, but thallium single-photon emission computed tomography and positron emission tomography scanning may help differentiate the two disorders. **(Levenson JL [ed]: APP Textbook of Psychosomatic Medicine: Psychiatric Care of the Medically Ill, 2nd Edition, Chapter 28, pp. 641–642)**

25.7 The personality type of a hospitalized patient may elicit various countertransference responses from the treating physician. A physician notices that she feels little connection with a patient and finds the patient difficult to engage. Which of the following personality types might elicit this countertransference response?

A. Masochistic.
B. Histrionic.
C. Paranoid.
D. Narcissistic.
E. Schizoid.

The correct response is option E: Schizoid.

A doctor may feel little connection with, and find it difficult to engage, a schizoid patient (option E). The masochistic patient (option A) usually produces anger, hate, and frustration in the physician, who also may feel helpless. The histrionic patient (option B) may produce anxiety and impatience in the physician or elicit erotic responses. The paranoid patient (option C) causes the doctor to feel angry, attacked, or accused. The narcissistic patient (option D) frequently produces anger and the desire to counterattack in the doctor, who also may feel inferior. **(Levenson JL [ed]: APP Textbook of Psychosomatic Medicine: Psychiatric Care of the Medically Ill, 2nd Edition, Chapter 4, pp. 52–54 and Table 4–1, p. 51)**

25.8   Which of the following statements is true about the use of electroencephalograms (EEGs) in psychiatric diagnosis?

   A. There are clear guidelines for use of EEGs in routine screening of psychiatric patients.
   B. An EEG is considered an invasive recording of electrical activity of the brain.
   C. An EEG can always diagnose epilepsy.
   D. An EEG can be helpful in diagnosing sleep disorders.
   E. Patients without epilepsy have a normal EEG.

The correct response is option D: An EEG can be helpful in diagnosing sleep disorders.

An abnormal EEG will consist of one or more of the following: 1) paroxysmal activity indicative of transient, episodic neuronal discharges as seen in epilepsy; 2) nonparoxysmal slowing of activity, as seen in delirium; 3) asymmetric activity as observed with mass lesions or infarction; or 4) sleep abnormalities consistent with sleep-wake disorders, including sleep apneas, narcolepsy (option D), and parasomnias such as rapid eye movement sleep behavior disorder.

The standard EEG is a noninvasive recording of electrical activity in the brain (option B). A normal EEG does not rule out the possibility of epilepsy; 20% of patients with epilepsy will have normal EEGs, and 2% of patients without epilepsy will have spike and wave formations (options C, E) (Engel 1992). Despite the fact that EEGs are widely available, noninvasive, inexpensive, and useful for diagnosing neurological disorders, EEGs have fairly limited utility in the differentiation of psychiatric disorders. No clear guidelines exist for the use of electroencephalographic evaluation in routine screening of the psychiatric patient (option A). **(Hales RE, Yudofsky SC, Roberts LW [eds]: APP Textbook of Psychiatry, 6th Edition, Chapter 4, p. 111)**

References

Appelbaum PS: Clinical practice. Assessment of patients' competence to consent to treatment. N Engl J Med 357(18):1834–1840, 2007 17978292

Appelbaum PS, Grisso T: Assessing patients' capacities to consent to treatment. N Engl J Med 319(25):1635–1638, 1988 3200278

Dougherty DD, Rauch SL: Neuroimaging in psychiatry, in Massachusetts General Hospital Psychiatry Update and Board Preparation, 2nd Edition. Edited by Stern TA, Herman JB. New York, McGraw-Hill, 2004, pp 227–232

Engel J Jr: The epilepsies, in Cecil Textbook of Medicine, 19th Edition, Vol 2. Edited by Wyngaarden JB, Smith LH, Bennett JC. Philadelphia, PA, WB Saunders, 1992, pp 2202–2213

Jellinger KA, Setinek U, Drlicek M, et al: Neuropathology and general autopsy findings in AIDS during the last 15 years. Acta Neuropathol 100(2):213–220, 2000 10963370

Joint Commission: Provision of care, treatment, and services, in Revised 2009 Accreditation Requirements as of March 26: Hospital Accreditation Program, Oakbrook Terrace, IL. Joint Commission Resources 2009:14–19, 2009

Kaplan JE, Benson C, Holmes KH, et al: Guidelines for prevention and treatment of opportunistic infections in HIV-infected adults and adolescents: recommendations from CDC, the National Institutes of Health, and the HIV Medicine Association of the Infectious Diseases Society of America. MMWR Recomm Rep 58(RR-4):1–207, 2009

Misono S, Weiss NS, Fann JR, et al: Incidence of suicide in persons with cancer. J Clin Oncol 26(29):4731–4738, 2008 18695257

Pirskanen-Matell R, Grützmeier S, Nennesmo I, et al: Impairment of short-term memory and Korsakoff syndrome are common in AIDS patients with cytomegalovirus encephalitis. Eur J Neurol 16(1):48–53, 2009 19087150

Powderly WG: Cryptococcal meningitis in HIV-infected patients. Curr Infect Dis Rep 2(4):352–357, 2000 11095877

Roth AJ, Massie MJ: Anxiety in palliative care, in Handbook of Psychiatry in Palliative Medicine, 2nd Edition. Edited by Chochinov HM, Breitbart W. New York, Oxford University Press, 2009, pp 69–80

Twycross RG, Lack SA: Therapeutics in Terminal Disease. London, Pitman, 1984

U.S. Department of Health and Human Services: Code of Federal Regulations, Title 42 (Public Health), Part 482 (Conditions of Participation for Hospitals), Section 13 (Patients' Rights), Standard e (Restraint for acute medical and surgical care). 71 FR 71426, Dec. 8, 2006. Available at: http://www.cms.gov/CFCsAndCoPs/downloads/finalpatientrightsrule.pdf. Accessed May 5, 2010.

CHAPTER 26

Psychiatric Interview

26.1 Which of the following is true regarding the use of outside information when gathering data on a patient?

A. It is safe to assume that medications previously taken by the patient were of therapeutic dose and duration and were prescribed for U.S. Food and Drug Administration–indicated psychiatric conditions.
B. If a patient has a diagnostic code written in his or her electronic health record, it is not necessary to verify the symptoms and chronology of that disorder before recommending treatment for it.
C. Psychiatrists may not contact a patient's relatives against his or her wishes, even in the setting of acute risk.
D. It would be rare for a patient's situation to evolve between a previous psychiatric evaluation and the current one.
E. In the event that a psychiatrist must obtain information from a patient's family member in an emergency situation, the psychiatrist must make every effort to not unnecessarily disclose confidential information.

The correct response is option E: In the event that a psychiatrist must obtain information from a patient's family member in an emergency situation, the psychiatrist must make every effort to not unnecessarily disclose confidential information.

Although most states allow psychiatrists to contact family members against the patient's objection in the setting of acute risk, the onus is on the psychiatrist to not violate the patient's privacy by unnecessarily providing confidential information to the family members (option E). A patient's previous medical records and sources of outside collateral information can offer important insights and perspectives that may inform diagnostic impressions and treatment planning. It is important to take a thorough history regarding previous medication trials, to evaluate the adequacy of the trials, and to also understand the indications for the medication trial (option A). It is similarly important to use previous diagnoses as a starting point for information gathering, rather than as definitive truth (option B).

349

States vary somewhat in regard to privacy legislation, but generally psychiatrists have the right to contact relatives over patient objection only in situations that involve acute risk (option C). Substance abuse, medication nonadherence, and psychosocial stressors are but a few of the possible factors that may make patients' presentations drastically differ between clinical encounters, even if only a short time has elapsed between encounters (option D). **(Hales RE, Yudofsky SC, Roberts LW [eds]: APP Textbook of Psychiatry, 6th Edition, Chapter 1, pp. 4–5)**

26.2. Which of the following describes the most appropriate approach to interviewing a patient with distinguishing sociological, religious, racial, or ethnic characteristics?

A. The examiner should draw on prior reading or experience with the subgroup of interest to appear as an expert.
B. It is best to ignore socioeconomic status, race, ethnicity, and sexual orientation, because these factors have little bearing on patients' experiences and symptoms.
C. To understand the relevance of the sociological characteristic to the patient's presenting complaint, the examiner should ask the patient for his or her perspective.
D. If the examiner shares a trait with the patient (such as race, religion, or sexual orientation), the examiner should proceed as if his or her experiences are the same as the patient's.
E. The "social" aspects of a patient's background are not clinically relevant.

The correct response is option C: To understand the relevance of the sociological characteristic to the patient's presenting complaint, the examiner should ask the patient for his or her perspective.

Exploring the ways that a person's social context influences their symptoms and experiences can inform the understanding of the patient (option E). Far from being irrelevant, these factors may significantly affect the presentation (option B). Different individuals experience social and cultural factors as different, and it behooves interviewers to find out from the patient his or her own perspective (option C) rather than making assumptions based on the examiner's prior experience (option A) or shared background (option D). **(Hales RE, Yudofsky SC, Roberts LW [eds]: APP Textbook of Psychiatry, 6th Edition, Chapter 1, pp. 8–9)**

26.3. A psychiatrist is interviewing a new patient in the emergency room. No previous health records are available on the patient, and no collateral informants are available. The patient exhibits psychomotor agitation, threatening behavior, and rapid/tangential speech. Which of the following would be a recommended early interview question?

A. "Have you ever used drugs or been admitted to a psychiatric unit?"
B. "You are too excited right now to be safe. Would you like to remain quietly in the room to get calm or would you prefer medication to help you?"
C. "How long have you been off your medications for bipolar disorder?"

D. "Is there a history of mental illness in your blood relatives?"
E. "Have you ever been in psychoanalytic treatment?"

The correct response is option B: "You are too excited right now to be safe. Would you like to remain quietly in the room to get calm or would you prefer medication to help you?"

Skilled clinicians adjust their interviewing techniques to both the patient and the clinical situation. In the case of an acutely unsafe patient in an emergency room setting, the initial task of the clinician is to ensure the patient's safety while preserving dignity. Option B accomplishes these goals in a straightforward way.

Double questions (option A) can be problematic because they require multiple answers; even if a patient answers "no," it is not clear whether he is denying the former, the latter, or both parts of the question. The interviewer needs to consider a broad differential diagnosis instead of reaching a conclusion regarding the patient's diagnosis and the events precipitating the presentation (option C). In the presentation described above, it would be important to rule out drug intoxication or withdrawal and delirium. Given the acuity of the presentation, questions about familial mental health history and prior psychoanalytic treatment are not relevant at this time (options D, E). **(Hales RE, Yudofsky SC, Roberts LW [eds]: APP Textbook of Psychiatry, 6th Edition, Chapter 1, pp. 14–17 and Table 1–3, p. 15)**

26.4. Which of the following terms refers to anything that prevents a patient from talking openly to an interviewer?

A. Resistance.
B. Countertransference.
C. Catatonia.
D. Affect.
E. Mood.

The correct response is option A: Resistance.

The psychiatric interviewer will frequently encounter *resistance,* which refers to anything that prevents the patient from talking openly to the interviewer (option A). Conscious resistance occurs when the patient knowingly neglects, distorts, or makes up important information. Unconscious resistance leads to similarly incomplete stories, but the mechanism is assessed to be out of the patient's awareness. *Countertransference* (option B) generally refers to the interviewer's own reactions to the patient. *Catatonia* (option C) is broadly defined as abnormality of movement or muscle tone associated with psychosis (Fisher 1989) and may be one specific syndrome preventing a patient from talking to an interviewer. *Affect* (option D) is the patient's expression of his or her emotional tone. *Mood* (option E) is the patient's predominant emotional state during the interview. **(Hales RE, Yudofsky SC, Roberts LW [eds]: APP Textbook of Psychiatry, 6th Edition, Chapter 1, pp. 7–8, 24;**

Yudofsky SC, Hales RE [eds]: APP Textbook of Neuropsychiatry and Behavioral Neuroscience, 5th Edition, Chapter 4, p. 152)

26.5. A psychiatrist is interviewing a patient to determine suitability for psychotherapy in an outpatient office setting. Which of the following is consistent with usual interviewing technique?

A. The examiner starts the interview with directive questioning.
B. The examiner in this situation should avoid the interview technique of confrontation, because it is likely to be experienced as an attack by a patient.
C. The examiner may reflect content and feelings to help the patient feel heard and to encourage the patient to continue speaking.
D. It is important to offer solutions early in the interview to develop positive transference; full understanding of the situation is not necessary before offering solutions.
E. The interviewer's eye contact and tone of voice are unlikely to be important in the building of the therapeutic alliance.

The correct response is option is C: The examiner may reflect content and feelings to help the patient feel heard and to encourage the patient to continue speaking.

It is recommended to use nondirective questioning during the initial phase of the interview to facilitate the patient telling his or her story (option A). The interview technique of confrontation (option B) refers to the interviewer pointing out discrepancies to the patient and assessing his or her response as a gauge of the patient's ability to work with conflict. It is a technique that can deepen the therapeutic relationship. Premature advice (option D) involves making suggestions without a full understanding of the patient's situation and is inadvisable. Poor eye contact may communicate lack of interest, and tone of voice may communicate negative judgment of the patient (option E). During the initial interview, therapeutic alliance is achieved with an interested and neutral demeanor. Psychiatrists may reflect content and feelings back to the patient to help the patient feel heard and encourage the patient to tell his or her story (option C). **(Hales RE, Yudofsky SC, Roberts LW [eds]: APP Textbook of Psychiatry, 6th Edition, Chapter 1, pp. 13–15 and Tables 1–2, 1–3, pp. 13, 15).**

Reference

Fisher CM: "Catatonia" due to disulfiram toxicity. Arch Neurol 46(7):798–804, 1989 2742552

CHAPTER 27

Psychoanalysis

27.1   What is a concordant countertransference reaction?

A. The therapist experiences the patient's feelings or emotional position.
B. The therapist empathizes with the feelings of someone in the patient's life.
C. The therapist feels frustrated with the patient due to the therapist's own conflict.
D. The therapist enacts a similar transference reaction with his or her own therapist.
E. The therapist feels that his or her emotions about the patient obscure his or her judgment.

The correct response is option A: The therapist experiences the patient's feelings or emotional position.

The psychodynamic psychotherapist observes his or her own emotional reactions and values and processes them as possible windows into the patient's experience. Frequently, the more intense and even embarrassing the therapist's responses, the more likely they are to reflect a crucial, hidden, conflicted state residing within the patient. There are generally two types of countertransference reactions (Racker 1968): concordant countertransference, in which the therapist experiences and empathizes with the patient's emotional position (option A), and complementary countertransference, in which the therapist experiences and empathizes with the feelings of an important person from the patient's life (option B). Often, countertransference is the result of events occurring in the therapist's life that may make him or her more sensitive to certain themes in the patient's associations (option E). Options C and D are incorrect because they reflect personal issues for the therapist and do not reflect empathy on the part of the therapist. **(Hales RE, Yudofsky SC, Roberts LW [eds]: APP Textbook of Psychiatry, 6th Edition, Chapter 30, pp. 1085, 1087 and Table 30–11, p. 1088)**

27.2   What defense mechanism is represented when children who have been abused become abusers themselves in adulthood?

A. Denial.
B. Displacement.
C. Reaction formation.
D. Identification with the aggressor.
E. Sublimation.

The correct response is option D: Identification with the aggressor.

Identification with the aggressor is the tendency to imitate what the patient perceives as the aggressive and intimidating manner of someone toward him or her (option D). Denial averts the patient's attention from painful ideas or feelings without making them completely unavailable to consciousness (option A). Displacement is changing the object of one's feelings to a safer one (option B). Reaction formation consists of exaggerating one emotional trend to help repress the opposite emotion (option C). Sublimation is a mature mechanism of defense that is the hoped-for, healthy, not conflicted evolution of primitive childhood impulses into a mature level of expression (option E). **(Hales RE, Yudofsky SC, Roberts LW [eds]: APP Textbook of Psychiatry, 6th Edition, Chapter 30, Table 30–10, p. 1086)**

27.3   A patient receives a bill that overcharges him for the most recent month of therapy. Which essential concept in psychodynamic psychotherapy is illustrated at the next appointment when this patient worries that his therapist is angry with him?

A. Countertransference.
B. Identification with the aggressor.
C. Transference.
D. Resistance.
E. Projection.

The correct response is option E: Projection.

The patient's defense mechanisms are an important source of resistance in psychotherapy. In 1936, Anna Freud, in *The Ego and the Mechanisms of Defense* (Freud 1966), outlined the functioning of many of these defense maneuvers. Since that time, the list of defense mechanisms has grown and been elaborated upon. *Projection* is a type of defense mechanism that involves the person experiencing an emotion as originating in the other person. In this situation, the patient is most likely angry with the therapist for overcharging him for the last session. Instead of realizing he is angry with his therapist, he believes that the therapist might be angry with him (option E). *Transference* refers to a patient's emotional reaction that stems from that patient's previous relationships (option C). The concept of *countertransference* refers to the therapist's feelings toward the patient (option A). *Identification with the aggressor* is a type of defense mechanism that involves the tendency of the patient to imitate the aggressive manner of a person toward that patient (option B). *Resistance* refers to all the forces in the patient, including defense mechanisms that keep painful feelings and memories outside of conscious awareness (option D). **(Hales RE, Yudofsky SC, Roberts LW [eds]: APP Textbook of Psychiatry, 6th Edition, Chapter 30, pp. 1083–1085 and Tables 30–8, 30–10, pp. 1083, 1086)**

27.4   What is the focus of the drive theory perspective of psychodynamic psychotherapy?

A. Wishes and feelings.
B. Defense mechanisms, cognitive style.
C. Regulation of self-esteem.
D. Internalized memories of interpersonal relationships.
E. Infant-caregiver attachment.

The correct response is option A: Wishes and feelings.

In psychodynamic listening, an important technique of psychodynamic psychotherapy, particular attention is paid to stories, present and past, about 1) feelings and wishes (drives); 2) the management of various feelings through the life cycle (e.g., defense mechanisms and cognitive style) and areas of healthy interaction with the world; 3) self-esteem regulation; and 4) interpersonal relationships. In psychodynamic psychotherapy, the focus of drive theory is wishes and feelings (option A). Ego function theory focuses on defense mechanisms and cognitive style (option B), whereas in self psychology emphasis is on regulation of self-esteem (option C). Internalized memories of interpersonal relationships are the focus of object relations theory (option D). The focus of attachment theory is infant-caregiver attachment (option E). **(Hales RE, Yudofsky SC, Roberts LW [eds]: APP Textbook of Psychiatry, 6th Edition, Chapter 30, p. 1074 and Table 30–3, p. 1075)**

27.5   Which of these defense mechanisms is considered to be "primitive"?

A. Repression.
B. Reaction formation.
C. Splitting.
D. Sublimation.
E. Intellectualization.

The correct response is option C: Splitting.

Since Anna Freud's *The Ego and the Mechanisms of Defense* (Freud 1966), the list of defense maneuvers has grown and been elaborated upon. The more primitive mechanisms of defense—splitting (option C), projection, projective identification, omnipotence, devaluing, primitive identification, and primitive idealization—are seen in severe personality disorders such as borderline personality disorder and in psychotic disorders. Repression (option A), reaction formation (option B), sublimation (option D), and intellectualization (option E) are some of the common defense mechanisms that are not considered primitive. **(Hales RE, Yudofsky SC, Roberts LW [eds]: APP Textbook of Psychiatry, 6th Edition, Chapter 30, p. 1085 and Table 30–9, p. 1086)**

References

Freud A: The Ego and the Mechanisms of Defense, Revised Edition. New York, International Universities Press, 1966

Racker H: Transference and Countertransference. New York, International Universities Press, 1968

CHAPTER 28

Psychological Testing

28.1 Which of the following terms refers to the ability of a test to produce stable scores when readministered at different times?

A. Content validity.
B. Criterion-related validity.
C. Alternate-form reliability.
D. Split-half reliability.
E. Test-retest reliability.

The correct response is option E: Test-retest reliability.

Test-retest reliability (option E) is the extent to which a test yields the same score when readministered under the same conditions at a later time. Alternate-form reliability (option C) is achieved when alternative forms of a test provide roughly equivalent scores for an individual, and split-half reliability (option D) is achieved when two separate subgroups of items on the test yield similar scores. Content validity (option A) is the extent to which a test's content can be said to adequately sample the area of interest, and criterion-related validity (option B) is the extent to which a test score correlates with an individual's ability in a particular area as measured by independent criteria or the ability of the test to make predictions about future behavior. **(Hales RE, Yudofsky SC, Roberts LW [eds]: APP Textbook of Psychiatry, 6th Edition, Chapter 3, pp. 62–63)**

28.2 In order for a test to demonstrate construct validity, which of the following conditions must apply?

A. The test score correlates with other measurements of the same area of activity.
B. The test measures a theoretical construct of interest, and scores on the test reflect this construct.
C. The test yields comparable scores at two proximate points in time.
D. Two forms of the same test yield comparable scores.
E. Subgroups of items yield scores comparable to those of other subgroups of items.

357

The correct response is option B: The test measures a theoretical construct of interest, and scores on the test reflect this construct.

Construct validity can be achieved only by demonstrating that the test specifically measures a theoretical construct of interest and that scores on the test are unrelated to similar areas. Establishing a test's validity requires demonstration that the test measures what it is intended to measure. Three major types of validity can be assessed: content validity, criterion-related validity, and construct validity. Content validity can be achieved only if the content of the test can be said to adequately sample the area of interest (option B). Criterion-related validity refers to the test's relationship to independent criteria of an individual's ability in a particular area (option A) (i.e., concurrent validity) or to the ability of the test to make predictions about future behavior (i.e., predictive validity). Test-retest reliability is achieved when a test yields comparable scores at two proximate points in time (option C). Alternate-form reliability is achieved when two forms of the same test yield comparable scores (option D). Split-form reliability refers to tests in which subgroups of items yield scores comparable to those of other subgroups of items (option E). **(Hales RE, Yudofsky SC, Roberts LW [eds]: APP Textbook of Psychiatry, 6th Edition, Chapter 3, pp. 62–63)**

28.3   For what assessment is the Minnesota Multiphasic Personality Inventory (MMPI) most useful?

A. Assessing affective disorders and personality symptoms and disorders.
B. Assessing thought disorders and personality symptoms and disorders.
C. Assessing personality symptoms and disorders only.
D. Assessing a variety of symptom patterns, including thought disorders, affective disorders, and personality symptoms.
E. Assessing a variety of symptom patterns but not personality disorders.

The correct response is option D: Assessing a variety of symptom patterns, including thought disorders, affective disorders, and personality symptoms.

Although labeled as a personality test, the MMPI was constructed to assess what are now categorized as symptom diagnoses and, to a lesser extent, a few dimensions of personality (option D). The MMPI-2 (Hathaway and McKinley 1989) and its more recent alternative, the MMPI-2 Restructured Form (Ben-Porath and Tellegen 2008/2011), are probably the most widely used assessment instruments in existence. There are several reasons for the MMPI's extensive use, including its efficiency, its extensive normative base, the use of validity scales that indicate the patient's test-taking attitude, and its impressive cross-cultural validation. The MMPI is an omnibus measure of symptomatology and assesses symptom diagnoses (i.e., affective disorders, thought disorders) in addition to personality symptoms. Options A, B, C, and E describe less comprehensive assessment. **(Hales RE, Yudofsky SC, Roberts LW [eds]: APP Textbook of Psychiatry, 6th Edition, Chapter 3, p. 64)**

28.4 The Beck Anxiety Inventory is a self-report questionnaire that is best used for which of the following?

A. Assessing whether a patient meets criteria for any mood disorder.
B. Assessing whether a patient meets criteria for panic disorder.
C. Differentiating between panic disorder and generalized anxiety disorder.
D. Distinguishing between somatic and nonsomatic symptoms of generalized anxiety disorder.
E. Discriminating between anxiety and depression.

The correct response is option E: Discriminating between anxiety and depression.

The Beck Anxiety Inventory (Beck et al. 1988) is a 21-item self-report questionnaire with a focus on somatic anxiety symptoms, such as heart pounding, nervousness, inability to relax, and dizziness or light-headedness. This measure takes approximately 5 minutes to complete and was designed specifically to discriminate between anxiety and depression (option E). There are a variety of other measures available to assess whether a patient meets criteria for any mood disorder (option A) or assessing whether a patient meets criteria for panic disorder (option B). The Beck Anxiety Inventory is not designed to differentiate between panic disorder and generalized anxiety disorder (option C) or to distinguish between somatic and nonsomatic symptoms of generalized anxiety disorder (option D). **(Hales RE, Yudofsky SC, Roberts LW [eds]: APP Textbook of Psychiatry, 6th Edition, Chapter 3, p. 70)**

28.5 A 22-year-old woman comes to you for treatment and reports a history of thinking about hurting herself. Which of the following is a general psychiatric assessment tool that also includes a specific measure for suicidal ideation?

A. Beck Hopelessness Scale.
B. University of Rhode Island Change Assessment.
C. Minnesota Multiphasic Personality Inventory—2.
D. Suicide Intent Scale.
E. Positive and Negative Syndrome Scale.

The correct response is option C: Minnesota Multiphasic Personality Inventory—2.

The revised Koss-Butcher critical item set on the MMPI-2 is a list of 22 items related specifically to depressed suicidal ideation (option C) (Butcher et al. 1989; Koss and Butcher 1973). The Beck Hopelessness Scale (option A) and the Suicide Intent Scale (option D) are self-report instruments specifically designed for assessment of known predictors of suicidal behavior. The University of Rhode Island Change Assessment (option B) is a measure developed to assess a patient's readiness to change in relation to the use of drugs, alcohol, and nicotine. The Positive and Negative Syndrome Scale (option E) assesses symptoms of disordered thinking. **(Hales RE, Yudofsky SC, Roberts LW [eds]: APP Textbook of Psychiatry, 6th Edition, Chapter 3, pp. 64–65, 70–71 and Table 3–2, pp. 66–69)**

28.6 A 72-year-old man is brought in by his family for evaluation because he has been having problems functioning at work and frequently misplaces objects around the house. After the patient receives neuroimaging, you also send him for neuropsychological testing. Which of the following neuropsychological instruments would yield the most useful information about this patient's executive functioning?

    A. WAIS-IV Digit Span Test.
    B. California Learning Test II.
    C. Token Test.
    D. Wisconsin Card Sorting Test.
    E. Judgment of Line Orientation Test.

The correct response is option D: Wisconsin Card Sorting Test.

The Wisconsin Card Sorting Test (Grant and Berg 1948) is a test of concept formation and cognitive flexibility. Subjects match cards according to feedback about the correctness of their sorts. A key feature is that after 10 correct sorts, the sorting principle changes without warning, and subjects must change their sorting strategy accordingly. Because of the lack of warning about the change, this test requires the ability to induce a sorting principle; to monitor the adequacy of this solution; and, when the solution is no longer applicable, to note the error, gain perspective, and arrive at a new solution (option D).

    The WAIS-IV Digit Span test is a measure of "attention span" that requires the patient to repeat a series of digits that increase in length (option A). The California Verbal Learning Test II (Delis et al. 2000) is a word-list learning test designed to assess the use of encoding strategies; both free recall and recognition memory are assessed (option B). The Token Test assesses language comprehension using multistep commands that increase in syntactic complexity (De Renzi and Faglioni 1978) (option C). Spatial perception in the most basic form can be examined with the Judgment of Line Orientation Test (Benton et al. 1994), which assesses the perception of angular relationships using matching of straight lines presented at the same angles (option E). **(Hales RE, Yudofsky SC, Roberts LW [eds]: APP Textbook of Psychiatry, 6th Edition, Chapter 3, pp. 75–80)**

References

Beck AT, Epstein N, Brown G, Steer RA: An inventory for measuring clinical anxiety: psychometric properties. J Consult Clin Psychol 56(6):893–897, 1988 3204199

Ben-Porath YS, Tellegen A: Minnesota Multiphasic Personality Inventory—2 Restructured Form: Manual for Administration, Scoring, and Interpretation. Minneapolis, University of Minnesota Press, 2008/2011

Benton A, Sivan A, Hamsher K: Contributions to Neuropsychological Assessment: A Clinical Manual, 2nd Edition. New York, Oxford University Press, 1994

Butcher JN, Dahlstrom WG, Graham JR, et al: Manual for the Restandardized Minnesota Multiphasic Personality Inventory (MMPI-2): An Administrative and Interpretive Guide. Minneapolis, University of Minnesota Press, 1989

Delis D, Kaplan E, Kramer JH, et al: California Verbal Learning Test, 2nd Edition (CVLT-II) Manual. San Antonio, TX, Psychological Corporation, 2000

De Renzi E, Faglioni P: Normative data and screening power of a shortened version of the Token Test. Cortex 14(1):41–49, 1978 16295108

Grant DA, Berg EA: A behavioral analysis of the degree of reinforcement and ease of shifting to new responses in a Weigl-type card-sorting problem. J Exp Psychol 38(4):404–411, 1948 18874598

Hathaway SR, McKinley JC: Minnesota Multiphasic Personality Inventory 2. Minneapolis, University of Minnesota Press, 1989

Koss MP, Butcher JN: A comparison of psychiatric patients' self-report with other sources of clinical information. J Res Pers 7:225–236, 1973

CHAPTER 29

Psychopharmacology

29.1 A 65-year-old woman with diabetes mellitus type 2, neuropathic pain, and normal renal function reports depressive symptoms that adversely affect her functioning. Which of the following antidepressants would be the best choice for this patient?

A. Bupropion.
B. Citalopram.
C. Duloxetine.
D. Fluoxetine.
E. Mirtazapine.

The correct response is option C: Duloxetine.

The serotonin-norepinephrine reuptake inhibitor duloxetine (option C) has been has product labeling that supports its use in the treatment of both major depression and neuropathic pain. Bupropion (option A), citalopram (option B), fluoxetine (option D), and mirtazapine (option E) do not have this designation. **(Hales RE, Yudofsky SC, Roberts LW [eds]: APP Textbook of Psychiatry, 6th Edition, Chapter 27, pp. 965–966)**

29.2 A 42-year-old woman in good physical health with mild depressive symptoms is eager to quit smoking. Which of the following antidepressants has been demonstrated to increase rates of smoking cessation?

A. Bupropion.
B. Fluoxetine.
C. Fluvoxamine.
D. Sertraline.
E. Venlafaxine.

The correct response is option A: Bupropion.

The norepinephrine-dopamine reuptake inhibitor bupropion (option A) has efficacy in the treatment of depression and as a smoking cessation aid. Fluoxetine (option B), fluvoxamine (option C), sertraline (option D), and venlafaxine (option E) do not have this designation. **(Hales RE, Yudofsky SC, Roberts LW [eds]: APP Textbook of Psychiatry, 6th Edition, Chapter 27, pp. 965–966)**

29.3   A 35-year-old man with generalized anxiety disorder treated with sertraline develops lethargy, confusion, restlessness, flushing, tremors, diaphoresis, and myoclonic jerks when he is started on an antibiotic. Which of the following antibiotic medications could have been responsible for these symptoms?

A. Erythromycin.
B. Ceftriaxone.
C. Ciprofloxacin.
D. Linezolid.
E. Trimethoprim/sulfamethoxazole.

The correct response is option D: Linezolid.

Serotonin syndrome results from excess serotonergic stimulation and can range in severity from mild to life threatening. Common symptoms include confusion, hemodynamic changes (hypertension, hypotension, and tachycardia), diaphoresis, tremor, and myoclonus. Even though patients might develop symptoms of serotonin syndrome in the context of monotherapy with a serotonergic agent, this scenario more commonly results from the simultaneous use of two or more serotonergic drugs. Besides its antibiotic effects, linezolid (option D) inhibits serotonin catabolism, which could increase the risk of serotonin syndrome. Erythromycin (option A), ceftriaxone (option B), ciprofloxacin (option C), and trimethoprim/sulfamethoxazole (option E) are neither directly nor indirectly serotonergic. **(Hales RE, Yudofsky SC, Roberts LW [eds]: APP Textbook of Psychiatry, 6th Edition, Chapter 27, pp. 971–972 and Tables 27–13, 27–14 p. 973)**

29.4   Following administration of a medication to treat agitation, a patient develops confusion, autonomic instability, and rigidity. Which of the following agents is most likely to have caused the patient's symptoms?

A. Diphenhydramine.
B. Clozapine.
C. Haloperidol.
D. Lorazepam.
E. Valproate.

The correct response is option C: Haloperidol.

In rare instances, patients taking antipsychotic medications, including haloperidol (option C), develop a potentially life-threatening disorder known as neuroleptic malignant syndrome (NMS). Generally, the second-generation antipsychotics such as clozapine (option B) have lower risk of NMS. Classic NMS signs include hyperthermia, generalized rigidity with tremors, altered consciousness with catatonia, and autonomic instability. Other features include muscle enzyme elevations (primarily creatine phosphokinase, median elevations 1,000 IU/L; Gurrera et al. 2011), myoglobinuria, leukocytosis, metabolic acidosis, hypoxia, and low serum iron levels. There are rare but documented cases of clozapine-induced NMS, but clozapine requires a slow titration and is therefore less useful for treating acute agitation. Valproate (option E), lorazepam (option D), and diphenhydramine (option A) are not known to cause NMS. **(Hales RE, Yudofsky SC, Roberts LW [eds]: APP Textbook of Psychiatry, 6th Edition, Chapter 9, pp. 278–279; Chapter 27, pp. 935–936, 949, 953–954)**

29.5   What is the primary mechanism of action of buspirone?

A. Direct binding to γ-aminobutyric acid (GABA) subtype A.
B. Serotonin reuptake inhibition.
C. Partial agonism of serotonin type 1A (5-HT$_{1A}$) receptor.
D. α_2 Agonism.
E. β-Blockade.

The correct response is option C: Partial agonism of serotonin type 1A (5-HT$_{1A}$) receptor.

Buspirone, a 5-HT$_{1A}$ receptor partial agonist (option C), is indicated for the treatment of generalized anxiety disorder. Because it does not affect GABA receptors or chloride ion channels, buspirone does not possess many of the major liabilities of benzodiazepines—namely, the potential for abuse, tolerance, and withdrawal. Buspirone is not cross-tolerant with benzodiazepines; thus, a rapid switch from benzodiazepine to buspirone is likely to precipitate benzodiazepine withdrawal and therefore is not indicated. The mechanisms of other medications that can be used in the management of anxiety are the action of benzodiazepines (option A), the action of SSRIs (option B), the action of clonidine (option D), and the action of β-blockers (option E). **(Hales RE, Yudofsky SC, Roberts LW [eds]: APP Textbook of Psychiatry, 6th Edition, Chapter 27, p. 979)**

29.6   Which of the following benzodiazepines would be the best choice for treating acute anxiety in a patient with liver failure?

A. Alprazolam.
B. Lorazepam.
C. Clonazepam.
D. Diazepam.
E. Chlordiazepoxide.

The correct response is option B: Lorazepam.

The choice of benzodiazepine is based primarily on pharmacokinetic properties, including half-life, rapidity of onset, metabolism, and potency. All benzodiazepines are metabolized by the liver, increasing the risk of sedation, confusion, and frank hepatic encephalopathy in patients with hepatic failure. In patients with liver failure, lorazepam (option B), temazepam, and oxazepam may be preferred because they undergo hepatic conjugation and renal excretion and have no active metabolites, whereas other benzodiazepines (options A, C, D, E) undergo hepatic microsomal metabolism and may have long-acting active metabolites, making them less good choices in the setting of hepatic failure. **(Hales RE, Yudofsky SC, Roberts LW [eds]: APP Textbook of Psychiatry, 6th Edition, Chapter 27, p. 979)**

29.7 An unconscious 34-year-old man with newly diagnosed schizoaffective disorder is brought to the emergency department. He is stuporous, has dysarthric speech, walks with an ataxic gait, and exhibits nystagmus and myoclonus on examination. An electrocardiogram (ECG) reveals inverted T waves, and his blood work is remarkable for preserved renal function and a lithium level of 5.2 mEq/L. Which of the following is the most appropriate treatment?

A. Dantrolene.
B. Forced diuresis.
C. Activated charcoal.
D. Potassium supplementation.
E. Hemodialysis.

The correct response is option E: Hemodialysis.

A patient with a serum lithium level greater than 4.0 mEq/L should undergo hemodialysis (option E). Acute lithium toxicity occurs at serum levels above 1.5 mEq/L and can involve moderate to severe gastrointestinal, neurological, and cardiovascular effects. Management of lithium toxicity includes discontinuation of lithium, supportive hospital care, and, in severe cases, hemodialysis.

Signs of mild to moderate lithium intoxication (lithium level=1.5–2.0 mEq/L) include gastrointestinal symptoms (e.g., nausea, vomiting, diarrhea, dry mouth) and neurological symptoms (ataxia, slurred speech, dizziness, nystagmus, lethargy, and muscle weakness). Signs of moderate to severe lithium toxicity (serum level=2.1–2.5 mEq/L) include gastrointestinal symptoms (anorexia, persistent nausea, vomiting), neurological symptoms (e.g., blurred vision, muscle fasciculations, choreoathetoid movements, seizure, delirium), and cardiovascular symptoms (ECG changes such as QTc prolongation, T-wave flattening, and arrhythmias, in addition to circulatory failure and/or syncope). Severe lithium intoxication (lithium level >2.5 mEq/L) can lead to generalized seizures, oliguria and renal failure, and possibly death.

Dantrolene can be part of the management of malignant hyperthermia, including NMS (option A). Forced diuresis (option B) is a treatment for poisoning or overdose in which patients are given fluids and the pH of the urine is altered to actively eliminate the substance, such as giving sodium bicarbonate to alkalinize the urine to improve elimination of salicylates; although giving intravenous fluids does improve excretion of lithium and is part of the management of lithium toxicity, this method would be insufficient in a case this severe. Activated charcoal can be used in some toxic overdoses to bind toxins for safer (less corrosive) emesis; however, activated charcoal has no role in lithium overdose because charcoal does not bind to lithium (option C) (Timmer and Sands 1999). There is nothing in this scenario to suggest coingestion, thus no justification for using activated charcoal alone. Potassium supplementation would not be indicated because the patient's T waves are inverted due to lithium toxicity, not because of hypokalemia (option D). **(Hales RE, Yudofsky SC, Roberts LW [eds]: APP Textbook of Psychiatry, 6th Edition, Chapter 27, pp. 958–961 and Tables 27–9, 27–10, pp. 959, 960)**

29.8   Which of the following antidepressants has been associated with dose-dependent QTc interval prolongation, resulting in a U.S. Food and Drug Administration (FDA) warning about its use?

   A. Bupropion.
   B. Citalopram.
   C. Duloxetine.
   D. Fluoxetine.
   E. Venlafaxine.

The correct response is option B: Citalopram.

In 2011, the FDA announced that there had been reports of citalopram causing dose-dependent QTc interval prolongation (option B) and torsades de pointes (Vieweg et al. 2012). The FDA advised that citalopram should no longer be prescribed at doses greater than 40 mg/day, and no greater than 20 mg/day for patients who have hepatic impairment, who are older than 60 years of age, who are poor metabolizers of cytochrome P450 2C19, or who are taking concomitant cimetidine. Citalopram should not be prescribed in patients with the congenital long QT syndrome. Caution is also advised in treating patients with other risk factors for QTc prolongation (e.g., hypocalcemia, hypomagnesemia, or with other QTc-prolonging drugs). No other antidepressants (options A, C, D, E) have specifically been found to cause QTc interval prolongation necessitating an FDA warning. **(Hales RE, Yudofsky SC, Roberts LW [eds]: APP Textbook of Psychiatry, 6th Edition, Chapter 27, pp. 972–974)**

29.9   Which of the following antipsychotics is approved by the FDA for vocal and motor tics in children and adults with Tourette's syndrome?

   A. Olanzapine.
   B. Risperidone.
   C. Haloperidol.
   D. Ziprasidone.
   E. Quetiapine.

The correct response is option C: Haloperidol.

Haloperidol (option C) and pimozide are the only medications that are approved by the FDA for vocal and motor tics in children and adults with Tourette's syndrome. Options A, B, D, and E do have some research to support use in treating Tourette's syndrome, but they do not have this indication. **(Hales RE, Yudofsky SC, Roberts LW [eds]: APP Textbook of Psychiatry, 6th Edition, Chapter 27, p. 936 and Table 27–3, pp. 937–942; Chapter 34, p. 1211)**

29.10 Which of the following antipsychotic medications is *least* likely to prolong the QTc interval?

A. Haloperidol.
B. Aripiprazole.
C. Thioridazine.
D. Ziprasidone.
E. Droperidol.

The correct response is option B: Aripiprazole.

All antipsychotics may prolong the QT interval, with the possible exception of aripiprazole (option B). Haloperidol (option A), droperidol (option E), thioridazine (option C), sertindole, and ziprasidone (option D) tend to produce greater magnitude QT prolongation than other agents (Glassman and Bigger 2001; Stöllberger et al. 2005). QT interval prolongation corrected for heart rate (QTc) greater than 500 msec is associated with increased risk of polymorphic sustained ventricular tachycardia (torsades de pointes), which can degenerate into ventricular fibrillation. **(Hales RE, Yudofsky SC, Roberts LW [eds]: APP Textbook of Psychiatry, 6th Edition, Chapter 27, p. 950)**

29.11 Weight gain is a common and problematic side effect of mood stabilizers. Which of the following mood stabilizers is associated with the greatest degree of weight gain?

A. Gabapentin.
B. Carbamazepine.
C. Topiramate.
D. Lamotrigine.
E. Valproate.

The correct response is option E: Valproate.

Weight gain is a common factor leading to noncompliance (Mendlewicz et al. 1999). Weight gain is especially a problem with valproate (option E), with an average weight gain of more than 8% of baseline body weight (Chengappa et al. 2002). Gabapentin (option A) causes a 1% weight gain (Wang et al. 2002). Although carbamazepine (option B) is also reported to cause weight gain, the incidence is less than with valproate (Corman et al. 1997). Lamotrigine (option D) has little effect on weight (Biton et al. 2001), whereas topiramate (option C) causes a weight loss of about 0.7% of body weight (Chengappa et al. 2002). **(Levenson JL [ed]: APP Textbook of Psychosomatic Medicine: Psychiatric Care of the Medically Ill, 2nd Edition, Chapter 38, p. 975)**

29.12 Which of the following atypical antipsychotics is associated with the lowest risk of extrapyramidal symptoms (EPS)?

A. Ziprasidone.
B. Quetiapine.
C. Aripiprazole.
D. Risperidone.
E. Asenapine.

The correct response is option B: Quetiapine.

Acute EPS—akathisia, akinesia, and dystonia—occur in up to 50%–75% of patients who take typical antipsychotics (Collaborative Working Group on Clinical Trial Evaluations 1998). High-potency typical antipsychotics are associated with higher rates of EPS than are low-potency agents. Among the currently available atypical antipsychotics, the hierarchy of EPS risk (greater to lesser) is ziprasidone (option A)>aripiprazole (option C)>risperidone (option D)=paliperidone (estimated)>asenapine (option E) (estimated)>iloperidone (estimated) >olanzapine>quetiapine (option B)>clozapine (Citrome 2009; Gao et al. 2008; Tandon 2002; Weber and McCormack 2009). Therefore of the choices given, quetiapine (option B), has the lowest risk of EPS. **(Levenson JL [ed]: APP Textbook of Psychosomatic Medicine: Psychiatric Care of the Medically Ill, 2nd Edition, Chapter 38, p. 976)**

29.13 Which of the following nonbenzodiazepine sedatives is a melatonin agonist?

A. Eszopiclone.
B. Zopiclone.
C. Ramelteon.
D. Zolpidem.
E. Zaleplon.

The correct response is option C: Ramelteon.

Ramelteon (option C), a melatonin agonist approved by the FDA for insomnia, demonstrated efficacy for insomnia with no next-morning residual effects, an adverse-effect profile similar to that of placebo, and no withdrawal symptoms upon discontinuation in a 6-month controlled clinical trial (Mayer et al. 2009). Eszopiclone, zopiclone, zolpidem, and zaleplon (options A, B, D, E) are all very well tolerated hypnotics with a short half-life and very few dose-related adverse effects, although they operate through a different mechanism. **(Levenson JL [ed]: APP Textbook of Psychosomatic Medicine: Psychiatric Care of the Medically Ill, 2nd Edition, Chapter 38, p. 981)**

29.14 A 36-year-old man with chronic schizophrenia has had minimal relief of symptoms with three antipsychotic trials. At best, he has experienced partial relief from positive symptoms of schizophrenia but no relief from negative symptoms of schizophrenia. You are considering recommending clozapine for him. What is the correct regimen of blood count monitoring for patients taking clozapine?

A. Weekly red blood cell counts during the first 3 months of treatment, followed by bimonthly counts.
B. Weekly red blood cell and white blood cell counts during the first 3 months of treatment, followed by bimonthly counts.
C. Weekly white blood cell counts during the first 6 months of treatment, followed by biweekly counts.
D. Weekly platelet counts during the first year of treatment and then monthly counts.
E. Bimonthly plasma cell counts.

The correct response is option C: Weekly white blood cell counts during the first 6 months of treatment, followed by biweekly counts.

Agranulocytosis has been estimated to occur in 0.8% of patients receiving clozapine during the first year of treatment, with a peak incidence at 3 months. Clozapine dispensing is linked to weekly white blood cell counts during the first 6 months of treatment and biweekly counts thereafter (option C). Treatment guidelines do not support checking red blood cell counts (options A, B), platelet counts (option D), or plasma cell counts (option E). **(Hales RE, Yudofsky SC, Roberts LW [eds]: APP Textbook of Psychiatry, 6th Edition, Chapter 27, p. 953 and Table 27–7, p. 954)**

29.15 A 29-year-old woman with chronic generalized anxiety disorder and a history of alcohol abuse has achieved partial remission with fluoxetine 60 mg/day. You are reluctant to increase the dose and are considering adding another medication for adjunctive treatment of her anxiety disorder. Which of the following medications would be appropriate in this case?

A. Aripiprazole.
B. Gabapentin.
C. Quetiapine.
D. Olanzapine.
E. Risperidone.

The correct response is option B: Gabapentin.

Gabapentin (option B) and pregabalin have somewhat limited evidence for efficacy in treating anxiety disorders, although they are sometimes used as an alternative to benzodiazepines, often as an adjunct to antidepressants. There is some, at present very limited, evidence that atypical antipsychotics (e.g., quetiapine, risperidone) may be efficacious as monotherapy or as an adjunct to antidepressants for treatment-resistant anxiety disorders (options A, C, D, E) (Depping et al. 2010). **(Hales RE, Yudofsky SC, Roberts LW [eds]: APP Textbook of Psychiatry, 6th Edition, Chapter 12, p. 425)**

29.16 A 56-year-old woman with chronic alcohol dependence has achieved periods of sobriety following residential treatment for up to a few months at a time. She attended 12-step groups regularly; however, these interventions have not been sufficient in keeping her from craving alcohol or from relapsing to alcohol when things get more stressful. You are considering a pharmacological option to help her manage her alcohol use disorder. With consideration for efficacy and tolerability, which of the following medications has the most evidence to support its use?

A. Acamprosate.
B. Bupropion.
C. Fluoxetine.
D. Naltrexone.
E. Oxcarbazepine.

The correct response is option D: Naltrexone.

A Cochrane review on pharmacological treatment of alcohol use disorders suggests optimum efficiency and tolerability with naltrexone (option D) (Rösner et al. 2010). Acamprosate (option A) has also been studied for this indication, but the evidence to support its use is less robust. Bupropion (option B), fluoxetine (option C), and oxcarbazepine (option E) may have value in treating comorbid psychiatric conditions, but they are not used in the treatment of chronic alcohol dependence. **(Hales RE, Yudofsky SC, Roberts LW [eds]: APP Textbook of Psychiatry, 6th Edition, Chapter 23, pp. 753–754 and Table 23–11, p. 753)**

29.17 A 73-year-old nursing home resident with moderate to severe dementia experiences intermittent episodes of agitation, most commonly at times when staff encourage and assist him with bathing and grooming. As a result of the agitation, the patient is not receiving optimal care, although the agitation is not so severe as to seriously compromise patient or staff safety. The patient is receiving sertraline 100 mg/day and donepezil 10 mg/day. You are considering prescribing risperidone 0.25 mg for use as needed to address periods of agitation. This is an off-label use of this medication. In this case, which of the following side effects is particularly important to discuss with the patient's next of kin prior to obtaining consent and prescribing the medication?

A. Constipation.
B. Death.
C. Headache.

D. Dizziness.

E. Xerostomia.

The correct response is option B: Death.

The FDA has issued a black box warning on off-label use of antipsychotic medications in elderly patients with dementia because of the increased risk of death (option B). Therefore, this is a key side effect to review with the patient's alternate decision maker. Constipation (option A), headache (option C), dizziness (option D), and xerostomia (option E) are all possible side effects with antipsychotics, but these are nonspecific to use of risperidone in this patient population and clearly are not as serious as death. **(Hales RE, Yudofsky SC, Roberts LW [eds]: APP Textbook of Psychiatry, 6th Edition, Chapter 27, p. 952)**

29.18 You are taking care of a 28-year-old man with schizophrenia who has had paranoid thoughts and feelings. You have been seeing him once a month for about 3 years and feel that he is starting to trust you; however, he has intermittently stopped taking the prescribed oral antipsychotic medication that you have prescribed. You have tried two different antipsychotics as well as clozapine. You have a discussion about long-acting injectable (LAI) neuroleptic medication. What is the major and significant issue to discuss with him about the LAI?

A. Whether he trusts that the LAI will be helpful.

B. Whether he wants to see another psychiatrist.

C. How his cultural background may affect his decision.

D. How his childhood might have led to the diagnosis of schizophrenia.

E. Why he could not tolerate clozapine.

The correct response is option A: Whether he trusts that the LAI will be helpful.

There is extensive literature about difficulties in using long-acting depot neuroleptics, mostly centered on the therapeutic alliance and problems with patients who become mistrustful or paranoid about such forms of treatment (option A). It is very important to help patients with schizophrenia adhere to their medication regimen, especially because it is often difficult to find the right type and dose of medication, as well as to watch for side effects. The therapeutic alliance is particularly important when a long-acting medication is being provided. Option B is relevant if the therapeutic alliance is broken. That this patient has been keeping appointments for 3 years implies that the therapeutic alliance is still strong. Option E is relevant if the prescriber is considering a repeat trial of clozapine or if the patient draws a parallel between using the LAI medication and his prior experience with clozapine. Cultural background (option C) and childhood experiences (option D) are not relevant to prescribing antipsychotic medications. **(Hales RE, Yudofsky SC, Roberts LW [eds]: APP Textbook of Psychiatry, 6th Edition, Chapter 9, p. 291; Chapter 27, Table 27–1, p. 931)**

29.19 An 8-year-old girl with difficulty attending at school and at home also has trouble remembering instructions. She gets into trouble for fidgeting in her seat and for talking with her peers when she is supposed to be paying attention in class. She exhibits involuntary movements of her eyebrows and hands that she is able to suppress for a short time. These movements are distressing and embarrassing for her. Which of the following treatment options for attention-deficit/hyperactivity disorder (ADHD) is most appropriate for this patient?

A. Amphetamine salts.
B. Fluoxetine.
C. Clonidine.
D. Gabapentin.
E. Methylphenidate.

The correct response is option C: Clonidine.

Clonidine has efficacy for management of ADHD and low likelihood of exacerbating tics (option C). Amphetamine salts (option A) and methylphenidate (option E) can be used to treat ADHD, but they have a higher likelihood of exacerbating tics. Fluoxetine (option B) and gabapentin (option D) have no role in treating ADHD. **(Hales RE, Yudofsky SC, Roberts LW [eds]: APP Textbook of Psychiatry, 6th Edition, Chapter 27, p. 986 and Table 27–17, pp. 982–984)**

29.20 A 67-year-old man with chronic paranoid schizophrenia had been stable on oral medications. He is hospitalized with an ileus and is placed on bowel rest with nothing through the mouth. The surgical team is worried that he will become psychotic when not taking medication. Which of the following medications would be appropriate in this case?

A. Olanzapine.
B. Aripiprazole.
C. Risperidone.
D. Asenapine.
E. Perphenazine.

The correct response is option D: Asenapine.

The only medication with a sublingual formulation is asenapine (option D). Olanzapine (option A), aripiprazole (option B), and risperidone (option C) do have orally dissolving tablet formulations, but these formulations are still enterically absorbed. Olanzapine has intramuscular options; however, these are not preferred over a sublingual option because of the pain involved in receiving an injection. Perphenazine (option E) does not have an orally dissolving tablet formulation or a sublingual formulation. **(Hales RE, Yudofsky SC, Roberts LW [eds]: APP Textbook of Psychiatry, 6th Edition, Chapter 27, p. 943 and Table 27–3, pp. 937–942)**

29.21 A 46-year-old man with bipolar II disorder has chronic migraines. His neurologist recently added an antiepileptic medication to his regimen. During his most recent clinic visit, he complained of feeling that his memory was worse On examination, he seemed to be experiencing more psychomotor retardation and difficulty with sequencing. You suspect that the new antiepileptic medication is to blame for these mental status findings. Which of the following is the medication that was most likely added by the neurologist?

A. Gabapentin.
B. Lamotrigine.
C. Valproate.
D. Topiramate.
E. Pregabalin.

The correct response is option D: Topiramate.

Valproate has been extensively used over several decades; thus, its adverse-effect profile is well characterized (DeVane 2003; Prevey et al. 1996). In a large 1-year placebo-controlled study in bipolar disorder, tremor and reported weight gain were the only symptoms more commonly seen with divalproex than with placebo (option C) (DeVane 2003). Gabapentin has a highly desirable side-effect profile that has been remarkably consistent among the controlled studies of diverse disease states. Sedation, drowsiness, and dizziness have always been reported, and ataxia, dry mouth, infection, and asthenia have been reported in at least one placebo-controlled study (option A). In general, the side effects commonly occurring with pregabalin treatment have been mild and not associated with a severity sufficient to warrant drug discontinuation. The most frequently reported symptoms have been dizziness, sedation, dry mouth, edema, blurred vision, weight gain, and concentration difficulty (option E). The most common side effects of topiramate in the large registration trials for migraine headache (which used total daily doses of 50, 100, and 200 mg) were paresthesias, fatigue, memory difficulties, concentration/attention problems, and mood problems (Bussone et al. 2006). In the monotherapy trials in adult mania, paresthesias, decreased appetite, dry mouth, and weight loss were more common with topiramate than placebo (Kushner et al. 2006). Overall, paresthesias and cognitive complaints are the most troublesome adverse events with topiramate (van Passel et al. 2006). A meta-analysis suggested that a dose-response relationship exists for dizziness, cognitive impairment, and fatigue (Zaccara et al. 2008). Topiramate may be associated with more cognitive impairment than some of the other new antiepileptic drugs (Martin et al. 1999; Meador et al. 2003). In controlled monotherapy trials of lamotrigine in the treatment of mood disorders, the drug has been associated with headache, changes in sleep habits, nausea, and dizziness (option B) (Bowden et al. 2004). Among the possible antiepileptic medications listed, topiramate has the highest risk of cognitive side effects (option D) (Javed et al. 2015). **(Schatzberg AF, Nemeroff CB [eds]: Essentials of Clinical Psychopharmacology, 3rd Edition, Chapter 27, p. 446; Chapter 29, pp. 488, 493; Chapter 31, pp. 502, 514–515; Seizure 29:34–40, 2015)**

References

Biton V, Mirza W, Montouris G, et al: Weight change associated with valproate and lamotrigine monotherapy in patients with epilepsy. Neurology 56(2):172–177, 2001 11160951

Bowden CL, Asnis GM, Ginsberg LD, et al: Safety and tolerability of lamotrigine for bipolar disorder. Drug Saf 27(3):173–184, 2004 14756579

Bussone G, Usai S, D'Amico D: Topiramate in migraine prophylaxis: data from a pooled analysis and open-label extension study. Neurol Sci 27 (suppl 2):159–163, 2006 16688622

Chengappa KN, Chalasani L, Brar JS, et al: Changes in body weight and body mass index among psychiatric patients receiving lithium, valproate, or topiramate: an open-label, nonrandomized chart review. Clin Ther 24(10):1576–1584, 2002 12462287

Citrome L: Iloperidone for schizophrenia: a review of the efficacy and safety profile for this newly commercialised second-generation antipsychotic. Int J Clin Pract 63(8):1237–1248, 2009 19624791

Collaborative Working Group on Clinical Trial Evaluations: Assessment of EPS and tardive dyskinesia in clinical trials. J Clin Psychiatry 59(Suppl 12):23–27, 1998 9766616

Corman CL, Leung NM, Guberman AH: Weight gain in epileptic patients during treatment with valproic acid: a retrospective study. Can J Neurol Sci 24(3):240–244, 1997 9276111

Depping AM, Komossa K, Kissling W, et al: Second-generation antipsychotics for anxiety disorders. Cochrane Database of Systematic Reviews 2010, Issue 12. Art. No.: KCD008120. DOI:10.1002/14651858.CD008120.pub2

DeVane CL: Pharmacokinetics, drug interactions and tolerability of valproate. Psychopharmacol Bull 37 (suppl 2):25–42, 2003 14624231

Gao K, Kemp DE, Ganocy SJ, et al: Antipsychotic-induced extrapyramidal side effects in bipolar disorder and schizophrenia: a systematic review. J Clin Psychopharmacol 28(2):203–209, 2008 18344731

Glassman AH, Bigger JT Jr: Antipsychotic drugs: prolonged QTc interval, torsade de pointes, and sudden death. Am J Psychiatry 158(11):1774–1782, 2001 11691681

Gurrera RJ, Caroff SN, Cohen A, et al: An international consensus study of neuroleptic malignant syndrome diagnostic criteria using the Delphi method. J Clin Psychiatry 72(9):1222–1228, 2011 21733489

Javed A, Cohen B, Detyniecki K, et al: Rates and predictors of patient-reported cognitive side effects of antiepileptic drugs: An extended follow-up. Seizure 29:34–40, 2015 26076842

Kushner SF, Khan A, Lane R, et al: Topiramate monotherapy in the management of acute mania: results of four double-blind placebo-controlled trials. Bipolar Disord 8(1):15–27, 2006 16411977

Martin R, Kuzniecky R, Ho S, et al: Cognitive effects of topiramate, gabapentin, and lamotrigine in healthy young adults. Neurology 52(2):321–327, 1999 9932951

Mayer G, Wang-Weigand S, Roth-Schechter B, et al: Efficacy and safety of 6-month nightly ramelteon administration in adults with chronic primary insomnia. Sleep 32(3):351–360, 2009 19294955

Meador KJ, Loring DW, Hulihan JF, et al; CAPSS-027 Study Group: Differential cognitive and behavioral effects of topiramate and valproate. Neurology 60(9):1483–1488, 2003 12743236

Mendlewicz J, Souery D, Rivelli SK: Short-term and long-term treatment for bipolar patients: beyond the guidelines. J Affect Disord 55(1):79–85, 1999 10512611

Prevey ML, Delaney RC, Cramer JA, et al: Effect of valproate on cognitive functioning: comparison with carbamazepine. The Department of Veteran Affairs Epilepsy Cooperative Study 264 Group. Arch Neurol 53(10):1008–1016, 1996 8859063

Rösner S, Hackl-Herrwerth A, Leucht S, et al: Opioid antagonists for alcohol dependence. Cochrane Database Syst Rev (12):CD001867, 2010 21154349

Stöllberger C, Huber JO, Finsterer J: Antipsychotic drugs and QT prolongation. Int Clin Psychopharmacol 20(5):243–251, 2005 16096514

Tandon R: Safety and tolerability: how do newer generation "atypical" antipsychotics compare? Psychiatr Q 73(4):297–311, 2002 12418358

Timmer RT, Sands JM: Lithium intoxication. J Am Soc Nephrol 10(3):666–674, 1999 10073618

van Passel L, Arif H, Hirsch LJ: Topiramate for the treatment of epilepsy and other nervous system disorders. Expert Rev Neurother 6(1):19–31, 2006 16466308

Vieweg WV, Hasnain M, Howland RH, et al: Citalopram, QTc interval prolongation, and torsade de pointes. How should we apply the recent FDA ruling? Am J Med 125(9):859–868, 2012 22748401

Wang PW, Santosa C, Schumacher M, et al: Gabapentin augmentation therapy in bipolar depression. Bipolar Disord 4(5):296–301, 2002 12479661

Weber J, McCormack PL: Asenapine. CNS Drugs 23(9):781–792, 2009 19689168

Zaccara G, Gangemi PF, Cincotta M: Central nervous system adverse effects of new antiepileptic drugs. A meta-analysis of placebo-controlled studies. Seizure 17(5):405–421, 2008 18262442

CHAPTER 30

Psychosocial Interventions

30.1   Which of the following psychosocial interventions has been shown to reduce relapse rates in patients with schizophrenia?

A. Personal therapy.
B. Compliance therapy.
C. Supported employment.
D. Family psychoeducation.
E. Social skills training.

The correct response is option D: Family psychoeducation.

The American Psychiatric Association recommends family psychoeducation (option D) for individuals with schizophrenia who are in regular contact with family members or significant others (Dixon et al. 2009). Family psychoeducation includes family support, education, crisis intervention, problem-solving skills training, and coping skills training. When delivered for 6–9 months, it can improve patients' and family members' knowledge of the illness, improve treatment adherence, improve social and vocational outcomes, increase perceptions of professional and social support, reduce relapse rates, and reduce family burden (Dixon et al. 2009). Personal and compliance therapies (options A, B), supported employment (option C), and social skills training (option E) have not been shown to reduce relapse rates. **(Hales RE, Yudofsky SC, Weiss L, et al [eds]: APP Textbook of Psychiatry, 6th Edition, Chapter 9, pp. 299–300)**

30.2   Which of the following is an example of a psychosocial intervention for a patient with schizophrenia?

A. Long-acting injectable antipsychotic.
B. Combination of antidepressant and antipsychotic medications.
C. Assertive community treatment.
D. Long-term hospitalization.
E. Psychological testing.

The correct response is option C: Assertive community treatment.

The American Psychiatric Association recommends several social interventions for patients with schizophrenia: assertive community treatment (option C), supported employment, and social skills training. Assertive community treatment is recommended particularly for individuals who are frequently hospitalized. The model uses a multidisciplinary team that includes a medication prescriber. Team members share a caseload, and there is a low patient-to-staff ratio. The team provides direct patient services, frequently contacts patients, and performs outreach to patients in the community (Dixon et al. 2010). Assertive community treatment has been shown to reduce hospitalization rates and homelessness among patients with schizophrenia (Dixon et al. 2009). Options A and B are psychopharmacological rather than psychosocial interventions. Long-term hospitalization (option D) and psychological testing (option E) are not indicated for all patients with schizophrenia. **(Hales RE, Yudofsky SC, Weiss L, et al [eds]: APP Textbook of Psychiatry, 6th Edition, Chapter 9, p. 300)**

30.3   What is the core principle of supported employment for patients with schizophrenia?

  A. All patients should work whether they want to or not.
  B. What the person does in terms of employment does not matter.
  C. Taking a long period of time to find a job is essential.
  D. Any person who wants to work should be offered assistance.
  E. Once the person has the job, he or she no longer needs assistance.

The correct response is option D: Any person who wants to work should be offered assistance.

The core principle of supported employment is that any person with schizophrenia who wants to work should be offered assistance in obtaining and maintaining employment (option D). The supported employment model uses individually tailored job development (emphasizing patient preference and choice; options A, B), a rapid job search (option C), ongoing job supports (option E), and integration of vocational and mental health services (Dixon et al. 2010). It is effective for helping persons with schizophrenia obtain competitive employment, earn more wages, and work more hours (Dixon et al. 2009). **(Hales RE, Yudofsky SC, Weiss L, et al [eds]: APP Textbook of Psychiatry, 6th Edition, Chapter 9, p. 300)**

30.4   Which of the following statements regarding 12-step mutual-help organizations (MHOs) is true?

  A. There is extensive randomized-control trial evidence to support their efficacy.
  B. They extend the benefits of professionally delivered treatment for substance use disorders (SUDs).
  C. The magnitude of benefit is significantly lower than that achieved with professional intervention efforts.

D. People with dual diagnoses are unlikely to benefit from attendance.

E. They are most beneficial as a short-term adjunct to outpatient professional intervention efforts.

The correct response is option B: They extend the benefits of professionally delivered treatment for substance use disorders (SUDs).

Naturalistic studies support the role of 12-step programs as an important adjunct to professional care, especially as continuing care, and in helping to protect against relapse. They extend the benefits of professional delivered treatment for SUDs (option B). Twelve-step MHOs are not ideally suited for efficacy research through randomized controlled trials, because real-world participation usually is self-initiated and voluntary (except when court mandated), and randomly assigning individuals to attend these groups (or not) would conflict with the purpose of the groups and the way they are typically used (option A). Twelve-step attendance provides recovery benefits that are on par with the magnitude of those seen with professional intervention efforts (option C) (Kaskutas 2009). Subgroups of patients, such as those with dual diagnoses, may benefit from participation in traditional MHOs, but these benefits may be enhanced by attending groups tailored to their specific needs (option D). Although even short-term attendance may provide some benefits, naturalistic studies suggest that 12-step groups can serve as an important adjunct to professional care, especially as continuing care (option E). **(Galanter M, Kleber HD, Brady KT [eds]: APP Textbook of Substance Abuse Treatment, 5th Edition, Chapter 38, pp. 580–581)**

30.5 Twelve-step facilitation (TSF) is a professionally delivered intervention designed to support engagement with MHOs such as Alcoholics Anonymous (AA). Which of the following patient characteristics is most important to consider when deciding whether to provide a standard or intensive referral to a 12-step group?

A. Age.

B. Gender.

C. Spiritual beliefs.

D. Prior experience with 12-step programs.

E. Comorbid psychiatric diagnosis.

The correct response is option D: Prior experience with 12-step programs.

Studies of which intensity of referral is most likely to benefit patients have reported that individuals with prior AA experience tend to have better outcomes when given brief advice, whereas outcomes among those with no or limited AA experience tend to be better (e.g., greater attendance rates) when more intensive referrals are provided (option D). Patient age (option A), gender (option B), spiritual beliefs (or lack thereof; option C), and presence of dual diagnosis (option E) all are important for the clinician to take into account when recommending a particular 12-step program to an individual patient. The available empirical evidence suggests that, in general, these patient subgroups can benefit from participation in traditional 12-step MHOs but that benefits may be enhanced by attending groups that are more tailored to their specific needs. **(Galanter M, Kleber HD, Brady KT [eds]: APP Textbook of Substance Abuse Treatment, 5th Edition, Chapter 38, pp. 581, 584)**

30.6   Which cognitive MHO mechanism of change is most strongly associated with recovery in adolescents?

A. Enhanced self-efficacy.
B. Identifying coping strategies.
C. Motivation for abstinence.
D. Increased religiosity.
E. Reduction in anger.

The correct response is option C: Motivation for abstinence.

MHOs, including AA, work both through mechanisms similar to those operating in professional treatment, including cognitive, affective, and social network mechanisms, and through mechanisms more specific to MHOs, such as 12-step activities and spiritual mechanisms. Both single- and multiple-mediator studies have been conducted to determine the relative importance of these factors in explaining AA's effects, as well as in identifying specific interventions that may be of special benefit to particular patient subgroups. Self-efficacy, coping strategies, and motivation for abstinence all are cognitive MHO mechanisms. Research in adolescents has found that motivation for abstinence mediates both the effect of early AA attendance after inpatient treatment and subsequent substance use outcomes (option C); self-efficacy and coping (options A, B) were not found to mediate these effects in adolescents (Kelly et al. 2000). Increased religiosity (option D) falls in the spiritual rather than cognitive mechanism category and is associated with better outcomes among patients with the most severe alcohol impairments. It has been hypothesized that 12-step groups exert their effects through mitigating unpleasant affective states, such as anger and depression. Affective (option E), rather than cognitive, strategies aimed at reducing anger have not been found to mediate the relationship between AA attendance and improved drinking outcomes (Kelly et al. 2010). **(Galanter M, Kleber HD, Brady KT [eds]: APP Textbook of Substance Abuse Treatment, 5th Edition, Chapter 38, pp. 586–589)**

30.7   MHO participation has been associated with which of the following?

A. Increased health care costs.
B. Increased patient reliance on professional services.
C. Abstinence rate one-third lower than that achieved by patients treated in cognitive-behavioral therapy (CBT) programs.
D. Improved outcomes in adults but not in adolescents.
E. Helping individuals change their social networks in support of recovery.

The correct response is option E: Helping individuals change their social networks in support of recovery.

MHOs, such as AA, work through mechanisms similar to those operating in professional treatment but work most powerfully by helping individuals change their social networks in support of recovery (option E). Mutual-help groups can be attended for as long as necessary at little or no cost (option A). Research has shown that involvement in 12-step organizations can reduce the need for more costly professional treatments (option B) while simultaneously improving outcomes. Patients treated in 12-step–oriented professional treatment programs have been shown to have a roughly one-third *higher* rate of abstinence than those treated in CBT programs (option C) (Humphreys and Moos 2001, 2007). Adolescents attending 12-step programs have been shown to achieve similar benefits to those found in adult participants (option D), including improved substance use outcomes and lower overall medical costs. **(Galanter M, Kleber HD, Brady KT [eds]: APP Textbook of Substance Abuse Treatment, 5th Edition, Chapter 38, pp. 582, 590)**

30.8 What was the clinical significance of the CASA Substance Abuse Research Demonstration (CASASARD) study?

A. Intensive Case Management (ICM) clients were significantly more likely to have completed treatment, be abstinent from substances, and be employed than those who received the usual screening and referral to treatment.
B. Drug courts showed significant reduction in drug and alcohol use and improved family relationships.
C. Brief motivational interviewing techniques increased tobacco quit rates 2%–8% compared to brief advice.
D. In substance-abusing individuals, approaches using therapeutic communities, psychosocial rehabilitation, 12-step programs, and enhancement of supportive relationships were all successful.
E. Adding a family-based treatment component to a family treatment drug court (FTDC) program was shown to improve the chances that an at-risk child would remain in the family.

The correct response is option A: Intensive Case Management (ICM) clients were significantly more likely to have completed treatment, be abstinent from substances, and be employed than those who received the usual screening and referral to treatment.

CASASARD was a model ICM program that provided substance-abusing women with longitudinal involvement with two case managers who performed a variety of functions. At 24 months, ICM clients were significantly more likely to have completed treatment, be abstinent from substances, and be employed than those who received the usual screening and referral to treatment (option A) (National Center on Addiction and Substance Abuse at Columbia University 2009). Data from the Multisite Adult Drug Court Evaluation showed significant reduction in drug and alcohol use and improved family relationships as a result of drug courts (option B) (Huddleston and Marlowe 2011). According to Fiore and Baker (2011), 70% of smokers visit a primary care physician annually, and recording smoking as a vital sign identifies over 80% of smokers at an office visit. In the health care setting, brief motivational interviewing techniques increase quit rates from 2% to 8% compared to brief advice (option C). In substance-abusing individuals, approaches using therapeutic communities, psychosocial rehabilitation, 12-step program, and enhancement of supportive relationships have all been successful (option D) (Hitchcock et al. 1995; Moos et al. 1999). Adding a family-based treatment component to an FTDC program has also been shown to improve the chances that an at-risk child will remain in the family (option E) (Oliveros and Kaufman 2011). **(Galanter M, Kleber HD, Brady KT [eds]: APP Textbook of Substance Abuse Treatment, 5th Edition, Chapter 35, pp. 532, 535–536, 539–540)**

30.9 Which of the following is true about group therapy for patients with SUDs?

A. Group therapy is used primarily in inpatient and residential settings.
B. Group therapy is only indicated for patients without co-occurring psychiatric disorders.
C. Group therapy may be problematic for use in managed care settings because of cost.
D. Group therapy is not helpful for the symptoms and adverse effects that are the consequences of substance abuse.
E. Group psychotherapy is the psychosocial treatment of choice for most patients with SUDs.

The correct response is option E: Group psychotherapy is the psychosocial treatment of choice for most patients with SUDs.

Because of its therapeutic effectiveness as well as its cost-effectiveness, group therapy plays an ever more important role as the psychosocial treatment of choice for most SUDs, including substance abuse and addiction (option E). Group psychotherapy can be used in a wide variety of treatment settings and can address many of the psychosocial factors involved in the etiology of substance abuse (option A). It can also be used to treat symptoms and adverse effects that are the consequences of substance abuse and dependence and can also treat co-occurring psychiatric disorders that are so common in individuals with SUDs (options B, D) (Flores and Brook 2011). The lower cost of group treatment is helpful in managed care settings (option C). **(Galanter M, Kleber HD, Brady KT [eds]: APP Textbook of Substance Abuse Treatment, 5th Edition, Chapter 31, p. 463)**

30.10 A 36-year-old woman with a severe alcohol use disorder and bipolar I disorder (three past hospitalizations for mania) has started attending AA meetings. She is trying to identify a sponsor. Which of the following traits in a sponsor might be most beneficial for this patient?

A. A sponsor with a similar co-occurring psychiatric disorder.
B. A sponsor with many years of sobriety and experience in AA.
C. A sponsor willing to regularly speak with the patient's psychiatrist about the patient by phone.
D. A sponsor with similar sociodemographic characteristics to the patient.
E. A sponsor who continues to attend meetings at a high frequency.

The correct response is option A: A sponsor with a similar co-occurring psychiatric disorder.

Careful choice of a sponsor can be pivotal in achieving success in 12-step group-based approaches to substance abuse treatment and is a goal of 12-step facilitation techniques. For patients with substance abuse and co-occurring psychiatric illness, finding a sponsor with a similar dual-diagnosis history can be beneficial (option A). Attending AA meetings in which attendees either are unfamiliar with psychiatric illness or discourage the use of psychotropic medications could be very disruptive to this patient with serious mental illness. A sponsor with a history of psychiatric diagnosis and treatment will likely be more open to the unique needs of the patient in question. Many years of sobriety and AA experience (option B) and high-frequency meeting attendance (option E) and similar sociodemographic characteristics (option D) may be useful traits in a sponsor, especially depending on the patient in question, but do not address the needs of the patient as specifically as having a similar co-occurring disorder. Communication between the psychiatrist and the patient's sponsor, if any, should be done with the patient present so as to maintain boundaries and respect the confidentiality of the patient's relationship with the sponsor (option C). **(Galanter M, Kleber HD, Brady KT [eds]: APP Textbook of Substance Abuse Treatment, 5th Edition, Chapter 28, p. 418)**

30.11 What is an effective target of contingency management (CM) treatment for substance abuse disorders as demonstrated by research studies?

A. Doing homework assignments in CBT.
B. Looking for a job.
C. Finding a sober friend.
D. Entering treatment.
E. Going to an AA meeting.

The correct response is option D: Entering treatment.

Paying cash rewards contingent on attendance of one treatment session increased the probability that patients would enter treatment (option D). Although there are many potentially suitable target behaviors for CM, most have not been researched (options B, C, E). Indeed, not every potentially suitable target behavior proved to be effective in research studies. For example, Carroll et al. (2012) found that reinforcing completion of homework assignments did not improve treatment outcomes of CBT (option A). **(Galanter M, Kleber HD, Brady KT [eds]: APP Textbook of Substance Abuse Treatment, 5th Edition, Chapter 29, pp. 423, 430 and Figure 29–1, p. 424)**

30.12 A company decides to adopt a CM strategy to curb alcohol use among its employees. Most employees who drink alcohol also smoke cigarettes. What is the recommended action for the company to take?

    A. To target only alcohol, because there is no clinically significant relationship between alcohol use and smoking cigarettes.

    B. To target abstinence from all substances to avoid "substitution," namely, increased smoking to compensate for stopping drinking.

    C. To target abstinence from all substances, which is the usual recommendation despite lack of clear research evidence.

    D. To target only smoking, because smoking and drinking are related, smoking cessation is the easier goal to achieve, and dual-substance interventions are not supported by the evidence base.

    E. To seek a non-CM intervention because CM interventions for SUDs are ineffective in company settings because of conflicting interests, including patient confidentiality and employees' fear of repercussion due to treatment failure.

The correct response is option C: To target abstinence from all substances, which is the usual recommendation despite lack of clear research evidence.

Abstinence from all drugs is the usual recommendation in CM interventions (option C). Dual drug targets make clinical sense and have evidence-based effectiveness in CM interventions (options A, D). Interestingly, single drug targets have not resulted in detectable increases of nontarget drug use (i.e., "substitution"; option B). Contingency CM studies have been successfully conducted with employees of companies (option E). **(Galanter M, Kleber HD, Brady KT [eds]: APP Textbook of Substance Abuse Treatment, 5th Edition, Chapter 29, pp. 429, 431)**

References

Carroll KM, Nich C, Shi JM, et al: Efficacy of disulfiram and Twelve Step Facilitation in cocaine-dependent individuals maintained on methadone: a randomized placebo-controlled trial. Drug Alcohol Depend 126(1-2):224–231, 2012 22695473

Dixon L, Perkins D, Calmes C: Guideline Watch for the Practice Guideline for the Treatment of Patients With Schizophrenia. Arlington, VA, American Psychiatric Association, 2009

Dixon LB, Dickerson F, Bellack AS, et al; Schizophrenia Patient Outcomes Research Team (PORT): The 2009 schizophrenia PORT psychosocial treatment recommendations and summary statements. Schizophr Bull 36(1):48–70, 2010 19955389

Fiore MC, Baker TB: Clinical practice. Treating smokers in the health care setting. N Engl J Med 365(13):1222–1231, 2011 21991895

Flores PJ, Brook DW: Group Psychotherapy Approaches to Addiction and Substance Abuse. New York, American Group Psychotherapy Association, 2011

Hitchcock HC, Stainback RD, Roque GM: Effects of halfway house placement on retention of patients in substance abuse aftercare. Am J Drug Alcohol Abuse 21(3):379–390, 1995 7484986

Huddleston W, Marlowe D: Painting the Current Picture: A National Report on Drug Courts and Other Problem Solving Court Programs in the United States. Alexandria, VA, National Drug Court Institute, 2011. Available at: http://www.ndci.org/publications/painting-current-picture. Accessed January 19, 2013.

Humphreys K, Moos R: Can encouraging substance abuse patients to participate in self-help groups reduce demand for health care? A quasi-experimental study. Alcohol Clin Exp Res 25(5):711–716, 2001 11371720

Humphreys K, Moos RH: Encouraging posttreatment self-help group involvement to reduce demand for continuing care services: two-year clinical and utilization outcomes. Alcohol Clin Exp Res 31(1):64–68, 2007 17207103

Kaskutas LA: Alcoholics anonymous effectiveness: faith meets science. J Addict Dis 28(2):145–157, 2009 19340677

Kelly JF, Myers MG, Brown SA: A multivariate process model of adolescent 12-step attendance and substance use outcome following inpatient treatment. Psychol Addict Behav 14(4):376–389, 2000 11130156

Kelly JF, Stout RL, Tonigan JS, et al: Negative affect, relapse, and Alcoholics Anonymous (AA): does AA work by reducing anger? J Stud Alcohol Drugs 71(3):434–444, 2010 20409438

Moos RH, Moos BS, Andrassy JM: Outcomes of four treatment approaches in community residential programs for patients with substance use disorders. Psychiatr Serv 50(12):1577–1583, 1999 10577876

National Center on Addiction and Substance Abuse at Columbia University: CASASARDSM: Intensive Case Management for Substance-Dependent Women Receiving Temporary Assistance for Needy Families: A CASA White Paper. New York, National Center on Addiction and Substance Abuse at Columbia University, 2009. Available at http://www.casacolumbia.org/templates/publications_reports.aspx. Accessed February 25, 2013.

Oliveros A, Kaufman J: Addressing substance abuse treatment needs of parents involved with the child welfare system. Child Welfare 90(1):25–41, 2011 21950173

CHAPTER 31

Psychotherapies

31.1   In research on the treatment of personality disorders (PDs), which of the following is the most robust predictor of treatment outcome?

A. Therapeutic alliance.
B. Duration of therapy.
C. Therapeutic modality.
D. Socioeconomic factors.
E. Self-harm history.

The correct response is option A: Therapeutic alliance.

It is sometimes difficult to determine a priori which patient will benefit from what treatment and with whom, but one factor—therapeutic alliance (option A)—has stood out in the research literature as the most robust predictor of outcome (Horvath et al. 2011; Safran et al. 2011). There are a number of evidence-based, effective brief therapies, so duration of therapy (option B) would not be the most robust predictor of treatment outcome. Additionally, various therapeutic modalities (option C) have a strong evidence base of efficacy. Socioeconomic factors (option D) and self-harm history (option E), although important to address in therapy, do not preclude a beneficial treatment outcome. (**Oldham JM, Skodol AE, Bender DS [eds]: APP Textbook of Personality Disorders, 2nd Edition, Chapter 9, p. 189**)

31.2   When providing therapy to a person with borderline PD (BPD), which of the following approaches carries the greatest risk of rupturing the therapeutic alliance?

A. Supportive psychotherapy.
B. Cognitive-behavioral therapy (CBT).
C. Psychoeducation.
D. Medication management.
E. Transference interpretations.

The correct response is option E: Transference interpretations.

The most challenging therapist intervention with patients with BPD is making a transference interpretation, because examination of transference most intensely challenges the patient's personality difficulties (option E). Supportive therapy (option A), CBT (option B), psychoeducation (option C), and medication management (option D) are typically less emotionally intense than the examination of transference issues. Bond et al. (1998) demonstrated with a group of patients with PDs in long-term treatment that for those patients whose alliance was weak, transference interpretations caused further impairment to the alliance. **(Oldham JM, Skodol AE, Bender DS [eds]: APP Textbook of Personality Disorders, 2nd Edition, Chapter 9, pp. 208–209)**

31.3 During an inpatient hospitalization of a patient with BPD, the treatment team encounters escalating conflict with each other about the treatment. Which of the following is the recommended action?

A. Transfer the patient to a different unit.
B. Change the attending psychiatrist.
C. Have team members independently assess the patient and contribute opinions.
D. Request a second opinion to decide on treatment.
E. Hold a team meeting to communicate and have a common united approach.

The correct response is option E: Hold a team meeting to communicate and have a common united approach.

Conflict between team members as a result of splitting by the patient is common among inpatient teams when treating BPD. Skilled teams will recognize the development of splitting and meet regularly to communicate and to configure a common united treatment approach (option E). The central consideration regarding the alliance in this treatment context is that there is always a team of individuals responsible for the patient. With patients who exhibit borderline pathology, splitting tendencies frequently are quite pronounced. In these cases, communication and close collaboration among the members of a team are vital during every phase of the hospital treatment. Options A, B, C, and D would not address the underlying PD pathology and could in fact reinforce the splitting behavior. **(Oldham JM, Skodol AE, Bender DS [eds]: APP Textbook of Personality Disorders, 2nd Edition, Chapter 9, pp. 211–212)**

31.4 What is a typical way that patients with PDs reveal their pathology that can facilitate group treatment?

A. Describing in words.
B. Demonstrating in interpersonal actions.
C. Dealing with internally.
D. Defending against subconsciously.
E. Deliberating carefully.

The correct response is option B: Demonstrating in interpersonal actions.

Patients with PDs are more likely than patients with various other psychiatric illnesses to demonstrate their pathology in interpersonal exchanges rather than describing it in words, making group therapy especially useful (option B). Patients may be unable to describe (option A), be unaware of, or be unwilling to disclose of their interpersonal limitations and pathology, which may better be noticed as it manifests interpersonally. Dealing internally (option C), defending against subconsciously (option D), and deliberating carefully (option E) are all intrapersonal processes and more mature ways of coping, which do not primarily manifest in an interpersonal relationship context characteristic in PD pathology. Patients with PDs may not be intrapersonally distressed by their internal world, but they are more distressed by limitations in interpersonal interactions with others and the external world. **(Oldham JM, Skodol AE, Bender DS [eds]: APP Textbook of Personality Disorders, 2nd Edition, Chapter 13, p. 283)**

31.5   What is the role of the therapist when a patient is identified as a difficult group member?

A. Ask the patient to leave the group.
B. Discern whether the individual's behavior may be serving a defensive function for the group.
C. Ask the patient during the group why he or she is being difficult so that the group can contribute to the discussion.
D. Avoid bringing attention to the problem so that the patient's feelings are not hurt.
E. Invite the patient to join an alternative group to see if the problems continue.

The correct response is option B: Discern whether the individual's behavior may be serving a defensive function for the group.

At times "difficult" patients in group therapy can engage in behaviors that serve a defensive function for the group (option B). Asking a patient to leave the group (option A) or to join another group (option E) will not resolve the problem if the individual's behavior is serving a defensive function for the group. Care should be taken not to further "scapegoat" an individual during the group by identifying him or her as "difficult" (option C); however, difficult behavior should not be ignored if it is impairing the group's ability to function (option D). **(Oldham JM, Skodol AE, Bender DS [eds]: APP Textbook of Personality Disorders, 2nd Edition, Chapter 13, pp. 283–284)**

31.6   Which of the following is a typical characteristic focus of dialectical behavior therapy (DBT)?

A. Suicidal and self-injurious behaviors.
B. Countertransference.
C. Defense mechanisms.

D. Insecure attachment.

E. Socioeconomic status.

The correct response is option A: Suicidal and self-injurious behaviors.

DBT has been shown to reduce suicidal and self-injurious behavior for patients with BPD (option A) (Chapman 2006). DBT targets these behaviors by teaching a series of skills including distress tolerance, interpersonal effectiveness, emotion regulation, and mindfulness. Countertransference (option B) and defense mechanisms (option C) are focuses and typical features of psychodynamic and psychoanalytic therapy, whereas DBT is a multimodal cognitive-behavioral treatment for BPD. Insecure attachment (option D) refers to attachment theory (Bretherton 1992) and is characteristic of psychodynamic and developmental therapy, not a typical focus of DBT. Socioeconomic status (option E) is not a focus of DBT. (*Developmental Psychology* **28(5):759–775, 1992; Oldham JM, Skodol AE, Bender DS [eds]: APP Textbook of Personality Disorders, 2nd Edition, Chapter 10, pp. 225–226; Chapter 13, pp. 286, 293)**

31.7 Which core component is least consistently found in psychoeducational programs?

A. Education.

B. Problem solving.

C. Social support.

D. Skills training.

E. Bibliotherapy.

The correct response is option B: Problem solving.

Psychoeducation programs serve to 1) educate patients and family members about a particular disorder (option A), 2) teach coping skills and individual and family skills (option D), 3) provide ongoing support to the patient and/or to family members (option C), and 4) offer a problem-solving forum. Not all programs that are designated "psychoeducation" or "family psychoeducation" include all four components listed above, and problem solving (option B) is the component least consistently found in psychoeducational programs. Bibliotherapy (option E), or the recommending or providing of books and reading material, is a common form or component of education of patients and family members. **(Oldham JM, Skodol AE, Bender DS [eds]: APP Textbook of Personality Disorders, 2nd Edition, Chapter 14, pp. 305, 307)**

31.8 In which psychoeducation program does the patient assume the role of coteacher to inform and educate those people important to him or her?

A. Gunderson's Multifamily Groups.

B. Systems Training for Emotional Predictability and Problem Solving (STEPPS).

C. Family Connections.

D. DBT–Family Skills Training (DBT-FST).

E. Certified Peer Specialist Program.

The correct response is option B: Systems Training for Emotional Predictability and Problem Solving (STEPPS).

An essential feature of the STEPPS program (option B) is a systems component that encompasses the patient's environment and important individuals in the patient's life with whom he or she has regular contact. The patient assumes the role of coteacher to inform these individuals about the disorder and also to educate them on skills that are helpful to manage one's emotions more effectively. Family and significant others thus become an integral part of the treatment and are encouraged to attend education and skill sessions to learn ways to support the patient's treatment and to reinforce his or her newly acquired skills. In Gunderson's Multifamily Groups (option A), relatives from one or several families of patients meet with a group leader. Patients rarely participate, and when they do they are not coleaders or coteachers. Family Connections (option C) is a no-cost family education program developed specifically for family members, and patients do not attend. DBT-FST (option D) incorporates family members and patients as learners, so patients are not coteachers. In the Certified Peer Specialist Program (option E), individuals with personal experience in mental illness who have received specific training serve as mentors and advocates to other patients who are further behind in their recovery. **(Oldham JM, Skodol AE, Bender DS [eds]: APP Textbook of Personality Disorders, 2nd Edition, Chapter 14, pp. 315–318)**

31.9 "Attentiveness to thinking and feeling in self and others" defines which of the following terms?

A. Transference.

B. Countertransference.

C. Mentalizing.

D. Psychological mindedness.

E. Mindfulness.

The correct response is option C: Mentalizing.

In plain language, mentalizing (option C) can be characterized as attentiveness to thinking and feeling in self and others—or, in shorthand, as holding mind in mind. *Mentalizing* is technically defined as the natural human imaginative capacity to perceive and interpret behavior in self and others as conjoined with intentional mental states, such as desires, motives, feelings, and beliefs. Transference (option A) and countertransference (option B) are core psychodynamic principles that are not related to the question. *Psychological mindedness* (option D) relates to an individual's capacity for introspection and self-examination. *Mindfulness* relates to present-centered attention (option E). **(Hales RE, Yudofsky SC, Roberts**

LW [eds]: APP Textbook of Psychiatry, 6th Edition, Chapter 30, pp. 1069, 1073; Chapter 31, pp. 1095, 1098)

31.10 The concept of therapeutic alliance is attributed to which of the following people?

A. Gerald Adler.
B. Heinz Kohut.
C. Otto Kernberg.
D. Sigmund Freud.
E. Donald Winnicott.

The correct response is option D: Sigmund Freud.

The concept of the therapeutic alliance is often traced back to Sigmund Freud, who observed very early in his work the need to convey interest in and sympathy to the patient to engage him or her in a collaborative treatment endeavor (Meissner 1996; Safran and Muran 2000). Freud (1912/1958) also delineated an aspect of the transference—the unobjectionable positive transference—which is an attachment that should *not* be analyzed because it serves as the motivation for the patient to collaborate. This is an early precursor to the modern empirical evidence showing that alliance is related to treatment outcome across modalities. **(Oldham JM, Skodol AE, Bender DS [eds]: APP Textbook of Personality Disorders, 2nd Edition, Chapter 9, p. 190)**

31.11 Which of the following psychological mechanisms is/are most central to a psychoanalytic understanding of severe PDs?

A. Repression and reaction formation.
B. Splitting and projective identification.
C. Humor and sublimation.
D. A neurotic level of personality organization.
E. A significant absence of reality testing.

The correct response is option B: Splitting and projective identification.

Primitive defense mechanisms are central features of severe PDs. These primitive defense mechanisms include splitting and projective identification (option B), along with idealization-devaluation, primitive denial, and omnipotent control. Repression and reaction formation (option A) are neurotic defenses; dominance of these mechanisms characterizes the neurotic level of personality organization (option D). Humor and sublimation (option C) are mature defense mechanisms. Patients with severe PDs generally do not have significant absence of reality testing (option E). **(Oldham JM, Skodol AE, Bender DS [eds]: APP Textbook of Personality Disorders, 2nd Edition, Chapter 10, pp. 222–223)**

31.12 Which of the following describes the current American Psychiatric Association (APA) treatment guideline for patients with BPD?

    A. Pharmacotherapy only.
    B. Primary treatment of pharmacotherapy with adjunctive psychotherapy.
    C. Primary treatment of CBT.
    D. Primary treatment of psychotherapy with adjunctive, symptom-targeted pharmacotherapy.
    E. Pharmacotherapy with psychotherapy for anxiety, depressive, or substance abuse disorders as indicated.

The correct response is option D: Primary treatment of psychotherapy with adjunctive, symptom-targeted pharmacotherapy.

According to the American Psychiatric Association (2001) guideline for the treatment of patients with BPD and the subsequent guideline watch (Oldham 2005), psychotherapy is needed to attain and maintain lasting improvement in their personality, interpersonal problems, and overall functioning. Therefore, psychotherapy (not pharmacotherapy; option B) is considered the primary treatment. Pharmacotherapy alone (option A) is not considered the most effective treatment, but a meta-analysis has shown that it plays an important adjunctive role in decreasing the severity of anger, anxiety, impulsivity, and cognitive-perceptual disturbances (Ingenhoven et al. 2010). Therefore, the APA consensus is that patients will benefit most from a combination of these treatments (option D). Primary treatment with CBT (option C) is not recommended because a persuasive review of data from approximately 24 randomized controlled trials of BPD demonstrated clear and compelling evidence that several forms of psychotherapy, including CBT and DBT, help patients with BPD (Leichsenring et al. 2011). Pharmacotherapy with psychotherapy for anxiety, depressive, or substance abuse disorders (option E) does not address the defining features of PD—that is, an overarching pattern of distorted and maladaptive thinking about oneself and impaired interpersonal relationships. **(Oldham JM, Skodol AE, Bender DS [eds]: APP Textbook of Personality Disorders, 2nd Edition, Chapter 12, pp. 262–263; Chapter 15, p. 334)**

31.13 Which of the following is a newer form of CBT that is currently being explored and adapted to treatment of PDs?

    A. Dialectical behavior therapy.
    B. Psychodynamic therapy.
    C. Acceptance and commitment therapy.
    D. Interpersonal therapy.
    E. Schema-focused therapy.

The correct response is option C: Acceptance and commitment therapy.

Acceptance and commitment therapy (option C) (Hayes and Smith 2005) is one of a new wave of cognitive-behavioral interventions that use acceptance and mindfulness strategies to decrease psychological symptoms. Given the empirical evidence on the effectiveness for several disorders, the application of this approach to PDs is being developed and tested. DBT (option A), interpersonal psychotherapy (option D), and schema-focused therapy (option E) are well-established forms of CBT. Psychodynamic therapy (option B) is a well-established intervention that is separate and distinct from CBT. **(Oldham JM, Skodol AE, Bender DS [eds]: APP Textbook of Personality Disorders, 2nd Edition, Chapter 11, p. 241; Chapter 12, p. 268)**

31.14 Which of the following therapeutic strategies is likely to be employed during a brief psychodynamic therapy session?

A. The therapist emphasizes that change cannot occur until the patient develops full insight into his or her drives.
B. The therapist focuses on historical patterns within the therapeutic relationship.
C. The therapist takes a passive role in the therapeutic process.
D. The therapist involves himself or herself in the core conflictual relationship patterns.
E. The therapist uses interpretation as the chief therapeutic tool.

The correct response is option D: The therapist involves himself or herself in the core conflictual relationship patterns.

In brief psychodynamic therapy, change is catalyzed by the involvement of the therapist in core relationship patterns (option D), breaking the cycles of repetition by providing responses different from those anticipated by patients (Levenson 1995). Although psychodynamic brief therapies retain the theoretical and conceptual heritage of psychoanalysis, there are some important operational modifications. Brief dynamic therapists do not rely on interpretation (option E), lengthy exploration of the past (option B), or the development of insight (option A) as necessary sources of change. By the therapist limiting the work to a circumscribed "here-and-now" focus and attending to the "core conflictual relationship themes" (Luborsky and Mark 1991), and being active in the therapeutic process (option C), short-term psychodynamic therapy can accelerate the rate of change and decrease the number of treatment sessions. **(Hales RE, Yudofsky SC, Roberts LW [eds]: APP Textbook of Psychiatry, 6th Edition, Chapter 29, pp. 1039–1041)**

31.15 A patient in psychodynamic psychotherapy describes being angry with his boss, upon whom he is dependent for employment and financial stability. However, instead of expressing the anger to his boss, he screamed at one of his children over a minor offense later in the day. What defense mechanism is illustrated?

A. Denial.
B. Displacement.

C. Reaction formation.

D. Repression.

E. Sublimation.

The correct response is option B: Displacement.

Displacement is changing the object of one's feelings to a safer one (option B). *Denial* averts the patient's attention from painful ideas or feelings without making them completely unavailable to consciousness (option A). *Reaction formation* consists of exaggerating one emotional trend to help repress the opposite emotion (option C). *Repression* involves actively pushing painful memories, feelings, and impulses out of awareness (option D). *Sublimation* is a mature mechanism of defense that involves the evolution of primitive impulses into a mature level of expression (option E). **(Hales RE, Yudofsky SC, Roberts LW [eds]: APP Textbook of Psychiatry, 6th Edition, Chapter 30, pp. 1084–1085 and Tables 30–9, 30–10, p. 1086)**

31.16 What is the focus of the object relations perspective of psychodynamic psychotherapy?

A. Wishes and feelings.

B. Maladaptive cognitive defense mechanisms.

C. Regulation of self-esteem.

D. Internalized memories of interpersonal relationships.

E. Infant-caregiver attachment.

The correct response is option D: Internalized memories of interpersonal relationships.

Object relations theory focuses on internalized memories of interpersonal relationships (option D). Drive theory focuses on wishes and feelings (option A). Ego function theory focuses on defense mechanisms (option B). The self-psychology model focuses on regulation of self-esteem (option C). Attachment theory focuses on infant-caregiver attachment (option E). **(Hales RE, Yudofsky SC, Roberts LW [eds]: APP Textbook of Psychiatry, 6th Edition, Chapter 30, p. 1074 and Table 30–3, p. 1075)**

31.17 During a session in a couple's treatment, the husband voices concerns about rejection from his wife and his tendency to avoid intimate interactions with her. He reports that his overall functioning at work and with interpersonal relationships is positive. Which of the following would be a reason for the therapist to use solution-focused brief therapy?

A. The problem is clearly a result of only one party.

B. The couple is invested in exploring childhood and formative experiences.

C. The husband is interested in a formulation of his personality.

D. The husband can identify problem-free areas of his life where the symptom does not occur.

E. The couple has multiple presenting concerns.

The correct response is option D: The husband can identify problem-free areas of his life where the symptom does not occur.

Solution-focused brief therapies start from the premise that people are changing all the time, enacting solution patterns as well as problem ones (Ratner et al. 2012). One important idea underlying this theory is that patients have certain areas of their lives in which problems do not exist at all (option D). When patients cannot reach their goals, they at some point identify that they have a problem. This reification becomes self-fulfilling: the more patients focus on their problems, the more troubled they feel and act. Equally important, such a problem focus blinds patients to the occasions in which they do, in fact, reach their goals. The aim of solution-focused brief therapy is to break this self-fulfilling conceptualization. The therapist accomplishes this by focusing on solution patterns rather than on problems. Thus, in the initial assessment therapists ask patients to identify positive presession changes and occasions during which problems either do not occur or occur less often or less intensely (Walter and Peller 1992). Enacting these exceptions to problem patterns—doing more of what is already working (de Shazer 1988; O'Hanlon and Weiner-Davis 1989)—is the focus of therapy, not an analysis of childhood experiences (option B) or personality development (option C). Because the therapy is not initiating new behavior and thought patterns but rather building on existing ones, it tends to be highly targeted on one concern (option E) (Steenbarger 2012) and, in this case, to focus on the system (option A). **(Hales RE, Yudofsky SC, Roberts LW [eds]: APP Textbook of Psychiatry, 6th Edition, Chapter 29, p. 1048)**

31.18 Which of the following is a true statement about brief psychotherapies?

A. The brief therapies are similar in both duration and focus on the present.
B. All of the brief therapies stress in-session experience as central to change.
C. All of the brief therapies are manualized.
D. All of the brief therapies set limits on the number of sessions at the outset of treatment.
E. In all brief therapies, it is the therapist who maintains the treatment focus from session to session.

The correct response is option E: In all brief therapies, it is the therapist who maintains the treatment focus from session to session.

Brief therapies can be conceptualized along a continuum, ranging from highly abbreviated and highly structured contextual therapies to more exploratory relational treatments (option A). In all of these treatments, the therapist maintains the treatment focus from session to session (option E). The major schools of brief therapy differ in scope, degree of structure (option C), use of time in treatment (option D), and nature of the therapist activity to create change (option B). **(Hales RE, Yudofsky SC, Roberts LW [eds]: APP Textbook of Psychiatry, 6th Edition, Chapter 29, pp. 1050–1053)**

31.19 Which of the following terms refers to a therapist's emotional reaction to a patient that emanates from the therapist's own past?

    A. Countertransference.
    B. Identification with the aggressor.
    C. Transference.
    D. Resistance.
    E. Projection.

The correct response is option A: Countertransference.

Countertransference refers to the therapist's feelings toward the patient that may come from the therapist's own past (option A). *Identification with the aggressor* is a type of defense mechanism that involves the tendency of the patient to imitate the aggressive manner of a person toward that patient (option B). *Transference* refers to the pressures that either the therapist or patient feels to act in a certain way that stems from that patient's previous relationships (option C). *Resistance* refers to all of the forces in the patient, including defense mechanisms that keep painful feelings and memories outside of conscious awareness (option D). *Projection* is a type of defense mechanism that involves the person experiencing his or her emotion as originating in the other person (option E). **(Hales RE, Yudofsky SC, Roberts LW [eds]: APP Textbook of Psychiatry, 6th Edition, Chapter 30, pp. 1072–1073, 1082–1085 and Table 30–10 p. 1086)**

31.20 Mentalization-based therapy (MBT) was originally developed for the treatment of which of the following conditions?

    A. Borderline PD.
    B. Major depressive disorder.
    C. Anxiety disorders.
    D. Substance use disorders.
    E. Psychotic disorders.

The correct response is option A: Borderline PD.

MBT was originally developed for the treatment of BPD (option A). The core symptoms of BPD—emotional dysregulation, impulsivity, self-destructive behavior, and unstable relationships—are embedded in highly insecure (i.e., preoccupied and disorganized) attachment relationships and severe mentalizing impairments. More specifically, patients with BPD show marked impairments in the explicit, internal, and cognitive facets of mentalizing: they are reactive to external-behavioral cues (e.g., a grimace or a yawn), they have difficulty linking such cues appropriately to internal mental states, and they are subject to implicit mentalizing and emotional contagion concomitant with impaired capacity for explicit, reflective thinking (Fonagy and Luyten 2009). Although potentially useful in the other forms of psychopathology listed, MBT was not developed specifically for use with major depressive disorder (option B), anxiety disorders (option C), substance use disorders (option D), or psychotic disorders (option E). **(Hales RE, Yudofsky SC, Roberts LW [eds]: APP Textbook of Psychiatry, 6th Edition, Chapter 31, p. 1105)**

31.21 What is the "negative cognitive triad" of depression proposed by Beck and colleagues in the cognitive model?

A. Self, world/environment, and future.
B. Stimulus, response, reward versus punishment.
C. Misperception, error in logic, misattribution.
D. Cognition distortion, depression, reinforcing behavior.
E. Dysphoric mood, maladaptive behavior, negative cognition.

The correct response is option A: Self, world/environment, and future.

Beck and colleagues (Beck 1976) proposed that people with depression are prone to cognitive distortions in three major areas: self, world/environment, and future (i.e., the "negative cognitive triad") (option A). The cognitive model for psychotherapy is grounded on the theory that there are characteristic errors in information processing in psychiatric disorders and that these alterations in thought processes are closely linked to emotional reactions and dysfunctional behavior patterns (Alford and Beck 1997; Beck 1976; Clark et al. 1999). For example, people with anxiety disorders habitually overestimate the danger or risk in situations. Cognitive distortions such as misperceptions, errors in logic, and misattributions are thought to lead to dysphoric moods and are distinct from the negative cognitive triad (option C). Furthermore, a vicious cycle is perpetuated when the behavioral response confirms and amplifies negatively distorted cognitions, but neither reinforcing behavior (option D) nor maladaptive behavior (option E) is included in the negative cognitive triad. Finally, stimulus, response, and reward versus punishment (option B) are concepts related to behavior therapy and not the cognitive model. **(Hales RE, Yudofsky SC, Roberts LW [eds]: APP Textbook of Psychiatry, 6th Edition, Chapter 32, pp. 1120–1121)**

31.22 Exposure and response prevention (ERP), a specialized CBT technique, has been shown to be most effective and widely used for which disorder?

A. Posttraumatic stress disorder.
B. Acute stress disorder.
C. Panic disorder.
D. Social phobia.
E. Obsessive-compulsive disorder.

The correct response is option E: Obsessive-compulsive disorder.

ERP, a treatment that is primarily behavioral in focus, is the best-established therapy for obsessive-compulsive disorder, either alone or (more typically) combined with CBT in comprehensive treatment packages (option E) (James and Blackburn 1995; Salkovskis and Westbrook 1989; Simpson et al. 2006). Although the technique has been used for posttraumatic stress disorder (option A), acute stress disorder (option B), panic disorder (option C), and social phobia (option D), ERP has not emerged as the most effective technique with these disorders. **(Hales RE, Yudofsky SC, Roberts LW [eds]: APP Textbook of Psychiatry, 6th Edition, Chapter 32, pp. 1151–1153)**

31.23 Which of the following is a component of a CBT case conceptualization?

A. Selecting a manual to allow the therapist to use a standard approach to treatment.
B. Choosing CBT interventions based on a unique working hypothesis of the patient.
C. Adhering to and maintaining the same formulation throughout the duration of treatment.
D. Identifying fantasies and linking them to developmental history.
E. Describing the connections between thoughts, emotions, and early relationships.

The correct response is option B: Choosing CBT interventions based on a unique working hypothesis of the patient.

Assessment for CBT begins with completion of a standard history and mental status examination. Although special attention is paid to cognitive and behavioral elements, a full biopsychosocial evaluation is completed and used in formulating the treatment plan (option B). The case conceptualization contains the following elements: 1) an outline of the most salient aspects of the history and mental status examination; 2) detailing of at least three examples from the patient's life of the relationship between events, automatic thoughts, emotions, and behaviors; 3) identification of important schemas; 4) listing of strengths; 5) a working hypothesis that weaves together all of the information in numbers 1–4 with the cognitive and behavioral theories that most closely fit the patient's diagnosis and symptoms; and 6) a treatment plan that is based on the working hypothesis. Although a manual is typically selected to guide treatment, the plan is adapted to each patient (option A). The conceptualization is continually developed throughout therapy and may be augmented or revised as new information is collected and treatment methods are tested (option C). Case conceptualization from a CBT perspective is distinct from a psychodynamic perspective in that fantasies linked to developmental history (option D) or connecting thoughts, emotions, and childhood relationships (option E) are not included. **(Hales RE, Yudofsky SC, Roberts LW [eds]: APP Textbook of Psychiatry, 6th Edition, Chapter 32, p. 1128)**

31.24 Under which of the following circumstances might transference be discussed in supportive psychotherapy?

A. A negative transference interferes with treatment.
B. A positive transference becomes apparent.
C. The therapist experiences countertransference.
D. The patient's attitudes toward his mother are displaced onto the therapist.
E. The patient mistakes the therapeutic relationship for a real relationship.

The correct response is option A: A negative transference interferes with treatment.

In psychotherapy at the supportive end of the psychotherapy continuum, transference can be used to guide therapeutic interventions. However, transference is not generally discussed unless negative transference threatens to disrupt treatment. Positive transference reactions (option B) and countertransference (option C) generally are not explored but rather are simply accepted. Negative reactions must always be investigated, however, because they may compromise the treatment (option A) (Winston and Winston 2002). The real relationship (option E) is paramount and based on overt mutuality in the conduct of therapy. In addition, the patient's attitudes toward his mother are not specifically explored (option D) unless the patient evinces a negative transference that interferes with treatment. **(Hales RE, Yudofsky SC, Roberts LW [eds]: APP Textbook of Psychiatry, 6th Edition, Chapter 33, pp. 1175–1176)**

31.25 Which of the following has been shown to predict a positive outcome in both brief supportive psychotherapy and supportive-expressive psychotherapy?

A. An absence of countertransference.
B. A positive transference.
C. Frequent discussions about the therapeutic relationship.
D. A strong therapeutic alliance.
E. A relaxed patient-therapist relationship in which both participants feel free to express negative emotions.

The correct response is option D: A strong therapeutic alliance.

Bordin (1979) operationalized the therapeutic alliance concept as the degree of agreement between patient and therapist concerning the tasks and goals of psychotherapy and the quality of the bond between them. Outcome research in psychotherapy supports the idea that the quality of the therapeutic alliance is the best predictor of treatment outcome (Horvath and Symonds 1991). Specifically, there is evidence that in brief supportive and supportive-expressive psychotherapies, an early and strong therapeutic alliance is predictive of positive outcome (option D) (Hellerstein et al. 1998; Luborsky 1984). Other relationship variables, such as absence of countertransference (option A), positive transference (option B), frequent discussions (option C), and relaxed nature (option E), either have not been measured or have not consistently emerged as predictors of outcome. **(Hales RE, Yudofsky SC, Roberts LW [eds]: APP Textbook of Psychiatry, 6th Edition, Chapter 33, p. 1178)**

31.26 How might supportive psychotherapy be beneficial to patients with substance use disorders?

A. Helping patients admit to being powerless over their substance use.
B. Helping patients discover their spiritual side.
C. Helping patients make amends to those they have harmed.
D. Helping patients rediscover old hobbies.
E. Helping patients develop coping strategies to control their substance use.

The correct response is option E: Helping patients develop coping strategies to control their substance use.

Patients with substance use disorders can benefit from supportive psychotherapy, which can help them develop coping strategies to control or reduce substance use and diminish anxiety and dysphoria (option E). The therapist must actively strive to maintain a positive therapeutic alliance so that the patient can remain in treatment and actively contribute to the work of therapy. Newer evidence-based strategies such as relapse prevention (Marlatt and Gordon 1985) and motivational interviewing (Rollnick and Miller 1995) should be integrated into supportive psychotherapy, along with 12-step programs and group psychotherapy. Helping patients admit to being powerless over their substance use (option A), discover their spirituality (option B), and make amends to those they have harmed (option C) are general principles of 12-step programs that may be incorporated into supportive psychotherapy. Patients can be taught to rediscover old hobbies as part of their coping strategies; however, this factor alone is not considered beneficial (option D). **(Hales RE, Yudofsky SC, Roberts LW [eds]: APP Textbook of Psychiatry, 6th Edition, Chapter 33, pp. 1179–1180)**

31.27 Which two specific psychotherapies have been shown to be very effective in treatment of depressive disorders?

A. Dialectical behavior therapy (DBT) and cognitive-behavioral therapy (CBT).
B. Mentalization-based therapy (MBT) and interpersonal psychotherapy (IPT).
C. MBT and CBT.
D. MBT and DBT.
E. IPT and CBT.

The correct response is option E: IPT and CBT.

Research has shown that two specific psychotherapies, IPT and CBT (option E), are very effective in treating depressive disorders. IPT is a manual-based approach that is time limited and focuses on relationships (Weissman et al. 2000). CBT is also well manualized, time limited, and focused on the individuals' thoughts and perspectives toward themselves and their environment (Beck 2011). DBT and MBT have not shown the same effectiveness for depressive disorders (options A–D). DBT is more often recommended for the treatment of affect regulation, self-harm, and suicidal behaviors, and MBT is recommended for interpersonal challenges seen in PDs. **(Hales RE, Yudofsky SC, Roberts LW [eds]: APP Textbook of Psychiatry, 6th Edition, Chapter 11, p. 372)**

31.28 Which treatment component is considered most effective and linked to greatest symptom reduction for patients with an anxiety disorder?

A. Transference interpretations.
B. Exposure to anxiety-provoking situations.
C. Avoidance of anxiety-provoking situations.
D. Focus on therapeutic boundaries.
E. Supportive reassurance.

The correct response is option B: Exposure to anxiety-provoking situations.

CBT has the most robust evidence for efficacy among the psychosocial interventions for anxiety disorders. More specifically, exposure therapy is a key treatment component that focuses on the individual approaching the anxiety-provoking situation and preventing the response of avoidance (option B). Avoidance of anxiety-provoking situations (option C) enhances the functionally limiting symptom of avoidance in persons with anxiety disorders. Although supportive reassurance (option E) is an element of all therapies, it is more descriptive of supportive psychotherapy and not a specific element of CBT and does not help a patient learn to tolerate and reinterpret his or her fear and physical symptoms of anxiety. Transference interpretations (option A) are part of psychodynamic psychotherapy and psychoanalysis and do not have as robust evidence as CBT. A focus on therapeutic boundaries (option D) is not a common focus of CBT for anxiety disorders; it is more characteristically a therapeutic focus in psychodynamic therapy and with treatment of PDs. **(Hales RE, Yudofsky SC, Roberts LW [eds]: APP Textbook of Psychiatry, 6th Edition, Chapter 12, p. 421)**

References

Alford BA, Beck AT: The Integrative Power of Cognitive Therapy. New York, Guilford, 1997

American Psychiatric Association Practice Guidelines: Practice guideline for the treatment of patients with borderline personality disorder. Am J Psychiatry 158(10)(Suppl):1–52, 2001 11665545

Beck AT: Cognitive Therapy and the Emotional Disorders. New York, International Universities Press, 1976

Beck JS: Cognitive Behavior Therapy: Basics and Beyond. New York, Guilford, 2011

Bond M, Banon E, Grenier M: Differential effects of interventions on the therapeutic alliance with patients with personality disorders. J Psychother Pract Res 7(4):301–318, 1998 9752641

Bordin ES: The generalizability of the psychoanalytic concept of the working alliance. Psychotherapy 16:252–260, 1979

Bretherton I: The origins of attachment theory: John Bowlby and Mary Ainsworth. Dev Psychol 28(5):759–775, 1992

Chapman AL: Dialectical behavior therapy: current indications and unique elements. Psychiatry (Edgmont) 3(9):62–68, 2006 20975829

Clark DA, Beck AT, Alford BA: Scientific Foundations of Cognitive Theory and Therapy of Depression. New York, Wiley, 1999

de Shazer S: Clues: Investigating Solutions in Brief Therapy. New York, WW Norton, 1988

Fonagy P, Luyten P: A developmental, mentalization-based approach to the understanding and treatment of borderline personality disorder. Dev Psychopathol 21(4):1355–1381, 2009 19825272

Freud S: The dynamics of transference (1912), in The Standard Edition of the Complete Psychological Works of Sigmund Freud, Vol 12. Translated and edited by Strachey J. London, Hogarth Press, 1958, pp 99–108

Hayes S, Smith S: Get Out of Your Mind and Into Your Life: The New Acceptance and Commitment Therapy. Oakland, CA, New Harbinger Publications, 2005

Hellerstein DJ, Rosenthal RN, Pinsker H, et al: A randomized prospective study comparing supportive and dynamic therapies. Outcome and alliance. J Psychother Pract Res 7(4):261–271, 1998 9752637

Horvath AO, Symonds BD: Relation between working alliance and outcome in psychotherapy: a meta-analysis. J Couns Psychol 38:139–149, 1991

Horvath AO, Del Re AC, Flückiger C, Symonds D: Alliance in individual psychotherapy. Psychotherapy (Chic) 48(1):9–16, 2011 21401269

Ingenhoven T, Lafay P, Rinne T, et al: Effectiveness of pharmacotherapy for severe personality disorders: meta-analyses of randomized controlled trials. J Clin Psychiatry 71(1):14–25, 2010 19778496

James IA, Blackburn IM: Cognitive therapy with obsessive-compulsive disorder. Br J Psychiatry 166(4):444–450, 1995 7795914

Leichsenring F, Leibing E, Kruse J, et al: Borderline personality disorder. Lancet 377(9759):74–84, 2011 21195251

Levenson H: Time-Limited Dynamic Psychotherapy: A Guide to Clinical Practice. New York, Basic Books, 1995

Luborsky L: Principles of Psychoanalytic Psychotherapy: A Manual for Supportive-Expressive Treatment. New York, Basic Books, 1984

Luborsky L, Mark D: Short-term supportive-expressive psychoanalytic psychotherapy, in Handbook of Short-Term Dynamic Psychotherapy. Edited by Crits-Christoph P, Barber JP. New York, Basic Books, 1991, pp 110–136

Marlatt GA, Gordon JR: Relapse Prevention: Maintenance Strategies in the Treatment of Addictive Behaviors. New York, Guilford, 1985

Meissner WW: The Therapeutic Alliance. New Haven, CT, Yale University Press, 1996

O'Hanlon W, Weiner-Davis J: In Search of Solution: A New Direction in Psychotherapy. New York, WW Norton, 1989

Oldham JM: Guideline watch: practice guideline for the treatment of patients with borderline personality disorder. Focus 3:396–400, 2005

Ratner H, George E, Iveson C: Solution Focused Brief Therapy: 100 Key Points and Techniques. New York, Routledge, 2012

Rollnick S, Miller WR: What is motivational interviewing? Behav Cogn Psychother 23:325–334, 1995

Safran JD, Muran JC: Negotiating the Therapeutic Alliance. New York, Guilford, 2000

Safran JD, Muran JC, Eubanks-Carter C: Repairing alliance ruptures. Psychotherapy (Chic) 48(1):80–87, 2011 21401278

Salkovskis PM, Westbrook D: Behaviour therapy and obsessional ruminations: can failure be turned into success? Behav Res Ther 27(2):149–160, 1989 2930440

Simpson HB, Huppert JD, Petkova E, et al: Response versus remission in obsessive-compulsive disorder. J Clin Psychiatry 67(2):269–276, 2006 16566623

Steenbarger BN: Solution-focused brief therapy: doing what works, in The Art and Science of Brief Psychotherapies: An Illustrated Guide, 2nd Edition. Edited by Dewan MJ, Steenbarger BN, Greenberg RP. Washington, DC, American Psychiatric Publishing, 2012, pp 121–155

Walter JL, Peller JE: Becoming Solution-Focused in Brief Therapy. New York, Brunner/Mazel, 1992

Weissman MM, Markowitz JC, Klerman G: Comprehensive Guide to Interpersonal Psychotherapy. New York, Basic Books, 2000

Winston A, Winston B: Handbook of Integrated Short-Term Psychotherapy. Washington, DC, American Psychiatric Press, 2002

CHAPTER 32

Research/Biostatistics

32.1 Which of the following is a true statement regarding case-control studies?

A. Results of a case-control study are considered as definitive as those of a randomized controlled trial (RCT).
B. Control groups should include subjects with the disease of interest.
C. A comparison is made prospectively between two identical populations, one exposed to the factor of interest and the other not.
D. Case-control studies generally cost less than a prospective RCT.
E. Case-control studies are not very valuable sources of data.

The correct response is option D: Case-control studies generally cost less than a prospective RCT.

Epidemiologists developed case-control designs to aid them in searching for factors that might cause a given illness by comparing rates of exposure for potential risk factors in persons who have the illness (the case subjects) with those in the same population who presumably are not ill (the control subjects) (option B). Results of a case-control study are not considered as definitive as those of an RCT (option A), in which a comparison is made prospectively between two identical populations, one exposed to the factor of interest and the other not (option C); however, case-control studies are invaluable for several reasons (option E): 1) many factors, such as patients' genotypes, cannot be assigned randomly; 2) several factors, such as genetic and environmental risks, can be examined simultaneously; and 3) case-control studies generally cost less than a prospective RCT (option D). (*American Journal of Psychiatry* **169(8):785–789, 2012**)

32.2 Which of the following best describes Phase II of a human clinical trial?

A. Testing of multiple doses of a drug for bioavailability, pharmacokinetics, and side effects.
B. Dose-finding studies in patients with a given disorder.
C. Pivotal double-blind trials for demonstrating efficacy and safety/tolerability.

D. Trials to help clarify potential uses of a drug.

E. Assessment of drug bioavailability, metabolism, and toxicity.

The correct response is option B: Dose-finding studies in patients with a given disorder.

Drug development is a highly complex process that involves multiple steps of preclinical and clinical pharmacological refinement and testing. Preclinical studies include assessing drug bioavailability, metabolism, and toxicity (option E); effects on known biological targets (e.g., receptor binding); and performance in various animal models of pathology. After sufficient data are obtained in animal studies, drug testing in humans can begin. In the United States, human clinical trials are divided into four phases: Phase I involves testing multiple doses of a drug for bioavailability, pharmacokinetics, and side effects (option A). Phase II studies are dose-finding studies in patients with a given disorder (option B); they can be open-label or double-blind trials. Phase III generally includes pivotal double-blind trials for demonstrating efficacy and safety/tolerability (option C). Phase IV trials, which take place after a drug has received U.S. Food and Drug Administration (FDA) approval and is on the market, are conducted to help clarify potential uses of the drug (option D). **(Schatzberg AF, Nemeroff CB: APP Textbook of Psychopharmacology, 4th Edition, Chapter 11, p. 243)**

32.3   Which of the following statements is true regarding use of placebo controls in pharmacology research?

A. Placebo controls are not necessary if treatment is randomized.

B. Placebo response is consistent across patient groups.

C. For most psychiatric disorders, no treatment can be considered effective without a placebo control.

D. A placebo group is not needed to accurately assess a new drug's value if it is equivalent to the standard treatment.

E. Demonstrating statistical superiority to placebo is sufficient to convey a drug's clinical relevance.

The correct response is option C: For most psychiatric disorders, no treatment can be considered effective without a placebo control.

Following Phase II studies, placebo and treatment randomization trials are necessary. Treatment randomization addresses unknown prognostic factors but cannot compensate for variable placebo responsiveness (option A). For most psychiatric disorders, no treatment can be considered effective without a placebo control (option C) because placebo response rates vary widely across patient groups (option B). A placebo group is needed to accurately assess a new drug's value, even if a new drug is equivalent to the standard treatment (option D). Without calibrating a study group's placebo response rate, new and old drugs might appear equally effective when, in fact, neither was having any effect. Differences in drug-placebo improvement rates are a necessary condition to establish utility; however, merely demonstrating statistical superiority to placebo may not be sufficient to convey a drug's clinical relevance (option E). (*American Journal of Psychiatry* **156(6):829–836, p. 830, 1999**)

32.4   Which of the following is the mode in this list of test scores: 3, 4, 5, 5, 5, 6, 6, 7, 9, 10?

A. 2.049.
B. 6.
C. 5.
D. 5.5.
E. 7.

The correct response is option C: 5.

The most frequently occurring score is referred to as the *mode*. The mode of the distribution above is 5 (option C), because that score occurs more frequently (three times) than any other score. The use of the mode to describe a distribution has several advantages. The mode is easy to calculate and interpret. It may also be used to describe any distribution, regardless of whether the measure is categorical or numerical. The *median* is the midpoint of the distribution: the point at or below which 50% of the cases fall. The median is determined by arranging scores in order from lowest to highest. For distributions with an odd number (N) of scores, the median is the middlemost score (i.e., the score at $[(N+1)/2]$ in order); for distributions with an even number of scores, the median is the score midway between the scores at $[N/2]$ and $[(N/2)+1]$ in order. The median for the distribution of the 10 test scores is 5.5 (option D), because that is the midpoint between 5 (the fifth ordered score) and 6 (the sixth ordered score). The median is generally considered to be more informative about the "typical" score than is the mode. In contrast to the mean, the median is less sensitive to extreme scores. The *mean* is a third method for describing a distribution of scores, stated in terms of the arithmetic average. This is referred to as the mean. The mean is calculated by summing the scores and dividing by the number of scores. The mean for the distribution of the 10 test scores above is 6 (60/10) (option B). The mean can be thought of as the "balance point" of a distribution. As any number in the distribution is changed, the value of the mean changes as well. Thus, the mean, unlike the median and mode, takes into account the value of every score. The *range* (10−3=7; option E) is the difference between the largest and the smallest scores in the distribution. The advantages of the range include its ease of computation and its simplicity of interpretation. The *standard deviation* of the 10 test scores is the square root of the variance (4.2, the average squared deviation from the mean), which is 2.049 (option A). (**Mitchell JE, Crosby RD, Wonderlich SA, Adson DE: Elements of Clinical Research in Psychiatry, Chapter 5, pp. 46–49**)

32.5 The investigation by which of the following individuals led to the creation of institutional review boards?

A. Walter Mondale.
B. Andrew Ivy.
C. Henry Beecher.
D. Benjamin Rush.
E. Samuel Woodward.

The correct response is option C: Henry Beecher.

Deficiencies in the protection of research subjects were brought to the public eye with the publication in 1966, in the *New England Journal of Medicine,* of Henry Beecher's controversial article "Ethics in Clinical Research" (Beecher 1966). Beecher mentioned at the beginning of his article that an examination of 100 consecutive human studies published in 1964 in what he characterized as "an excellent journal" revealed that 12 of them seemed to be unethical. For the article, he had originally compiled 50 examples of research involving questionable ethics; in only two of these studies was consent mentioned. In the final version of his article, he provided 22 examples (the list was shortened for publication) of research published in respected journals by prominent researchers that had involved very significant risks to nonconsenting research subjects. In light of Beecher's disclosures (option C), significant public pressure was brought to bear on the National Institutes of Health (NIH) to regulate those involved in biomedical research. During 1966, NIH established guidelines covering all federally funded research involving human experimentation. With these guidelines, calling for review by a "committee of institutional associates," we see the beginnings of institutional review boards.

Walter Mondale (option A) was a senator from Minnesota who worked to establish a commission to study the social and ethical implications of advances in the biomedical field. Andrew Ivy (option B) was instrumental in the promulgation of the Nuremberg Code (document addressing the protection of human subjects in research during the modern era). Benjamin Rush (option D) was a Founding Father of the United States who led a successful campaign in 1792 for Pennsylvania to build a separate mental ward where the patients could be kept in more humane conditions. Samuel Woodward (option E) was the first president of the Association of Medical Superintendents of American Institutions for the Insane, which was renamed the American Psychiatric Association in 1921. **(Mitchell JE, Crosby RD, Wonderlich SA, Adson DE: Elements of Clinical Research in Psychiatry, Chapter 8, pp. 92, 96–98)**

32.6   A psychiatrist wants to learn more about the patients treated in her practice by performing structured diagnostic interviews at intake on all patients over the course of 1 year. These data are recorded, along with results from measures of depression and anxiety, at intake and at all subsequent visits. At the end of the year, she has a database of 150 patients. In the statistical analysis, which of the following is a *descriptive* statistical analysis?

A. Testing hypotheses regarding treatment decisions.
B. Testing hypotheses regarding outcomes for patients with different diagnoses.
C. Calculating whether men have more diagnoses of schizophrenia than women.
D. Deciding whether male patients have different anxiety disorders than female patients.
E. Calculating the percentage of patients in her practice who have mood disorders.

The correct response is option E: Calculating the percentage of patients in her practice who have mood disorders.

Statistics is a collection of methods for summarizing, displaying, and analyzing numerical data, often for the purposes of decision making. *Descriptive* statistics are methods for organizing, summarizing, and communicating data. The purpose of descriptive statistics is to characterize and delineate a specific data set; there is no attempt to make inferences beyond the available data. Thus, the psychiatrist may calculate the mean number of diagnoses of schizophrenia, the percentage of patients with a mood disorder (option E), or the correlation of depression and anxiety scores at intake, or may create a frequency distribution of anxiety disorders. These are examples of descriptive statistics because they describe or summarize some aspect of the data. *Inferential* statistics, in contrast, are methods of analyzing data to arrive at conclusions extending beyond the immediate data. Inferential statistics are typically used as a basis for decision making or hypothesis testing (options A–D). The psychiatrist may wish to know whether female patients have significantly fewer or greater diagnoses of schizophrenia than do male patients, or whether patients with a somatic symptom disorder have significantly poorer outcomes in terms of reduction of depression and anxiety symptoms than do patients without a somatic symptom disorder. These are examples that rely on inferential statistics, because the conclusions that the psychiatrist will make extend beyond the immediate sample of patients that has been measured. (**Mitchell JE, Crosby RD, Wonderlich SA, Adson DE: Elements of Clinical Research in Psychiatry, Chapter 5, pp. 45–46**)

Reference

Beecher HK: Ethics and clinical research. N Engl J Med 274(24):1354–1360, 1966 5327352

CHAPTER 33

Schizophrenia Spectrum and Other Psychotic Disorders

33.1 Which of the following symptoms is associated with a worse prognosis in schizophrenia?

A. Hallucinations.
B. Disorganization.
C. Delusions.
D. Paranoia.
E. Mood lability.

The correct response is option B: Disorganization.

Although disorganization is considered by many to be a positive symptom, factor analyses suggest that disorganization is distinct from delusions and hallucinations. Disorganization encompasses conceptual disorganization, disorientation, posturing and mannerisms, bizarre behavior, stereotyped thinking, difficulties with abstract thinking, poor attention, and inappropriate affect (Ventura et al. 2010). Disorganization is more socially impairing than hallucinations (option A) or delusions (option C) and is associated with a worse prognosis (option B). Although individuals may learn to ignore hallucinations or to avoid talking about or acting on delusions, disorganization is harder to mask. Disorganization also correlates with deficits in attention/vigilance, reasoning and problem solving, processing speed, and IQ (Ventura et al. 2010). Many patients learn to cope with their paranoia (option D) and learn to manage their mood lability (option E). **(Hales RE, Yudofsky SC, Roberts LW [eds]: APP Textbook of Psychiatry, 6th Edition, Chapter 9, p. 275)**

33.2 Which of the following is a risk factor for suicide among patients with schizo-phrenia?

A. Older age at symptom onset.
B. Low premorbid functioning.
C. Reduced awareness of symptoms.
D. Female sex.
E. High personal expectations.

The correct response is option E: High personal expectations.

Risk factors for suicide among people with schizophrenia include younger age, younger (not older) age at symptom onset (option A), and high (not low) premorbid functioning (option B). Additional risk factors include high personal expectations (option E), awareness that life's expectations are unlikely to be met, awareness of symptoms (especially if aware of delusions, anhedonia, asociality, blunted affect; option C), and a negative attitude toward or noncompliance with treatment. As in the general population, male (not female) sex (option D), unmarried status, living alone, being unemployed, and having access to lethal means are also risk factors for suicide among individuals with schizophrenia (Siris 2001). **(Hales RE, Yudofsky SC, Roberts LW [eds]: APP Textbook of Psychiatry, 6th Edition, Chapter 9, p. 276)**

33.3 Which of the following symptoms would be most likely to fluctuate when a patient has reached the chronic-residual stage of schizophrenia?

A. Anhedonia.
B. Social withdrawal.
C. Cognitive symptoms.
D. Stereotyped thinking.
E. Hallucinations.

The correct response is option E: Hallucinations.

The natural history of schizophrenia is characterized by four stages of illness: the premorbid, prodromal, progressive, and chronic-residual stages. All stages are characterized by specific symptoms and functional deficits that progress as patients move through the illness stages and worsen in severity. The progressive stage of schizophrenia can be said to begin when overt psychotic symptoms develop. Five to 10 years after entering the progressive stage of schizophrenia, patients typically enter what may be called the chronic-residual stage, which is characterized not by inexorable progression but rather by the persistence of residual symptoms and disability. Notably, the preponderance of the evidence suggests that once the progressive stage is reached, cognitive symptoms (option C) and negative symptoms remain relatively stable, with positive symptoms, such as hallucinations (option E), being the most likely to fluctuate significantly. Anhedonia (option A), social withdrawal (option B), and stereotyped thinking (option D) are examples of negative symptoms. **(Hales RE, Yudofsky SC, Roberts LW [eds]: APP Textbook of Psychiatry, 6th Edition, Chapter 9, pp. 275, 288, 291–292)**

33.4 Antipsychotic medication is most likely to improve which of the following schizophrenia symptoms?

A. Social withdrawal.
B. Stereotyped thinking.
C. Muscle rigidity.
D. Disorganization.
E. Autonomic instability.

The correct response is option D: Disorganization.

Antipsychotics have a robust effect on the core positive symptoms and disorganization (option D) that are characteristic of schizophrenia (Tandon 2011). Research has shown that patients with schizophrenia who achieve remission when taking antipsychotic drugs and then consistently continue to take the drugs are about three times less likely to relapse than patients who stop taking the drugs (Hogarty et al. 1976).

Social withdrawal (option A) and stereotyped thinking (option B) are negative symptoms and are unlikely to be affected by antipsychotics. Many antipsychotics cause muscle rigidity (option C) as a side effect. Occasionally, antipsychotics cause neuroleptic malignant syndrome, a life-threatening emergency that includes autonomic instability (option E). **(Hales RE, Yudofsky SC, Roberts LW [eds]: APP Textbook of Psychiatry, 6th Edition, Chapter 9, pp. 293–296)**

33.5 Which of the following has been found in neuroimaging studies of patients with schizophrenia?

A. Decreased size of lateral and third ventricles.
B. Increased prefrontal cortex.
C. Increased superior temporal lobe.
D. Increased thalamic volume.
E. Decreased volume in the hippocampus.

The correct response is option E: Decreased volume in the hippocampus.

Schizophrenia is associated with signs of abnormal development at the macroscopic level, and studies using computed tomography (CT) and magnetic resonance imaging (MRI) consistently show structural brain abnormalities. The most reproducible findings are a slight overall decrease in brain volume and an increase (not decrease) in size of ventricles (option A). Localized findings are less reproducible, but among the most robust are decreased size of the hippocampus (option E), superior temporal lobe (option C), prefrontal cortex (option B), and thalamus (option D). Many of these deficits are present at first psychotic break and in nonaffected relatives with high genetic risk for schizophrenia, suggesting that they contribute to susceptibility to disease rather than result from disease and treatment (Fornito et al. 2009; Vita et al. 2006). **(Hales RE, Yudofsky SC, Roberts LW [eds]: APP Textbook of Psychiatry, 6th Edition, Chapter 9, p. 303)**

33.6   Which of the following distinguishes between brief psychotic disorder and schizophreniform disorder?

    A. Delusions are present in brief psychotic disorder but not in schizophreniform disorder.
    B. Duration of the disturbance is less than 1 month in brief psychotic disorder and less than 6 months in schizophreniform disorder.
    C. Brief psychotic disorder cannot occur with catatonia.
    D. Schizophreniform disorder symptoms last less than 1 month.
    E. Presence of stressors rules out a diagnosis of brief psychotic disorder.

The correct response is option B: Duration of the disturbance is less than 1 month in brief psychotic disorder and less than 6 months in schizophreniform disorder.

Unlike for schizophreniform disorder, in brief psychotic disorder, delusions, hallucinations, or disorganized speech last for more than 1 day but resolve within 1 month (option B). Catatonic features may be present (option C) and are a specifier in DSM-5 (American Psychiatric Association 2013). Other DSM-5 specifiers include with or without marked stressor(s) (option E). Schizophreniform disorder, like schizophrenia, is characterized by two or more of the following core symptoms: delusions (option A), hallucinations, disorganized speech, disorganized or catatonic behavior, and negative symptoms. The duration of an episode of schizophreniform disorder is between 1 and 6 months (option D). **(Hales RE, Yudofsky SC, Roberts LW [eds]: APP Textbook of Psychiatry, 6th Edition, Chapter 9, pp. 283–285)**

33.7   Which of the following is a true statement regarding delusional disorder?

    A. Symptoms are present for less than 1 month.
    B. Hallucinations are prominent.
    C. Individuals tend to behave and appear appropriately when their delusions are not being discussed or acted upon.
    D. Functioning is markedly impaired.
    E. Hallucinations are not typically related to delusional content.

The correct response is option C: Individuals tend to behave and appear appropriately when their delusions are not being discussed or acted upon.

Delusional disorder is characterized by one or more delusions that are present for longer than 1 month (option A). If hallucinations are present, they are not prominent (option B) and are related to the content of the delusions (option E). For a diagnosis of delusional disorder, functioning should not be markedly impaired (option D) and behavior not obviously odd (apart from the impact of the delusions). Individuals with delusional disorder tend to behave and appear appropriately when their delusions are not being discussed or acted upon (option C). **(Hales RE, Yudofsky SC, Roberts LW [eds]: APP Textbook of Psychiatry, 6th Edition, Chapter 9, pp. 285–286)**

33.8   Which of the following is a DSM-5 diagnostic criterion for schizoaffective disorder?

A. Delusions or hallucinations must occur for 2 or more weeks in the absence of a major mood episode during the lifetime duration of the illness.
B. Delusions or other psychotic symptoms occur exclusively during manic or depressive episodes.
C. Major mood episodes must be present for one quarter of the total duration of illness.
D. Social and occupational functioning must be impaired.
E. Major mood symptoms must occur for 2 or more weeks in the absence of delusions or hallucinations.

The correct response is option A: Delusions or hallucinations must occur for 2 or more weeks in the absence of a major mood episode during the lifetime duration of the illness.

The presence of delusions or hallucinations in the absence of major mood symptoms is characteristic of schizoaffective disorder (option E). Schizoaffective disorder is diagnosed when the core symptom criteria for schizophrenia co-occur with a manic or major depressive episode but are preceded or followed by at least 2 weeks of delusions or hallucinations without a major mood episode (option A). If delusions or other psychotic symptoms occur exclusively during manic or depressive episodes, then the diagnosis is bipolar or major depressive disorder with psychotic features (option B). To meet DSM-5 criteria for schizoaffective disorder, major mood episodes must be present for at least half the total duration of the illness (option C). Impaired social or occupational functioning is not a diagnostic criterion (option D), reflecting a belief that schizoaffective disorder has a somewhat better prognosis than schizophrenia. **(Hales RE, Yudofsky SC, Roberts LW [eds]: APP Textbook of Psychiatry, 6th Edition, Chapter 9, p. 287)**

References

American Psychiatric Association: Diagnostic and Statistical Manual of Mental Disorders, 5th Edition. Arlington, VA, American Psychiatric Association, 2013
Fornito A, Yücel M, Pantelis C: Reconciling neuroimaging and neuropathological findings in schizophrenia and bipolar disorder. Curr Opin Psychiatry 22(3):312–319, 2009 19365187
Hogarty GE, Ulrich RF, Mussare F, Aristigueta N: Drug discontinuation among long term, successfully maintained schizophrenic outpatients. Dis Nerv Syst 37(9):494–500, 1976 971653
Siris SG: Suicide and schizophrenia. J Psychopharmacol 15(2):127–135, 2001 11448086
Tandon R: Antipsychotics in the treatment of schizophrenia: an overview. J Clin Psychiatry 72(Suppl 1):4–8, 2011 22217436

Ventura J, Thames AD, Wood RC, et al: Disorganization and reality distortion in schizophrenia: a meta-analysis of the relationship between positive symptoms and neurocognitive deficits. Schizophr Res 121(1-3):1–14, 2010 20579855

Vita A, De Peri L, Silenzi C, Dieci M: Brain morphology in first-episode schizophrenia: a meta-analysis of quantitative magnetic resonance imaging studies. Schizophr Res 82(1):75–88, 2006 16377156

CHAPTER 34

Sexual Dysfunction/ Gender Dysphoria

Sexual Dysfunction

34.1   A 22-year-old man is diagnosed with schizophrenia and treated with risperidone titrated up to 3 mg twice a day. After 2 weeks, he reports clear thinking and cessation of auditory hallucinations; however, he is bothered by the fact that his ejaculation is delayed. What is the best first course of action in this case?

A. Lower the dose of risperidone.
B. Add aripiprazole.
C. Switch to perphenazine.
D. Switch to haloperidol.
E. Add sildenafil.

The correct response is option A: Lower the dose of risperidone.

Antipsychotic agents, especially the traditional antipsychotics (options C, D) and risperidone, are associated with delayed ejaculation. This side effect can usually be managed by dose reduction (option A) or drug substitution. Drugs such as quetiapine, ziprasidone, and aripiprazole have a lower incidence of delayed ejaculation. With antipsychotic-induced sexual dysfunction, most clinicians would first attempt dose reduction or shift to a prolactin-sparing antipsychotic. Additionally, there have been isolated case reports of various antidotes (e.g., sildenafil; option E) to reverse antipsychotic-induced sexual dysfunction, although these agents have not been studied in controlled trials. Polypharmacy increases the risk of drug-drug interactions and should be minimized or avoided if possible (option B). **(Hales RE, Yudofsky SC, Roberts LW [eds]: APP Textbook of Psychiatry, 6th Edition, Chapter 20, p. 657, 673–674; Chapter 27, p. 930)**

34.2 In a 50-year-old obese man who smokes and presents with erectile dysfunction, which of the following clinical tests would you prioritize?

A. Nocturnal tumescence.
B. Nerve conduction studies.
C. A lipid panel.
D. Testosterone level.
E. A complete blood count.

The correct response is option C: A lipid panel.

The extent to which a clinician pursues possible medical etiologies of erectile problems is dependent on the patient's age, his overall health status and risk factors, and the presentation of the problem. Population surveys have found relationships between the presence of erectile dysfunction in men ages 40 and older with aging, vascular disease, smoking, and inactivity. Studies of serum lipid profiles are indicated because the onset of erectile problems in men ages 40 and older is highly predictive of future coronary artery disease (option C). Because the patient does not complain of peripheral neuropathy, nerve conduction studies such as somatosensory evoked potentials are not indicated (option B). If a patient had a history compatible with low sexual desire, either bioavailable testosterone or free testosterone level should be obtained to rule out hypogonadism (option D). Measurement of nocturnal tumescence can help in the differential diagnosis of psychogenic impotence on the assumption that full erections during rapid eye movement sleep indicate the probable diagnosis (option A). Anemia and other abnormalities of a complete blood count have not been associated with erectile dysfunction (option E). Other factors to be considered in the differential diagnosis are major depressive and anxiety disorders, both of which can be associated with erectile problems. Some clinicians would also routinely order serum glucose and thyroid-stimulating hormone levels. If one suspects a possible vascular etiology, Doppler ultrasonography and intracavernosal injection of a vasoactive drug can be employed, as well as more invasive procedures such as dynamic infusion cavernosometry. **(Hales RE, Yudofsky SC, Roberts LW [eds]: APP Textbook of Psychiatry, 6th Edition, Chapter 20, pp. 658–659)**

34.3 How is the diagnosis of substance/medication-induced sexual dysfunction usually made?

A. By noting that sexual dysfunction occurs with 25%–50% of occasions of sexual activity.
B. By noting that the sexual difficulties increase when the medication is withdrawn and disappear upon reintroduction of the medication.
C. By noting that sexual dysfunction occurs with 50%–75% of occasions of sexual activity.
D. By noting a close temporal relationship between the initiation of a medication or dose increase and the occurrence of the sexual problem.

E. By noting that sexual function is unchanged from baseline prior to initiating pharmacotherapy.

The correct response is option D: By noting a close temporal relationship between the initiation of a medication or dose increase and the occurrence of the sexual problem.

The diagnosis of a substance/medication-induced sexual dysfunction is usually made by noting a close temporal relationship between the initiation or dose increase of a medication and the occurrence of the sexual problem (option D, not option E). The diagnosis is substantiated if the difficulty resolves when the medication is withdrawn and reappears when it is reintroduced (option B). The frequency of sexual dysfunction (options A, C), although not used in the diagnosis of substance/medication-induced sexual dysfunction, does indicate the severity of the illness. The DSM-5 diagnostic criteria for substance/medication–induced sexual dysfunction include severity specifiers to indicate the frequency of sexual dysfunction: mild if dysfunction occurs on 25%–50% of occasions of sexual activity, moderate if on 50%–75% of occasions, and severe if on 75% or more of occasions (American Psychiatric Association 2013). Fortunately, most medication-induced sexual side effects appear shortly after beginning the medication and dissipate quickly upon medication discontinuation. Because many psychiatric disorders are themselves associated with sexual dysfunction, it is important to establish a pretreatment baseline of sexual function prior to initiating pharmacotherapy. **(Hales RE, Yudofsky SC, Roberts LW [eds]: APP Textbook of Psychiatry, 6th Edition, Chapter 20, pp. 672–673)**

34.4   A 30-year-old woman comes to your office and reports that she is there only because her mother pleaded with her to see you. She tells you that although she has a good social network with friends of both sexes, she has never had any feelings of sexual arousal in response to men or women, does not have any erotic fantasies, and has little interest in sexual activity. She has found other like-minded individuals, and she and her friends accept themselves as asexual. Which of the following best describes her diagnosis?

A. Female sexual interest/arousal disorder, early onset, mild.
B. Female sexual interest/arousal disorder, early onset, severe.
C. Sexual aversion disorder.
D. No diagnosis, because she does not have the minimum number of symptoms required (Criterion A) for female sexual interest/arousal disorder.
E. No diagnosis, because she does not have clinically significant distress or impairment.

The correct response is option E: No diagnosis, because she does not have clinically significant distress or impairment.

Criterion A indicators for female sexual interest/arousal disorder include 1) absent/reduced interest in sexual activity; 2) absent/reduced sexual/erotic thoughts or fantasies; 3) no/reduced initiation of sexual activity, and typically unreceptive to a partner's attempts to initiate; 4) absent/reduced sexual excitement/pleasure during sexual activity in almost all or all (approximately 75%–100%) sexual encounters (in identified situations or contexts or, if generalized, in all contexts); 5) absent/reduced sexual interest/arousal in response to any internal or external sexual/erotic cues (e.g., written, verbal, visual); and 6) absent/reduced genital or nongenital sensations during sexual activity in almost all or all (approximately 75%–100%) sexual encounters (in identified situations or contexts or, if generalized, in all contexts). Female sexual interest/arousal disorder is defined by having at least three of six Criterion A indicators for at least about 6 months, as well as distress over the symptoms. Although this patient has met three of six criteria for longer than 6 months (option D), she is not distressed by her symptoms (option E). The severity of female sexual interest/arousal disorder—mild (option A), moderate, or severe (option B) is defined by the severity of the distress. The diagnosis of sexual aversion disorder (option C), which was present in DSM-IV-TR (American Psychiatric Association 2000), no longer exists because it was used infrequently and there was little research to support it. **(DSM-5, Sexual Dysfunctions, p. 433)**

34.5   Which of these statements is most correct about sexual dysfunctions that occur in the context of other social, medical, or psychiatric factors?

A. If the sexual symptoms are fully explainable by another psychiatric diagnosis, you should *not* give a sexual dysfunction diagnosis.
B. If the person has a concurrent medical condition that contributes to his or her sexual symptoms, you should give a psychiatric diagnosis.
C. If the sexual symptoms are fully explainable by the use of or discontinuation from a drug or other substance, you should *not* give a psychiatric diagnosis.
D. If the sexual symptoms are fully explainable by relationship distress or partner violence, you should diagnose a sexual dysfunction with a specifier for relationship factors.
E. Only the three most significant contributing factors/specifiers should be included.

The correct response is option A: If the sexual symptoms are fully explainable by another psychiatric diagnosis, you should *not* give a sexual dysfunction diagnosis.

Sexual symptoms that are fully explainable by another psychiatric condition, such as a major depressive episode, do not constitute a sexual dysfunction (option A). A diagnosis of sexual dysfunction is also withheld if a concurrent medical condition can explain or account for a patient's symptoms (option B). If the symptoms can be explained by substance use or discontinuation, the patient would qualify for a substance/medication-induced sexual dysfunction (option C). Symptoms that are fully explainable by relationship distress, partner violence, or other significant stressors also preclude a diagnosis of a sexual dysfunction (option D). There is no limit on the number of specifiers that may be used (option E). **(DSM-5, Sexual Dysfunctions, pp. 423–424)**

34.6   Which of the following statements is most correct with regard to the diagnosis of male hypoactive sexual desire disorder?

   A. The individual must have a low or absent desire for sex, as well as deficient or absent sexual thoughts and fantasies.
   B. The prevalence rates of low desire across cultures are remarkably consistent.
   C. A severity of "mild" is given if the presence of the symptoms is "rare to occasional."
   D. The symptoms must be present for a minimum of 3 months.
   E. A pattern of noninitiation of sexual activity is always a valid indicator of low or absent desire for sex.

The correct response is option A: The individual must have a low or absent desire for sex, as well as deficient or absent sexual thoughts and fantasies.

According to Criterion A, male hypoactive sexual desire disorder involves "persistent or recurrently deficient (or absent) sexual/erotic thoughts or fantasies and desire for sexual activity" (option A) for at least 6 months (option D). The severity is based on the level of distress experienced by the patient rather than the frequency of symptoms (option C). The prevalence of low sexual desire varies broadly across cultures (e.g., 12.5% in Northern European men and 28% in Southeast Asian men) (option B). A pattern of noninitiation of sexual activity is not considered to be an indication of low or absent desire for sex if the man prefers to have his partner initiate sexual activity (option E). **(DSM-5, Sexual Dysfunctions, pp. 440–442)**

Gender Dysphoria

34.7   Which of the following refers to the "watchful waiting" approach to gender dysphoria in children?

   A. Deferring treatment until the child declares his or her sexual orientation.
   B. Deferring treatment until the child undergoes puberty.
   C. Treatment whose primary goal is for the child and family to function optimally while waiting to see if the child's gender dysphoria continues into adolescence.
   D. Treatment whose primary goal is to contain symptoms until they make it difficult for the child to function at home or at school.
   E. Deferring treatment until the child asks to be treated.

The correct response is option C: Treatment whose primary goal is for the child and family to function optimally while waiting to see if the child's gender dysphoria continues into adolescence.

The "watchful waiting" approach (de Vries and Cohen-Kettenis 2012) supports careful observation of how gender dysphoria develops in the first stages of puberty (option C). This approach involves psychotherapeutic management of emotional, behavioral, and family problems in order to minimize their impact on the child's gender dysphoria and his or her functioning at home and in school (option D). The treatment follows a family and parent assessment, as well as an extensive psychodiagnostic assessment of the child. Treatment should not be deferred until a child asks for help (option E), undergoes puberty (option B), or declares his or her sexual orientation (option A). The watchful waiting approach is useful because a majority of children with gender dysphoria will not continue to have gender dysphoria as adults or even adolescents. **(Hales RE, Yudofsky SC, Roberts LW [eds]: APP Textbook of Psychiatry, 6th Edition, Chapter 21, p. 691)**

34.8   What is the beginning phase of the treatment of adult gender dysphoria?

A. Hormone therapy.
B. Bilateral orchiectomy in men and bilateral mastectomy and optional hysterectomy in women.
C. Encouraging the patient to live in the world in the cross-gender role.
D. Cognitive therapy designed to minimize the patient's dissatisfaction with his or her birth gender.
E. Referral to an endocrinologist and a surgeon.

The correct response is option C: Encouraging the patient to live in the world in the cross-gender role.

The course of treatment usually begins with the patient living in the world in the cross-gender role before surgical reassignment (option C). The exact nature of the cross-gender role will vary from patient to patient, but males typically crossdress, have electrolysis, and practice female behaviors, whereas women cut their hair and bind or conceal their breasts. Some patients change their identity to the opposite gender on official documents and at work. Hormone treatment should begin only after patients have successfully lived in their cross-gender roles and their treatment teams find no contraindications to their gender reassignment (options A, E). More invasive procedures, such as orchiectomy for men and bilateral mastectomy and optional hysterectomy for women, are pursued following hormone treatment (option B). Patients are encouraged to live in the cross-gender role rather than minimize the patient's dissatisfaction with his or her birth gender (option D). **(Hales RE, Yudofsky SC, Roberts LW [eds]: APP Textbook of Psychiatry, 6th Edition, Chapter 21, pp. 694–695)**

34.9   Which of the following is a true statement about adolescents with gender dysphoria?

A. Childhood gender dysphoria usually persists into adolescence.
B. Adolescent patients generally do not require endocrinological screening unless there is suspicion of a hormonal disorder.

C. Early surgical intervention is recommended because of better outcomes in terms of healing and scarring.
D. If the behavior has persisted from childhood into adolescence, it is likely to persist into adulthood.
E. Adolescent patients do not require a psychiatric examination unless a specific psychiatric problem is suspected.

The correct response is option D: If the behavior has persisted from childhood into adolescence, it is likely to persist into adulthood.

Most childhood gender dysphoria does not persist into adolescence (option A) (Zucker et al. 2012), although gender dysphoria that persists into adolescence often persists into adulthood (option D). Because the majority of childhood gender dysphoria resolves in adolescence, physical interventions are not recommended for children (option C) but are increasingly considered appropriate for adolescents with persistent symptoms (de Vries et al. 2011; Hembree et al. 2009). Adolescents with gender dysphoria require a thorough psychiatric examination (option E) and screening by an endocrinologist (option B), and may benefit from individual and family therapy. **(Hales RE, Yudofsky SC, Roberts LW [eds]: APP Textbook of Psychiatry, 6th Edition, Chapter 21, pp. 692–693)**

34.10 In DSM 5, which of the following statements is true about the words gender and transgender?

A. Gender refers to the biological indicators of male or female seen in an individual.
B. Gender refers to the individual's initial assignment of male or female, usually given at birth.
C. Gender refers to the individual's lived role in society or identification as male or female.
D. A transgender individual is someone who has undergone a social transition from male to female or female to male.
E. A transgender individual is someone who has sought sex reassignment treatment of some kind.

The correct response is option C: Gender refers to the individual's lived role in society or identification as male or female.

The words sex, gender, transgender, and transsexual are complex and should be used properly. In general, *sex* refers to biology (options A, B), and *gender* refers to a lived role or experience (option C). *Transgender* describes individuals who experience gender incongruence and/or dysphoria but do not necessarily seek out sex reassignment or social transition (options D, E). The term *transsexual* applies to individuals who have sought or undergone role transition or sex reassignment. **(DSM-5, Gender Dysphoria, p. 451)**

34.11 Which of the following is true for adults suffering from gender dysphoria?

A. There can be a specifier added for a posttransition phase of the disorder.
B. For this diagnosis to be made, the individual must seek some kind of sex reassignment treatment.
C. For this diagnosis to be made, the individual must have a strong desire to be the other gender or must insist that he or she is the other gender.
D. For this diagnosis to be made, there must be an associated disorder of sex development.
E. For this diagnosis to be made, the individual must engage in cross-dressing behavior.

The correct response is option A: There can be a specifier added for a posttransition phase of the disorder.

The diagnosis of gender dysphoria can include a posttransition specifier, indicating that the original dysphoria has largely been treated (option A). The diagnosis requires that the patient wishes to be viewed as the other gender, not necessarily that he or she wants to be the other gender (option C). The diagnosis does not require the patient to seek gender reassignment (option B) or cross-dress (option E). The disorders of sex development are congenital conditions in which the development of chromosomal, gonadal, or anatomical sex is atypical and not required for a diagnosis of gender dysphoria (option D). **(DSM-5, Gender Dysphoria, pp. 452–453)**

34.12 Which of the following *must* be present to make a diagnosis of gender dysphoria in children?

A. There must be a co-occurring disorder of sex development.
B. There must be a strong desire to be the other gender or an insistence that the person is the other gender.
C. There must be a strong dislike of one's sexual anatomy.
D. The child must have stated a wish to change gender.
E. There must be a strong desire for the primary and/or secondary sex characteristics that match the experienced gender.

The correct response is option B: There must be a strong desire to be the other gender or an insistence that the person is the other gender.

Gender dysphoria in children, unlike in adults, must be accompanied by the strong desire to be the other gender or an insistence that one is the other gender (option B). The inclusion of this criterion in DSM-5 makes the diagnosis more conservative. The strong desire does not need to be explicitly stated (option D), given that social and/or cultural factors may inhibit this expression. There may be a strong dislike of one's sexual anatomy (option C) or a strong desire for sex characteristics that match the experienced gender (option E), but these are not necessary factors for diagnosis. A disorder of sex development may co-occur but is not necessary for diagnosis (option A). **(DSM-5, Gender Dysphoria, p. 452)**

References

American Psychiatric Association: Diagnostic and Statistical Manual of Mental Disorders, 4th Edition, Text Revision. Washington, DC, American Psychiatric Association, 2000

American Psychiatric Association: Diagnostic and Statistical Manual of Mental Disorders, 5th Edition. Arlington, VA, American Psychiatric Association, 2013

de Vries ALC, Cohen-Kettenis PT: Clinical management of gender dysphoria in children and adolescents: the Dutch approach. J Homosex 59(3):301–320, 2012 22455322

de Vries ALC, Steensma TD, Doreleijers TAH, Cohen-Kettenis PT: Puberty suppression in adolescents with gender identity disorder: a prospective follow-up study. J Sex Med 8(8):2276–2283, 2011 20646177

Hembree WC, Cohen-Kettenis P, Delemarre-van de Waal HA, et al; Endocrine Society: Endocrine treatment of transsexual persons: an Endocrine Society clinical practice guideline. J Clin Endocrinol Metab 94(9):3132–3154, 2009 19509099

Zucker KJ, Wood H, Singh D, Bradley SJ: A developmental, biopsychosocial model for the treatment of children with gender identity disorder. J Homosex 59(3):369–397, 2012 22455326

CHAPTER 35

Sleep-Wake Disorders

35.1 Which of the following best characterizes the electroencephalogram (EEG) tracing of rapid eye movement (REM) sleep?

A. Low-voltage fast activity.
B. Delta waves.
C. Theta waves.
D. High-voltage slow activity.
E. Nonspecific changes.

The correct response is option A: Low-voltage fast activity.

The EEG tracing of REM sleep is characterized by a low-voltage, fast-frequency pattern (option A) and not by nonspecific changes (option E). A slow, high-voltage tracing is characteristic of non-REM (NREM) sleep (option D). Theta waves (option C) are also characteristic of NREM sleep, present at the onset of Stage 1 (NREM 1, abbreviated as N1) and Stage 2 (N2) sleep. Delta waves (option B) usually arise during Stage 3 (N3) sleep. **(Hales RE, Yudofsky SC, Roberts LW [eds]: APP Textbook of Psychiatry, 6th Edition, Chapter 19, Table 19–2, p. 614)**

35.2 Rapid eye movement (REM) sleep behavior disorder is characterized by which of the following?

A. Episode occurrence during the first part of the sleep period.
B. Muscle atonia during REM sleep.
C. Open eyes during REM sleep.
D. Shortened episodes of REM sleep.
E. Loss of muscle atonia during REM sleep.

The correct response is option E: Loss of muscle atonia during REM sleep.

Except for some skeletal muscles (e.g., eyes, diaphragm), we are paralyzed while we dream. Failure of muscle inhibition during REM sleep (option E) leads to acting out of dreams, sometimes with violent behaviors—such as punching, kicking, and tackling—that are likely to injure the patient or bed partner. REM sleep behavior disorder may herald neurodegenerative disease or be induced by commonly used medications (Arnulf 2012; Mahowald and Schenck 2004; Mahowald et al. 2011). In contrast to sleepwalkers, whose eyes are open and whose arousal events typically occur in the first part of the sleep period (option C), individuals with REM sleep behavior disorder enact their dreams (option B) with eyes closed during the second half of the sleep period (option A), when REM sleep episodes increase in length and intensity (option D). **(Hales RE, Yudofsky SC, Roberts LW [eds]: APP Textbook of Psychiatry, 6th Edition, Chapter 19, p. 638)**

35.3 Which of the following symptoms is characteristic of patients with NREM sleep arousal disorder?

A. Cataplexy.
B. Chronic insomnia.
C. Sleepwalking with eyes closed.
D. Total or partial amnesia for nighttime events.
E. Passive behavior.

The correct response is option D: Total or partial amnesia for nighttime events.

NREM sleep arousal disorder symptoms exist on a continuum: confusional arousals (sitting up, eyes open, talking), sleep terrors (usually beginning with a blood-curdling scream), and sleepwalking all can occur in the same patient. During episodes, frontal lobes are "offline"; patients appear to be awake, with open eyes (option C), and may be able to converse, but awareness is not present. Sleepwalkers have climbed or fallen out of windows, jumped off roofs, driven cars, and attacked those who got in their way or tried to wake them (option E). In the morning, sleepwalkers are partially or totally amnestic for nighttime events (option D). Cataplexy is a symptom of narcolepsy (option A). Chronic insomnia is not a symptom of NREM sleep arousal disorder (option B). **(Hales RE, Yudofsky SC, Roberts LW [eds]: APP Textbook of Psychiatry, 6th Edition, Chapter 19, pp. 636, 639)**

35.4 Which of the following commonly prescribed hypnotic medications is a melatonin agonist?

A. Zaleplon.
B. Temazepam.
C. Ramelteon.
D. Eszopiclone.
E. Doxepin.

The correct response is option C: Ramelteon.

Ramelteon is a melatonin agonist (option C). Zaleplon (option A), zolpidem, and eszopiclone (option D) are nonbenzodiazepine γ-aminobutyric acid (GABA) agonists; temazepam (option B) is a benzodiazepine GABA agonist; and doxepin (option E) is an antihistamine. **(Hales RE, Yudofsky SC, Roberts LW [eds]: APP Textbook of Psychiatry, 6th Edition, Chapter 19, Table 19–3, p. 615)**

35.5   A 48-year-old woman with uterine fibroids and mild hypertension reports symptoms of waking discomfort, occasional pain, and the urge to move her legs that occur almost every night. The discomfort is somewhat relieved by leg movement. Which of the following would be an appropriate initial treatment for this patient?

A. Pramipexole.
B. Oxycodone.
C. Gabapentin.
D. Iron replacement if necessary.
E. Zolpidem.

The correct response is option D: Iron replacement if necessary.

For all patients with restless legs syndrome, the clinician should obtain a serum ferritin level, which provides a measure of body iron stores. Iron needs to be replaced if levels are 50 ng/mL or less (although 50 ng/mL will be reported as "normal" by laboratories). Some experts replace iron at levels well above that level, since cerebrospinal fluid ferritin levels can be lower than peripheral values. The causes of low levels need to be identified (e.g., diet). Given this patient's history of uterine fibroids, iron depletion is the most likely cause of restless legs syndrome (option D). Typically, ferrous sulfate 325 mg with 100 mg vitamin C (which promotes absorption) is taken twice a day if tolerated. It should not be taken with meals. Ferritin levels should be retested every 3–4 months to avoid overtreatment. Medication classes that have been found useful for treating restless legs syndrome include opiates (e.g., oxycodone; option B), anticonvulsants (e.g., gabapentin; option C), benzodiazepines (e.g., clonazepam), and dopamine agonists (e.g., pramipexole; option A). Although still widely prescribed, dopamine agonists can cause symptom rebound and augmentation (Salas et al. 2010); for this reason, some sleep clinicians prefer to avoid prescribing these agents. GABA$_A$ α_1-agonists such as zolpidem have not been found to be useful for restless leg syndrome (option E). **(Hales RE, Yudofsky SC, Roberts LW [eds]: APP Textbook of Psychiatry, 6th Edition, Chapter 19, pp. 623–624, 635)**

35.6   Which of the following brain structures controls circadian rhythms?

A. Locus coeruleus.
B. Pineal gland.
C. Mesopontine junction.
D. Pedunculopontine nucleus.
E. Suprachiasmatic nucleus.

The correct response is option E: Suprachiasmatic nucleus.

Circadian rhythms are controlled by the suprachiasmatic nucleus (option E) of the anterior hypothalamus, and the circadian clock controls many internal rhythms, including the sleep-wake cycle, which it keeps in tune with the day-night pattern of the external environment. Circadian rhythms are genetically determined and persist even in the absence of external time cues such as the day-night cycle. The pineal gland (option B) produces melatonin in response to timing information from the suprachiasmatic nucleus. The locus coeruleus (option A) produces norepinephrine, which promotes wakefulness. The mesopontine junction (option C) is a region that includes several nuclei involved in arousal and wakefulness but does not set circadian rhythms. The pedunculopontine nucleus (option D) is part of the reticular activating system, which is also involved in arousal and sleep-wake transitions but does not control circadian rhythms. **(Hales RE, Yudofsky SC, Roberts LW [eds]: APP Textbook of Psychiatry, 6th Edition, Chapter 19, pp. 608–609, 611–612)**

References

Arnulf I: REM sleep behavior disorder: motor manifestations and pathophysiology. Mov Disord 27(6):677–689, 2012 22447623

Mahowald MW, Schenck CH: Rem sleep without atonia—from cats to humans. Arch Ital Biol 142(4):469–478, 2004 15493548

Mahowald MW, Cramer Bornemann MA, Schenck CH: State dissociation, human behavior, and consciousness. Curr Top Med Chem 11(19):2392–2402, 2011 21906025

Salas RE, Gamaldo CE, Allen RP: Update in restless legs syndrome. Curr Opin Neurol 23(4):401–406, 2010 20581683

CHAPTER 36

Somatic Symptom and Related Disorders

36.1 Which of the following statements about illness anxiety disorder is true?

A. Patients with this diagnosis bear no relationship to patients diagnosed with hypochondriasis.

B. A person with this disorder has no significant somatic symptoms.

C. A negative medical workup usually alleviates the anxiety of patients with this disorder.

D. A history of parental overprotection has not been associated with the development of this disorder.

E. Given the delusional basis for the disorder, it can be expected that pharmacotherapy with antipsychotic medication may have some utility.

The correct response is option B: A person with this disorder has no significant somatic symptoms.

Illness anxiety disorder is a new diagnosis introduced to DSM-5 (American Psychiatric Association 2013) that defines a disorder based on maladaptive behaviors related to a preoccupation with having or acquiring a medical illness. A key feature is the absence of significant somatic symptoms (option B), and a predominant response to this preoccupation is anxiety (not psychosis; option E). Two predominant types of illness anxiety disorder are recognized in DSM-5: care-seeking type (in which medical care is frequently used) and care-avoidant type (in which medical care is rarely accessed). This diagnosis is expected to capture a minority of patients previously diagnosed with hypochondriasis (option A), which is not included as a DSM-5 diagnosis. Patients with illness anxiety disorder are most commonly encountered in medical settings but may present to psychiatrists for treatment of anxiety. These patients' excessive concerns about undiagnosed disease are unlikely to be alleviated by medical reassurance or negative diagnostic tests (option C). A history of parental overprotection has been associated with the development of illness anxiety disorder (option D). **(Hales RE, Yudofsky SC, Roberts LW [eds]: APP Textbook of Psychiatry, 6th Edition, Chapter 16, pp. 537–539)**

36.2   A patient with illness anxiety disorder would most likely benefit from which of the following?

A. Medical hospitalization.
B. Pharmacotherapy with antipsychotics.
C. Pharmacotherapy with selective serotonin reuptake inhibitors (SSRIs).
D. Additional medical tests.
E. Psychiatric hospitalization.

The correct response is option C: Pharmacotherapy with selective serotonin reuptake inhibitors (SSRIs).

Treatment of illness anxiety disorder has yet to be thoroughly researched, but research on and clinical experience with hypochondriasis remains relevant. Because illness anxiety disorder shares many features with other anxiety disorders, it can be expected that SSRI pharmacotherapy (not antipsychotic therapy; option B) may have some utility. In patients with hypochondriasis, research has suggested that SSRI treatment (option C) is useful for either acute or long-term treatment, with significant proportions of patients achieving remission (Schweitzer et al. 2011). Stoudemire (1988) suggested an approach featuring consistent treatment, generally by the same primary physician, with supportive, regularly scheduled office visits not focused on the evaluation of symptoms. Hospitalization (options A, E), medical tests (option D), and medications with addictive potential are to be avoided if possible. Psychotherapeutic approaches may be enhanced greatly by effective pharmacotherapy. Cognitive-behavioral therapy (CBT) was found to be effective in a 2004 study in which 57% of CBT-treated patients showed a reduction in hypochondriacal beliefs at 12-month follow-up (Barsky and Ahern 2004). **(Hales RE, Yudofsky SC, Roberts LW [eds]: APP Textbook of Psychiatry, 6th Edition, Chapter 16, pp. 539–540)**

36.3   After a medical illness is ruled out, how should treatment of factitious disorder be approached?

A. The physician should aggressively confront the patient with the fact that no legitimate medical illness is present.
B. The treatment team should confront the patient with the diagnosis of factitious disorder.
C. The treatment team should confront the patient with his or her deception after conferring with hospital administration.
D. The physician should inform the patient of a treatment plan and attempt to enlist him or her in that plan, with minimal expectation that the patient will "confess" to the deception.
E. The physician should inform the patient of a treatment plan and attempt to enlist him or her in that plan, resorting to psychiatric admission only if the patient refuses to acknowledge the deception.

The correct response is option D: The physician should inform the patient of a treatment plan and attempt to enlist him or her in that plan, with minimal expectation that the patient will "confess" to the deception.

Once the contribution of general medical illness has been factored out, the patient must be informed of a change in the treatment plan, and an attempt must be made to enlist him or her in that plan (option D). The literature generally refers to this process (perhaps alluding to its countertransference aspects) as containing an element of "confrontation." There is now general agreement that treatment begins at this point and that it is best done indirectly, with minimal expectation that the patient "confess" or acknowledge the deception (option E). It is a delicate process, with patients frequently leaving the hospital against medical advice or otherwise leaving treatment. Guziec et al. (1994) aptly likened this process to making a psychodynamic interpretation. Eisendrath (1989) described techniques for reducing confrontation (options A–C), such as using inexact interpretations, therapeutic double binds, and other strategic and face-saving techniques to allow the patient tacitly to relinquish the factitious signs and symptoms. **(Hales RE, Yudofsky SC, Roberts LW [eds]: APP Textbook of Psychiatry, 6th Edition, Chapter 16, p. 551)**

36.4   What percentage of neurology outpatients has been found to have a history of conversion symptoms?

   A. 4%–15%.
   B. 25%–40%.
   C. 50%.
   D. 1%–3%.
   E. 75%–90%.

The correct response is option A: 4%–15%.

Approximately 4%–15% of neurology outpatients, 5%–24% of psychiatric outpatients, 5%–14% of general hospital patients, and 1%–3% of outpatient psychiatric referrals have a history of conversion symptoms (Cloninger 1994; Ford 1983; Stone et al. 2010; Toone 1990). **(Hales RE, Yudofsky SC, Roberts LW [eds]: APP Textbook of Psychiatry, 6th Edition, Chapter 16, p. 543)**

36.5   Which of the following is the most active symptomatic phase for somatization disorder?

   A. Childhood.
   B. Adolescence.
   C. Early adulthood.
   D. Middle age.
   E. Old age.

The correct response is option C: Early adulthood.

Although an extensive literature on the natural history of somatic symptom disorder is not yet available, the DSM-IV/DSM-IV-TR diagnosis of somatization disorder (American Psychiatric Association 1994, 2000) was well studied over decades, and it can be assumed that some of its observed natural history will continue to be relevant for patients with somatic symptom disorder. Robins and O'Neal (1953) found somatization disorder to be unusual in children younger than 9 years (option A). In most cases, characteristic symptoms begin during adolescence (option B), and the criteria are satisfied by the mid-20s. Somatization disorder, a chronic illness with fluctuations in the frequency and diversity of symptoms, was previously thought to remit only in rare cases. The most active symptomatic phase is usually early adulthood (option C), but aging (options D, E) does not lead to total remission. Early longitudinal prospective studies showed that 80%–90% of patients diagnosed with somatization disorder retained the diagnosis over many years (Cloninger et al. 1986). However, newer studies have yielded much higher rates of remission, suggesting that up to 50% of patients experience remission within 1 year (Creed and Barsky 2004). **(Hales RE, Yudofsky SC, Roberts LW [eds]: APP Textbook of Psychiatry, 6th Edition, Chapter 16, pp. 534–535)**

36.6   Which of the following complications of somatization disorder (DSM-5 somatic symptom disorder) are likely to be preventable if the disorder is recognized and symptoms managed appropriately?

A. Surgical procedures and drug dependence.
B. Marital discord and occupational dysfunction.
C. Separations and divorces.
D. Suicide attempts and completions.
E. Drug addiction and mortality.

The correct response is option A: Surgical procedures and drug dependence.

The most frequent and important complications of somatization disorder are repeated surgical operations, drug dependence, suicide attempts, and marital separation or divorce, according to Goodwin and Guze (1996), who suggested that surgical operations and drug dependence (option A) are preventable if the disorder is recognized and the symptoms are managed appropriately. Generally, because of awareness that somatization disorder is an alternative explanation for various pains and other symptoms, invasive techniques (which have the potential to cause iatrogenic illness) can be withheld or postponed when objective indications are absent or equivocal. There is no evidence of excess mortality in patients with somatization disorder (option E). Avoiding the prescribing of habit-forming or addictive substances for persistent or recurrent complaints of pain should be paramount in the mind of the treating physician. Suicide attempts are common, but completed suicide is not (option D). It is unclear whether marital or occupational dysfunction can be minimized through psychotherapy (options B, C). **(Hales RE, Yudofsky SC, Roberts LW [eds]: APP Textbook of Psychiatry, 6th Edition, Chapter 16, p. 535)**

36.7 Which of the following is a true statement about the DSM-5 diagnostic criteria for somatic symptom disorder?

A. A minimum number of symptoms must be present to qualify for the diagnosis.
B. The requirement that the symptoms be medically unexplained has been eliminated.
C. The criteria no longer stipulate that the patient's somatic symptoms be accompanied by abnormal thoughts, feelings, or behaviors.
D. Somatic symptom disorder is no longer defined by the presence of somatic symptoms.
E. The DSM-5 diagnosis of somatic symptom disorder replaces and incorporates the previous DSM-IV/DSM-IV-TR diagnoses of hypochondriasis and pain disorder.

The correct response is option B: The requirement that the symptoms be medically unexplained has been eliminated.

The DSM-5 diagnosis of somatic symptom disorder replaces the previous DSM-IV/DSM-IV-TR diagnoses of somatization disorder and undifferentiated somatoform disorder (not hypochondriasis and pain disorder; option E). Somatic symptom disorder is defined by the presence of somatic symptoms, as in the older classifications (option D). However, the DSM-5 criteria for somatic symptom disorder do not require that the symptoms be medically unexplained (option B). No specific numbers or types of symptoms are needed to meet the diagnosis (option A). Rather, the additional core feature of this diagnosis is presence of abnormal thoughts, feelings, and behaviors associated with the somatic symptoms (option C). **(Hales RE, Yudofsky SC, Roberts LW [eds]: APP Textbook of Psychiatry, 6th Edition, Chapter 16, pp. 532–533)**

36.8 In patients with somatization disorder (DSM-5 somatic symptom disorder), which of the following, when combined with a psychiatric consultation, was found to be more effective in improving symptoms and functioning than a psychiatric consultation alone?

A. Cognitive-behavioral therapy (CBT).
B. Hospitalization for a more in-depth medical evaluation.
C. Supportive psychotherapy.
D. Psychoanalytic psychotherapy.
E. Dynamic psychotherapy.

The correct response is option A: Cognitive-behavioral therapy (CBT).

In 2001, the National Institute of Mental Health funded a single-blind, active-control, parallel-assignment interventional study of CBT for somatization disorder in the primary care setting. In this study, Allen et al. (2006) found that CBT (vs. supportive psychotherapy [option C], psychoanalytic psychotherapy [option D], and dynamic psychotherapy [option E]) with psychiatric consultation was more effective in improving symptoms and functioning than psychiatric consultation alone (option A). Somatization disorder is difficult to treat, and there appears to be no single superior treatment approach. In short, patients require an empathic, supportive, and functional approach to address their suffering; physicians should, however, be cautious about ordering repetitive, unnecessary, and invasive medical/surgical workups, which can cause iatrogenic illness. Primary care physicians generally can manage patients with somatization disorder adequately, but the expertise of a consulting psychiatrist has been shown to be useful. In a prospective, randomized, controlled study, Smith et al. (1986) found a reduction in health care costs for patients with somatization disorder who received a psychiatric consultation as opposed to those who did not receive a consultation. Reduced expenditures were largely the result of decreased rates of hospitalization. These gains were accomplished with no decrement in medical status or in patient satisfaction, suggesting that many of the evaluations and treatments otherwise provided to patients with somatization disorder are unnecessary (option B). **(Hales RE, Yudofsky SC, Roberts LW [eds]: APP Textbook of Psychiatry, 6th Edition, Chapter 16, pp. 536–537)**

36.9   Which of the following is the *least* likely condition to be included in the differential diagnosis of illness anxiety disorder?

A. Adjustment disorder.
B. Generalized anxiety disorder.
C. Obsessive-compulsive disorder.
D. Major depressive disorder.
E. Schizophrenia.

The correct response is option E: Schizophrenia.

Illness anxiety disorder, a new diagnosis in DSM-5, is characterized by a preoccupation with having or acquiring a serious illness. A key feature of the disorder is the absence of significant somatic symptoms; the patient's distress derives not from any specific physical complaints but rather from anxiety surrounding the possibility of having a dreaded illness. Various other conditions may share the diagnostic features of illness anxiety disorder, particularly mood and anxiety disorders. Adjustment disorder (option A) should be considered in patients whose symptoms have not met the criteria for duration or severity and are clearly in response to a specific event. This may be particularly relevant when the event leading to the adjustment disorder is health related. Generalized anxiety disorder (option B) typically involves persistent worrying about topics aside from those that are strictly health related. Obsessive-compulsive disorder (option C) would be expected to focus on a fear of getting the disease in the future as opposed to a focus on current symptoms and would also generally involve additional obsessions or compulsions. Because patients with major depressive disorder (option D) frequently report anxious and somatic preoccupations, depressive disorders may overlap with the symptoms of illness anxiety disorder; however, the former would include other mood, vegetative, and cognitive symptoms consistent with common mood disorders. Schizophrenia (option E) is likely to have a different set of symptoms, which would not easily be included in illness anxiety disorder. **(Hales RE, Yudofsky SC, Roberts LW [eds]: APP Textbook of Psychiatry, 6th Edition, Chapter 16, pp. 537–538)**

36.10 Research and clinical experience with illness anxiety disorder (DSM-IV/DSM-IV-TR hypochondriasis) suggest better outcomes for patients treated with which of the following approaches?

A. Reassurance by the treatment provider that the symptoms are not serious.
B. Medical evaluation and treatment only.
C. Psychiatric evaluation as a replacement for continued medical care.
D. Direct referral for psychiatric evaluation and treatment.
E. Early confrontation about the irrational fears of illness.

The correct response is option D: Direct referral for psychiatric evaluation and treatment.

Patients referred early for psychiatric evaluation and treatment (option D) of hypochondriasis appear to have a better prognosis than those receiving only medical evaluations and treatments (option B). As with other somatic symptom and related disorders, psychiatric referrals should be made with sensitivity and awareness of stigma related to mental illness (option E). Perhaps the best guideline to follow is for the referring physician to stress that the patient's distress is serious and that psychiatric evaluation will be a supplement to, not a replacement for (option C), continued medical care. Patients may feel dissatisfied by reassurance that their symptoms are "not serious" and may avoid psychiatric referral due to anger over being told that the symptoms "are all in their head" (option A). **(Hales RE, Yudofsky SC, Roberts LW [eds]: APP Textbook of Psychiatry, 6th Edition, Chapter 16, p. 539)**

36.11 Which of the following is a recommended treatment approach for illness anxiety disorder?

A. Gradual redirection of focus from interpersonal difficulties to symptoms during office visits.
B. Regular office visits focused on evaluation of symptoms.
C. Consistent treatment by the same primary care physician, with supportive, regularly scheduled office visits.
D. Extensive medical tests to clarify the clinical picture of the patient.
E. Supportive therapy to help the patient adjust to a state of chronic illness and disability.

The correct response is option C: Consistent treatment by the same primary care physician, with supportive, regularly scheduled office visits.

Treatment of illness anxiety disorder has yet to be thoroughly researched, but research on and clinical experience with hypochondriasis remains relevant. Stoudemire (1988) suggested an approach featuring consistent treatment, generally by the same primary physician, with supportive, regularly scheduled office visits (option C) not focused on the evaluation of symptoms (option B). Hospitalization, medical tests (option D), and medications with addictive potential are to be avoided if possible. During office visits, the clinical interview should gradually shift in content from symptoms to social and/or interpersonal difficulties (option A). Preventing adoption of the sick role and chronic invalidism should be a guiding principle for clinicians when treating patients with illness anxiety symptoms (option E). **(Hales RE, Yudofsky SC, Roberts LW [eds]: APP Textbook of Psychiatry, 6th Edition, Chapter 16, pp. 539–540)**

36.12 How does DSM-5 differ from DSM-IV/DSM-IV-TR in its conceptualization of conversion disorder?

A. In DSM-5, a patient's symptoms must be fully explainable by culturally sanctioned behavior.
B. In DSM-5, the requirement that symptoms be produced unintentionally has been eliminated.
C. In DSM-5, the symptoms must be temporally associated with an identifiable stressor.
D. In DSM-5, the requirement that symptoms be incompatible with any recognized neurological or medical condition has been removed.
E. In DSM-5, the symptoms may involve pain or sexual dysfunction in addition to motor or sensory dysfunction.

The correct response is option B: In DSM-5, the requirement that symptoms be produced unintentionally has been eliminated.

The essential feature of conversion disorder (functional neurological symptom disorder) is the presence of symptoms of altered motor or sensory function (not pain and sexual dysfunction; option E) that, as evidenced by clinical findings, are incompatible with any recognized neurological or medical condition and not better explained by another medical or mental disorder (options A, D). The DSM-5 criteria for conversion disorder explicitly require neurological examination findings that are inconsistent with known neurological disease. DSM-5 does not include a requirement that the symptoms be produced unintentionally (option B), because absence of feigning is difficult to determine reliably. Although the symptoms of conversion disorder often occur in association with an identifiable stressor, the DSM-IV-TR criterion that required identification of associated psychological factors has been removed (option C). **(Hales RE, Yudofsky SC, Roberts LW [eds]: APP Textbook of Psychiatry, 6th Edition, Chapter 16, pp. 540–542)**

36.13 Which of the following is a core feature of the DSM-5 diagnosis of psychological factors affecting other medical conditions?

A. Presence of both a medical condition and a mental disorder.
B. Preoccupation with having or acquiring a serious illness.
C. Clinical evidence of incompatibility between patients' symptoms and recognized medical conditions.
D. Documented falsification or self-induction of medical symptoms.
E. Presence of a psychological or behavioral factor that adversely affects a medical condition.

The correct response is option E: Presence of a psychological or behavioral factor that adversely affects a medical condition.

Medical conditions and comorbid mental disorders are present in many patients (option A), but the DSM-5 diagnosis is reserved for cases in which patient psychological factors are judged to have a clinically significant impact on a medical condition. The core feature of the diagnosis of psychological factors affecting other medical conditions is the presence of psychological or behavioral factors that adversely affect a medical condition (option E) by increasing the risk for suffering, disability, or death. The most common types of psychological factors include mental disorders, psychological symptoms, personality traits, coping styles, and maladaptive health behaviors. Culturally specific behaviors such as use of faith healers must be excluded when applying this diagnosis, because a variety of health practices exist as a normal pattern within certain cultures and represent attempts to treat illness rather than to perpetuate it. Preoccupation with having or acquiring a serious illness (option B) is a core feature of illness anxiety disorder. Incompatibility between symptoms and recognized medical conditions (option C) is a feature of conversion disorder. Falsification or self-induction of medical symptoms (option D) is a feature of factitious disorder or malingering. **(Hales RE, Yudofsky SC, Roberts LW [eds]: APP Textbook of Psychiatry, 6th Edition, Chapter 16, pp. 537, 540, 546–547)**

36.14 Which of the following is a true statement about conversion disorder?

A. The onset of conversion disorder is generally acute, but it may be characterized by gradually increasing symptomatology.
B. The typical course of individual conversion symptoms is generally lengthy.
C. Among patients whose symptoms disappear, 5%–10% will relapse within 1 year.
D. A factor traditionally associated with good prognosis is late onset.
E. There are no clear precipitants to an episode of conversion disorder.

The correct response is option A: The onset of conversion disorder is generally acute, but it may be characterized by gradually increasing symptomatology.

Onset of conversion disorder is generally acute, but it may be characterized by gradually increasing symptomatology (option A). The typical course of individual conversion symptoms is generally short (option B); half to nearly all patients show a disappearance of symptoms by the time of hospital discharge. However, 20%–25% will relapse within 1 year (option C). Factors traditionally associated with good prognosis include acute onset (option D), presence of clearly identifiable stress at the time of onset (option E), short interval between onset and institution of treatment, and good intelligence. **(Hales RE, Yudofsky SC, Roberts LW [eds]: APP Textbook of Psychiatry, 6th Edition, Chapter 16, p. 543)**

References

Allen LA, Woolfolk RL, Escobar JI, et al: Cognitive-behavioral therapy for somatization disorder: a randomized controlled trial. Arch Intern Med 166(14):1512–1518, 2006 16864762

American Psychiatric Association: Diagnostic and Statistical Manual of Mental Disorders, 4th Edition. Arlington, VA, American Psychiatric Association, 1994

American Psychiatric Association: Diagnostic and Statistical Manual of Mental Disorders, 4th Edition, Text Revision. Washington, DC, American Psychiatric Association, 2000

American Psychiatric Association: Diagnostic and Statistical Manual of Mental Disorders, 5th Edition. Arlington, VA, American Psychiatric Association, 2013

Barsky AJ, Ahern DK: Cognitive behavior therapy for hypochondriasis: a randomized controlled trial. JAMA 291(12):1464–1470, 2004 15039413

Cloninger CR: Somatoform and dissociative disorders, in The Medical Basis of Psychiatry, 2nd Edition. Edited by Winokur G, Clayton P. Philadelphia, PA, WB Saunders, 1994, pp 169–192

Cloninger CR, Martin RL, Guze SB, Clayton PJ: A prospective follow-up and family study of somatization in men and women. Am J Psychiatry 143(7):873–878, 1986 3717427

Creed F, Barsky A: A systematic review of the epidemiology of somatisation disorder and hypochondriasis. J Psychosom Res 56(4):391–408, 2004 15094023

Eisendrath SJ: Factitious physical disorders: treatment without confrontation. Psychosomatics 30(4):383–387, 1989 2798730

Ford CV: The Somatizing Disorders: Illness as a Way of Life. New York, Elsevier, 1983

Goodwin DW, Guze SB: Psychiatric Diagnoses, 5th Edition. New York, Oxford University Press, 1996

Guziec J, Lazarus A, Harding JJ: Case of a 29-year-old nurse with factitious disorder. The utility of psychiatric intervention on a general medical floor. Gen Hosp Psychiatry 16(1):47–53, 1994 8039685

Robins E, O'Neal P: Clinical features of hysteria in children, with a note on prognosis; a two to seventeen year follow-up study of 41 patients. Nerv Child 10(2):246–271, 1953 13087551

Schweitzer PJ, Zafar U, Pavlicova M, Fallon BA: Long-term follow-up of hypochondriasis after selective serotonin reuptake inhibitor treatment. J Clin Psychopharmacol 31(3):365–368, 2011 21508861

Smith GR Jr, Monson RA, Ray DC: Psychiatric consultation in somatization disorder. A randomized controlled study. N Engl J Med 314(22):1407–1413, 1986 3084975

Stone J, Carson A, Duncan R, et al: Who is referred to neurology clinics?--the diagnoses made in 3781 new patients. Clin Neurol Neurosurg 112(9):747–751, 2010 20646830

Stoudemire GA: Somatoform disorders, factitious disorders, and malingering, in The American Psychiatric Press Textbook of Psychiatry. Edited by Talbott JA, Hales RE, Yudofsky SC. Washington, DC, American Psychiatric Press, 1988, pp 533–556

Toone BK: Disorders of hysterical conversion, in Physical Symptoms and Psychological Illness. Edited by Bass C. London, Blackwell Scientific, 1990, pp 207–234

CHAPTER 37

Special Topics: Seclusion/ Risk Management/ Abuse and Neglect

37.1   Testimonial privilege statutes protect a patient from having his or her treating clinician testify about protected health information in court. There are several common exceptions to testimonial privilege statutes. Which of the following patient behaviors would constitute such an exception?

A. Perpetrating child abuse.
B. Engaging in an extramarital affair.
C. Driving while intoxicated.
D. Engaging in tax fraud.
E. Using illicit drugs.

The correct response is option A: Perpetrating child abuse.

Exceptions to testimonial privilege commonly involve cases of reported child abuse (option A), involuntary hospitalization, sexually violent predator commitments, court-ordered evaluations, cases in which a patient places his or her mental state in question as a claim or defense, criminal proceedings, child custody disputes, and child abuse proceedings. Depending on the details of the case, courts might well be interested in whether the patient was involved in an extramarital affair (option B), driving while intoxicated (option C), engaging in tax fraud (option D), or using illicit drugs (option E). The clinician might know this information but should not disclose it in court; these behaviors are not exceptions to the principle of testimonial privilege. **(Hales RE, Yudofsky SC, Roberts LW [eds]: APP Textbook of Psychiatry, 6th Edition, Chapter 6, p. 180 and Table 6–2, p. 181)**

37.2 If a patient commits suicide, which of the following circumstances renders the psychiatrist most vulnerable to a wrongful death claim?

A. The psychiatrist is never vulnerable to a wrongful death claim when a patient commits suicide.
B. The suicide was not foreseeable, and the psychiatrist did not implement precautions.
C. The suicide was not foreseeable, and the psychiatrist implemented reasonable precautions.
D. The suicide was foreseeable, and the psychiatrist implemented reasonable precautions.
E. A suicide contract between the clinician and patient was in place.

The correct response is option E: A suicide contract between the clinician and patient was in place.

Psychiatrists are not automatically liable whenever an outpatient commits suicide (*Speer v. United States* 1981). Instead, the reasonableness of the psychiatrist's efforts is determinative. A failure either to reasonably assess a patient's suicide risk or to implement an appropriate precautionary plan after the suicide potential becomes foreseeable is likely to render a practitioner liable if the patient is harmed because of a suicide attempt. Psychiatrists are always somewhat vulnerable to wrongful death claims when a patient commits suicide (option A); however, this vulnerability is reduced when the suicide was not foreseeable (options B, C) or when the psychiatrist implemented reasonable precautions (option D). Suicide prevention contracts created between the clinician and the patient attempt to develop an expressed understanding that the patient will call for help rather than act out suicidal thoughts or impulses. Suicide prevention contracts have no legal authority, and such agreements must not be used in place of adequate suicide assessment (Simon 1999) (option E). **(Hales RE, Yudofsky SC, Roberts LW [eds]: APP Textbook of Psychiatry, 6th Edition, Chapter 6, p. 185)**

37.3 A managed care company refuses to authorize payment for an extended hospital stay for a patient who is deemed violent by the hospital's doctors. Which of the following entities is most likely to carry the burden of liability if this patient commits a violent act soon after discharge?

A. The managed care company.
B. The psychiatric hospital.
C. The outpatient psychiatrist.
D. The inpatient psychiatrist.
E. The patient.

The correct response is option D: The inpatient psychiatrist.

Managed care companies can authorize payment for procedures, treatments, and hospital stays. Most psychiatric units, particularly in general hospitals, have become short-stay, acute-care psychiatric facilities, where only suicidal, homicidal, or gravely disabled patients with major psychiatric disorders pass strict precertification review for hospitalization (Tischler 1990). Close scrutiny by utilization reviewers often permits only short hospitalization for these patients (Wickizer et al. 1996). Clinicians can sometimes feel financial pressure to discharge a patient, but the decision to discharge or retain a patient rests with the inpatient psychiatrist (option D). The managed care company (option A) can only assess from a distance, whereas the inpatient psychiatrist has firsthand experience with the patient. The psychiatric hospital (option B) might put pressure on the psychiatrist to keep hospital stays short, but the inpatient psychiatrist makes the final decision to discharge the patient. The outpatient psychiatrist (option C) can potentially weigh in on the discharge decision, but the decision remains in the hands of the inpatient team. If a patient is discharged in an unstable state, it is the inpatient team that carries some responsibility, rather than the patient (option E), if the patient commits a violent act. **(Hales RE, Yudofsky SC, Roberts LW [eds]: APP Textbook of Psychiatry, 6th Edition, Chapter 6, pp. 188–189)**

37.4 A 33-year-old woman has been treated with psychodynamic psychotherapy for major depressive disorder and borderline personality disorder since age 20. She has been stable for many years. When her treating psychiatrist decides to retire from practice, he informs the patient and begins to help her prepare for his departure. As they discuss the issue in sessions over the ensuing several months, the patient becomes regressed and angry with him. He ultimately retires, transfers his patient's care to another psychiatrist (with whom she resumes treatment), and moves out of state. A month later, he learns that the patient is suing him for abandonment and receives a subpoena to appear in court. Why would this case *not* be considered patient abandonment?

A. The psychiatrist informed the patient with adequate notice that he was closing his practice.
B. The psychiatrist transferred his patient's care to another physician, and the situation was not an emergency.
C. Physicians can choose whom they serve.
D. The patient was clinically stable.
E. Retirement is a legitimate reason to stop treating patients.

The correct response is option B: The psychiatrist transferred his patient's care to another physician, and the situation was not an emergency.

According to accepted ethical standards in medicine, physicians are "free to choose whom to serve" (American Medical Association 2009; American Psychiatric Association 2009). Once an ongoing doctor-patient relationship has been established, however, the physician may not ethically abandon the patient (option C), regardless of the patient's clinical stability (option D). As a practical matter, this means that psychiatrists must arrange for clinical coverage when on vacation and must give adequate notice to patients when closing their practices (options A, E) (American Psychiatric Association 2009). It is not considered patient abandonment to transfer a patient's care to another physician if the treating psychiatrist is not able to provide necessary care and if the situation is not an emergency (option B). **(Hales RE, Yudofsky SC, Roberts LW [eds]: APP Textbook of Psychiatry, 6th Edition, Chapter 7, p. 211)**

37.5 Which of the following describes the importance of the psychiatrist's maintaining therapeutic boundaries?

A. Because boundaries are only important in treatment of psychiatric illness.
B. Because the psychiatrist can terminate treatment at any time.
C. Because sexual relationships with patients are acceptable in some circumstances.
D. Because of the intimacy of the psychotherapeutic relationship.
E. Because there are no time constraints or financial requirements imposed on the therapeutic encounter.

The correct response is option D: Because of the intimacy of the psychotherapeutic relationship.

Therapeutic boundaries are important in any type of clinical work (option A), but they are especially important in the intimacy of the psychotherapeutic relationship (option D). Such boundaries include temporal and spatial limits: therapeutic encounters typically occur at the physician's office during business hours, except in crisis situations (option E). Limits are also observed in the nature of the relationship, which involves the psychiatrist being paid for services and acting as a *fiduciary*, a professional who is worthy of the patient's trust. Nontherapeutic encounters, including business arrangements, social relationships, and sexual activity, are forbidden (option C). Within the therapeutic relationship, limits are also observed. The patient is encouraged to share intimate feelings, thoughts, and memories, whereas the physician generally avoids self-disclosure and adopts a posture of neutrality. Physical contact other than handshakes is avoided. Once an ongoing doctor-patient relationship has been established, the physician may not ethically abandon the patient (option B). **(Hales RE, Yudofsky SC, Roberts LW [eds]: APP Textbook of Psychiatry, 6th Edition, Chapter 7, pp. 210–211)**

37.6 There are many strategies for helping psychiatrists to ensure that role conflicts do not distort their professional judgments. Which of the following is *not* an appropriate safeguard against role conflicts?

A. Disclosure and documentation.
B. Focused supervision.
C. Oversight committees.
D. Medical education seminars sponsored by pharmaceutical companies.
E. Retrospective review.

The correct response is option D: Medical education seminars sponsored by pharmaceutical companies.

By virtue of their skills and training, psychiatrists are naturally invited to participate in a variety of roles in the medical community and in society. Psychiatrists are educators of medical students and residents, administrators of academic programs and health care systems, clinical researchers and basic scientists, and consultants to industry. Because the ethical duties required by one role may not align precisely with the duties of another role, psychiatrists in multiple roles often face ethical binds. The conflicts of interest that arise are not necessarily unethical, but they must be managed in a way that allows the psychiatrist to fulfill professionalism expectations and maintain a fiduciary relationship with patients. There are many strategies for helping to ensure that role conflicts do not distort the judgment of professionals, such as disclosure and documentation (option A), focused supervision (option B) and oversight committees (option C), retrospective review (option E), and other safeguards (Roberts and Dyer 2004). Medical education seminars sponsored by pharmaceutical companies may raise rather than safeguard against conflict of interest issues (option D). **(Hales RE, Yudofsky SC, Roberts LW [eds]: APP Textbook of Psychiatry, 6th Edition, Chapter 7, pp. 217–218)**

37.7   Which of the following is a true statement regarding the use of seclusion?

A. Seclusion is the direct application of physical force to an individual to restrict his or her freedom of movement.
B. Federal law permits the use of seclusion and restraint only as a last resort to protect the patient's safety and dignity.
C. Seclusion orders do not typically require specific time periods.
D. Once a patient has been placed in seclusion, no further review of the seclusion order is required.
E. Any mental health staff member can write orders to place a patient in seclusion if the patient is considered imminently dangerous to self or others.

The correct response is option B: Federal law permits the use of seclusion and restraint only as a last resort to protect the patient's safety and dignity.

Seclusion is the involuntary confinement of a person alone in a room where the person is physically prevented from leaving or the separation of the patient from others in a safe, contained, controlled environment. *Restraint* is the direct application of physical force to an individual, with or without the individual's permission, to restrict his or her freedom of movement (option A). Generally, the courts have held that seclusion and restraints are an intrusion on a patient's constitutionally protected interests and may be implemented only when a patient presents a risk of harm to self or others and no less restrictive alternative is available. Federal law permits the use of seclusion and restraint only as a last resort to protect the patient's safety and dignity and never for the convenience of the staff (option B). Some courts have also required the following: 1) Restraint and seclusion may be implemented only by a written order from an appropriate medical official (option E). 2) Orders must be confined to specific, time-limited periods (option C). 3) A patient's condition must be regularly reviewed and documented (option D). 4) Any extension of an original order must be reviewed and reauthorized.

Federal requirements permit qualified staff members to initiate seclusion or restraint for the safety and protection of the patient and staff only if they obtain an order from the licensed independent practitioner as soon as possible within 1 hour of initiation. Stringent requirements for face-to-face evaluation of the patient within 1 hour of initiation and for assessment, frequency of reassessment, monitoring, time-limited orders, notification of family members, discontinuation at the earliest possible opportunity, and debriefing with patient and staff members have been carefully defined by the Center for Medicare Services and The Joint Commission (2006). **(Hales RE, Yudofsky SC, Roberts LW [eds]: APP Textbook of Psychiatry, 6th Edition, Chapter 6, pp. 191–193)**

37.8   There are certain instances when a nonconsenting patient may have the privilege of confidentiality suspended based on the physician's overriding duties to others. In which of the following situations would suspension of confidentiality be most appropriate?

A. A patient admits to shoplifting numerous times.
B. A patient admits to use of intravenous heroin using a dirty needle.
C. A patient admits to frequent episodes of unprotected sex.
D. A patient admits to child abuse.
E. A patient admits to suicidal thoughts.

The correct response is option D: A patient admits to child abuse.

There are instances when a nonconsenting patient may have the privilege of confidentiality suspended based on the physician's overriding duties to others. These situations typically involve elder or child abuse (option D) or threatened violence. The notion that psychiatrists have "duty to protect" members of the public from the violent intentions of their patients was demonstrated by the legal case *Tarasoff v. Regents of the University of California* (1976). An important evolving trend is the application of the *Tarasoff* duty to cases involving sexual abuse by an alleged pedophile. Although options A, B, C, and E are clinically significant and could potentially place the patient and others at risk, they do not directly involve frankly threatened violence or abuse of children or elders and therefore do not meet criteria for suspension of confidentiality. **(Hales RE, Yudofsky SC, Roberts LW [eds]: APP Textbook of Psychiatry, 6th Edition, Chapter 6, p. 187; Chapter 7, pp. 216–217)**

37.9   Which of the following statements is most accurate regarding seclusion and restraint?

A. Legal regulation of seclusion and restraint has become less stringent over time.
B. Legal challenges to the use of seclusion and restraint are uncommon.
C. Most states have developed requirements designed to minimize and avoid the use of seclusion and restraint.

D. Federal requirements regarding seclusion and restraint may never be superseded.

E. Federal law does not include the use of drugs in the definition of restraint.

The correct response is option C: Most states have developed requirements designed to minimize and avoid the use of seclusion and restraint.

The legal regulation of seclusion and restraint has become increasingly more stringent (option A). Legal challenges to the use of seclusion and restraints have been made on behalf of institutionalized persons with mental illness or mental retardation (option B). Frequently, these lawsuits do not stand alone but are part of a challenge to a wide range of alleged abuses within a hospital (Recupero et al. 2011). Most states have enacted statutes regulating the use of restraints, normally specifying the circumstances in which restraints can be used. The Center for Medicare Services, The Joint Commission (2006), and most states have developed requirements designed to minimize and avoid the use of seclusion and restraint (option C) (Simon and Hales 2006). Where they apply, federal requirements establish a floor but may be superseded by more restrictive state laws (option D). As do many state laws, federal law includes the use of drugs in the definition of restraint (option E) (Simon and Hales 2006). **(Hales RE, Yudofsky SC, Roberts LW [eds]: APP Textbook of Psychiatry, 6th Edition, Chapter 6, pp. 191–193)**

37.10 Under which of the following circumstances is it permissible to treat an adult patient without obtaining informed consent?

A. The patient lacks decision-making capacity and has a surrogate decision maker.

B. The patient has been legally declared incompetent and has a guardian.

C. There is a medical emergency.

D. The treatment is in the patient's best interests.

E. It is never permissible to treat without informed consent.

The correct response is option C: There is a medical emergency.

An adult patient is presumed competent unless adjudicated incompetent or temporarily incapacitated because of a medical emergency (option C). When immediate treatment is necessary to save a life or prevent serious harm and it is not possible to obtain either the patient's consent or that of someone authorized to provide consent for the patient, the law typically presumes that the consent would have been granted (option E). When the patient lacks decision-making capacity or when the patient is legally declared incompetent, the treatment team must still obtain informed consent (options A, B), but from the surrogate decision maker rather than the patient. Whether a treatment is in the best interests of the patient is for the patient or the surrogate decision maker to decide (option D). **(Hales RE, Yudofsky SC, Roberts LW [eds]: APP Textbook of Psychiatry, 6th Edition, Chapter 6, pp. 177–179; Chapter 7, p. 213)**

37.11 Under what circumstances can a physician bypass informed consent because of "therapeutic privilege"?

A. The physician has more clinical knowledge than the patient, making the informed consent process unnecessary.
B. The physician knows confidential information about the patient, making the informed consent process unnecessary.
C. Complete disclosure of risks and alternatives might harm the patient's health and welfare.
D. The physician is the surrogate decision maker.
E. There is a medical emergency.

The correct response is option C: Complete disclosure of risks and alternatives might harm the patient's health and welfare.

Therapeutic privilege, an exception to the requirements of informed consent, means that a complete disclosure of possible risks and alternatives might have a deleterious impact on the patient's health and welfare (option C). Physicians almost always have more clinical knowledge than patients, which is why informed consent is necessary (option A). Psychiatrists often know confidential (or privileged) information, but this has no impact on the need for informed consent (option B). Physicians should never be the surrogate decision maker as long as there is not a medical emergency (option D). In a medical emergency, physicians can bypass informed consent; therapeutic privilege does not apply in such cases (option E). **(Hales RE, Yudofsky SC, Roberts LW [eds]: APP Textbook of Psychiatry, 6th Edition, Chapter 6, p. 179)**

37.12 According to the Health Insurance Portability and Accountability Act (HIPAA), under which of the following circumstances is it permissible for a provider to disclose a patient's health care information without prior patient authorization?

A. It is never permissible to disclose a patient's health care information without prior consent.
B. The patient's spouse asks for an update.
C. The patient's friend asks for an update.
D. A researcher is recruiting subjects for a clinical trial.
E. The requesting party is another clinician on the patient's treatment team.

The correct response is option E: The requesting party is another clinician on the patient's treatment team.

HIPAA limits disclosure of patient health information without patient authorization except as necessary for treatment (option E), payment, and health care operations. It is notable that HIPAA does permit some disclosing of health care information (option A), but this information should not be provided to a spouse, a friend, or clinical researchers without the patient's permission (options B–D).

(Hales RE, Yudofsky SC, Roberts LW [eds]: APP Textbook of Psychiatry, 6th Edition, Chapter 6, p. 180)

37.13 When state law regarding patient confidentiality disagrees with federal law, which regulation should the physician follow?

A. The more protective rule.
B. The less restrictive rule.
C. The state law.
D. The federal law.
E. Whatever a "reasonable physician" would do.

The correct response is option A: The more protective rule.

With regard to patient confidentiality, a provider should always follow the more protective rule (option A), which means abiding by the more protective state or federal law (options B–D). The "reasonable physician" standard does not apply (option E). **(Hales RE, Yudofsky SC, Roberts LW [eds]: APP Textbook of Psychiatry, 6th Edition, Chapter 6, p. 180)**

37.14 A patient who is deemed not competent to enter into a marriage contract refuses to take his prescribed psychotropic medications. What would be the most appropriate course of action for the treating clinician?

A. Medicate over objection because the patient is incompetent.
B. Identify a surrogate decision maker.
C. Transfer the patient to a higher level of care.
D. Ask the court to conduct another competency assessment.
E. Wait and see if the patient's decision changes.

The correct response is option D: Ask the court to conduct another competency assessment.

The legal designation of "incompetent" is applied to an individual who fails one of the mental tests of capacity and is therefore considered *by law* to be not mentally capable of performing a particular act or assuming a particular role. The adjudication of incompetence by a court is commonly subject or issue specific, and therefore another competency assessment is needed for this patient (option D). This patient has been determined by law to be not competent to enter into a marriage contract, but no determination has yet been made about his competency regarding taking medications (options A, B). For example, the fact that a psychiatric patient is adjudicated incompetent to drive does not automatically render that patient incompetent to do other things, such as give consent to treatment, testify as a witness, marry, or enter into a contract. Transferring the patient to a higher level of care (option C) does not directly address the problem of the patient's refusal of medications. Waiting to see if the patient's decision changes (option E) is not clinically appropriate because he is refusing treatment that is determined necessary at this time for his well-being. **(Hales RE, Yudofsky SC, Roberts LW [eds]: APP Textbook of Psychiatry, 6th Edition, Chapter 6, pp. 177–178)**

References

American Medical Association: Principles of Medical Ethics. Chicago, IL, American Medical Association, 2009. Available at: http://www.ama-assn.org/ama/pub/physician-resources/medical-ethics/code-medical-ethics/principles-medical-ethics.page. Accessed September 4, 2012.

American Psychiatric Association: Opinions of the Ethics Committee on the Principles of Medical Ethics. Washington, DC, American Psychiatric Association, 2009. Available at: http://www.psychiatry.org/practice/ethics/resources-standards. Accessed September 4, 2012.

Joint Commission: Comprehensive Accreditation Manual for Behavioral Healthcare Restraint and Seclusion Standards for Behavioral Health. Oak Brook Terrace, IL, Joint Commission, 2006

Recupero PR, Price M, Garvey KA, et al: Restraint and seclusion in psychiatric treatment settings: regulation, case law, and risk management. J Am Acad Psychiatry Law 39(4):465–476, 2011 22159974

Roberts LW, Dyer AR: Concise Guide to Ethics in Mental Health Care. Washington, DC, American Psychiatric Publishing, 2004

Simon RI: The suicide prevention contract: clinical, legal, and risk management issues. J Am Acad Psychiatry Law 27(3):445–450, 1999 10509943

Simon RI, Hales RE (eds): The American Psychiatric Publishing Textbook of Suicide Assessment and Management. Washington, DC, American Psychiatric Publishing, 2006

Speer v United States, 512 F.Supp. 670 (N.D. Tex. 1981), aff'd, Speer v United States, 675 F.2d 100 (5th Cir. 1982)

Tarasoff v Regents of the University of California, 17 Cal.3d 425, 551 P.2d 334; 131 Cal. Rptr. 14 (1976)

Tischler GL: Utilization management of mental health services by private third parties. Am J Psychiatry 147(8):967–973, 1990 2197885

Wickizer TM, Lessler D, Travis KM: Controlling inpatient psychiatric utilization through managed care. Am J Psychiatry 153(3):339–345, 1996 8610820

CHAPTER 38

Spirituality

38.1 Which of the following is not true of the research regarding Alcoholics Anonymous (AA) and spirituality?

A. Outpatient clients who attend AA meetings may report having had a spiritual awakening as a result of their AA attendance.
B. Spirituality is uniformly discussed in mainstream AA meetings regardless of differences in perceived AA group social dynamics.
C. Spirituality is measured by asking only about the extent that God is discussed in meetings.
D. Exposure to AA is associated with increased spirituality.
E. Gains in spiritual practices among AA members is a significant predictor of later abstinence.

The correct response is option C: Spirituality is measured by asking only about the extent that God is discussed in meetings.

The core AA literature (Alcoholics Anonymous 1981, 2001) posits that an individual will have a spiritual awakening as a result of working the 12 steps and that continued practice of spiritual principles will lead to sustained abstinence. In a series of three studies, spirituality was uniformly discussed in mainstream AA meetings regardless of differences in perceived AA group social dynamics (option B) (Horstmann and Tonigan 2000; Montgomery et al. 1993; Tonigan et al. 1995). In each of these studies, *spirituality* was defined using items asking to what extent God, spirituality, or a higher power was discussed in meetings and to what extent prayer and meditation were discussed (option C). In project MATCH, 27.6% of the outpatient clients who attended AA during the 12 weeks of treatment also reported having had a spiritual awakening as a result of their AA attendance (option A) (Project MATCH Research Group 1997, 1998). Strong evidence across diverse measures of religiousness and spirituality documents spiritual increases among AA members (option D). A meta-analysis of six well-conducted studies found gains in spiritual practices when combined across studies to be a significant predictor of later abstinence (option E). **(Galanter M, Kleber HD, Brady KT**

[eds]: APP Textbook of Substance Abuse Treatment, 5th Edition, Chapter 37, pp. 568–571 and Table 37–1, p. 569)

38.2   Which of the following is a true statement regarding the relationship between religion/spirituality and late-life depression?

A. Religious involvement is not a common coping behavior used by older adults.
B. Religious involvement has been shown to predict faster recovery from depression in older adults.
C. Religious coping has been found to have a positive association with depressive symptoms in older adults with or without medical illness.
D. Older men are more likely than older women to use religious involvement to cope with stress.
E. Older adults with medical illness who use religion to cope experience no improvement in depressive symptoms over time.

The correct response is option B: Religious involvement has been shown to predict faster recovery from depression in older adults.

Coping behavior may affect the prognosis of late-life depression. One of the coping behaviors most commonly used by recent generations of older adults is religious involvement (option A). In a study involving 100 middle-aged or elderly adults, one-third of men and nearly two-thirds of women (option D) used religious cognitions or behaviors to help them cope with a stressful period (Koenig et al. 1988). A number of investigators have reported inverse associations between religious coping and depressive symptoms in older adults with or without medical illness (option C) (Braam et al. 1997b; Idler 1987; Koenig 2007a; Koenig et al. 1992; Pressman et al. 1990). A study involving 850 hospitalized medically ill older adults found that those using religion to cope were less likely to be depressed and more likely to experience improvement in depressive symptoms over time (option E) (Koenig et al. 1992). Religious involvement also appears to be a predictor of faster recovery from depression in both community-dwelling and clinical samples of older adults (option B) (Braam et al. 1997a; Koenig 2007b; Koenig et al. 1998). **(Steffens DC, Blazer DG, Thakur ME [eds]: APP Textbook of Geriatric Psychiatry, 5th Edition, Chapter 9, pp. 248–249)**

38.3   Which of the following statements is true regarding the relationship between religious coping and bereavement course?

A. Personal religiosity has been shown in some cultures to decrease the negative psychological effects of losing a spouse.
B. There is no association between religious coping and resilience for individuals in the postloss period.
C. Patients with chronic grief are the most likely to use religious coping.

D. Resilient patients are less likely than other groups of bereaved patients to use religious coping.

E. Patients with chronic grief, resilience, and relief, are equally likely to use religious coping.

The correct response is option A: Personal religiosity has been shown in some cultures to decrease the negative psychological effects of losing a spouse.

Although a period of distress followed by gradual abatement may be the most common course following a loss, it is not the only pattern. Several prospective and retrospective studies have identified other common patterns, including resilience, relief, and chronic grief. Individuals identified as resilient demonstrate consistently low levels of depression or negative affect across the postloss period. Resilient individuals did not differ from common or chronic grief groups in either relationship quality or interviewer ratings of interpersonal skill or warmth (Bonanno et al. 2004; Ott et al. 2007), but they were more likely than the other groups to use religious coping (options B–E) (Ott et al. 2007). A study of elderly widowed adults discovered that personal religiosity (i.e., viewing religion as important and engaging in private prayer) decreased the negative psychological effects of losing a spouse (option A) (Momtaz et al. 2010). **(Steffens DC, Blazer DG, Thakur ME [eds]: APP Textbook of Geriatric Psychiatry, 5th Edition, Chapter 15, pp. 418–419)**

38.4   Which of the following statements is true regarding the role of religion and spirituality in therapist selection among older adults?

A. Older adults care more about therapist gender than religion.

B. Older adults feel more comfortable receiving care from practitioners who share the same race but not necessarily the same religion.

C. Spiritual concerns and values are not important factors in therapist selection among older adults.

D. Older adults feel more comfortable receiving care from practitioners who share the same religion.

The correct response is option D: Older adults feel more comfortable receiving care from practitioners who share the same religion.

Older adults have been shown to favor therapists who understood their existential and spiritual concerns and values (option D is correct; options B and C are incorrect), and as a result of their unique sociohistorical context, they often feel more comfortable receiving care from practitioners who share the same race, ethnicity, and religion (Bartels et al. 2004; Chen et al. 2006; Gum et al. 2010; Hinrichsen 2006; Snodgrass 2009) (option A). **(Steffens DC, Blazer DG, Thakur ME [eds]: APP Textbook of Geriatric Psychiatry, 5th Edition, Chapter 23, pp. 649–650)**

38.5   Which of the following is a true statement regarding the FICA religion/spirituality screening tool?

A. It was primarily developed for use with children and adolescents.
B. It was developed for evaluating families in the medical setting.
C. It involves assessment of ethics and value systems.
D. It is a self-assessment tool that the patient completes independently.
E. It is a tool for obtaining basic information about a patient's religious and spiritual experiences.

The correct response is option E: It is a tool for obtaining basic information about a patient's religious and spiritual experiences.

The screening mnemonic FICA—based on questions about faith, influence, community, and spiritual needs addressed—is simple and easy to use and remember and is a good tool for obtaining basic information about a patient's religious and spiritual experiences (option E). Primarily developed for and used in adult populations (option A), it can be used with parents and older children, provided that developmentally appropriate language is used by the interviewer (option D). These questions serve as a starting point to discuss past religious and spiritual experiences, current practices, satisfaction with religious and spiritual elements of life, and supportive resources (Caraballo et al. 2006; Puchalski and Romer 2000).

The mnemonic BELIEF—based on questions about belief, ethics (option C), lifestyle, involvement, education, and the future—was developed for evaluating families in the medical setting (option B) and is helpful in mental health settings as well. The examiner inquires about issues prompted by each letter of the word. This device is especially helpful in establishing trust and rapport for the future when matters of religious or spiritual significance might arise (McEvoy 2003). **(Dulcan M [ed]: Dulcan's Textbook of Child and Adolescent Psychiatry, Chapter 34, p. 526 and Tables 34–3, 34–4, p. 527)**

References

Alcoholics Anonymous: Twelve Steps and Twelve Traditions. New York, Alcoholics Anonymous World Services, 1981

Alcoholic Anonymous: Alcoholics Anonymous, 4th Edition. New York, Alcoholics Anonymous World Services, 2001

Bartels SJ, Coakley EH, Zubritsky C, et al; PRISM-E Investigators: Improving access to geriatric mental health services: a randomized trial comparing treatment engagement with integrated versus enhanced referral care for depression, anxiety, and at-risk alcohol use. Am J Psychiatry 161(8):1455–1462, 2004 15285973

Bonanno GA, Wortman CB, Nesse RM: Prospective patterns of resilience and maladjustment during widowhood. Psychol Aging 19(2):260–271, 2004 15222819

Braam AW, Beekman AT, Deeg DJ, et al: Religiosity as a protective or prognostic factor of depression in later life; results from a community survey in The Netherlands. Acta Psychiatr Scand 96(3):199–205, 1997a 9296551

Braam AW, Beekman AT, van Tilburg TG, et al: Religious involvement and depression in older Dutch citizens. Soc Psychiatry Psychiatr Epidemiol 32(5):284–291, 1997b 9257519

Chen H, Coakley EH, Cheal K, et al: Satisfaction with mental health services in older primary care patients. Am J Geriatr Psychiatry 14(4):371–379, 2006 16582046

Caraballo A, Hamid H, Lee JR, et al: A resident's guide to the cultural formulation, in Clinical Manual of Cultural Psychiatry. Edited by Lim RF. Washington, DC, American Psychiatric Publishing, 2006, pp 243–269

Connors G, Tonigan JS, Miller WR: Religiosity and responsiveness to alcoholism treatments: matching findings and causal chain analyses, in Project MATCH: A Priori Matching Hypotheses, Results and Mediating Mechanisms. Edited by Longabaugh R, Wirth PW. Rockville, MD, U.S. Government Printing Office, 2001

Gum AM, Iser L, Petkus A: Behavioral health service utilization and preferences of older adults receiving home-based aging services. Am J Geriatr Psychiatry 18(6):491–501, 2010 21217560

Hinrichsen GA: Why multicultural issues matter for practitioners working with older adults. Prof Psychol Res Pr 37(1):29–35, 2006

Horstmann MJ, Tonigan JS: Faith development in Alcoholics Anonymous: a study of two AA groups. Alcohol Treat Q 18(4):75–84, 2000

Idler EL: Religious involvement and the health of the elderly: some hypotheses and an initial test. Soc Forces 66(1):226–238, 1987

Koenig HG: Religion and depression in older medical inpatients. Am J Geriatr Psychiatry 15(4):282–291, 2007a 17384313

Koenig HG: Religion and remission of depression in medical inpatients with heart failure/pulmonary disease. J Nerv Ment Dis 195(5):389–395, 2007b 17502804

Koenig HG, Meador KG, Cohen HJ, Blazer DG: Depression in elderly hospitalized patients with medical illness. Arch Intern Med 148(9):1929–1936, 1988 3415405

Koenig HG, Cohen HJ, Blazer DG, et al: Religious coping and depression among elderly, hospitalized medically ill men. Am J Psychiatry 149(12):1693–1700, 1992 1443246

Koenig HG, George LK, Peterson BL: Religiosity and remission of depression in medically ill older patients. Am J Psychiatry 155(4):536–542, 1998 9546001

McEvoy M: Culture & spirituality as an integrated concept in pediatric care. MCN Am J Matern Child Nurs 28(1):39–43, quiz 44, 2003 12514355

Momtaz YA, Ibrahim R, Hamid TA, Yahaya N: Mediating effects of social and personal religiosity on the psychological well being of widowed elderly people. Omega (Westport) 61(2):145–162, 2010 20712141

Montgomery HA, Miller WR, Tonigan JS: Differences among AA groups: implications for research. J Stud Alcohol 54(4):502–504, 1993 8341051

Ott CH, Lueger RJ, Kelber ST, Prigerson HG: Spousal bereavement in older adults: common, resilient, and chronic grief with defining characteristics. J Nerv Ment Dis 195(4):332–341, 2007 17435484

Pressman P, Lyons JS, Larson DB, Strain JJ: Religious belief, depression, and ambulation status in elderly women with broken hips. Am J Psychiatry 147(6):758–760, 1990 2343920

Project MATCH Research Group: Matching Alcoholism Treatments to Client Heterogeneity: Project MATCH posttreatment drinking outcomes. J Stud Alcohol 58(1):7–29, 1997 8979210

Project MATCH Research Group: Matching Alcoholism Treatments to Client Heterogeneity: Project MATCH three-year drinking outcomes. Alcohol Clin Exp Res 22(6):1300–1311, 1998 9756046

Puchalski C, Romer AL: Taking a spiritual history allows clinicians to understand patients more fully. J Palliat Med 3(1):129–137, 2000 15859737

Snodgrass J: Toward holistic care: integrating spirituality and cognitive behavioral therapy for older adults. J Relig Spirit Aging 21(3):219–236, 2009

Tonigan JS, Ashcroft F, Miller WR: AA group dynamics and 12-step activity. J Stud Alcohol 56(6):616–621, 1995 8558892

CHAPTER 39

Substance-Related and Addictive Disorders

39.1 What is thought to be the mechanism of action of hallucinogens such as lysergic acid diethylamide (LSD)?

A. Antagonism of the adenosine A_{2A} receptor.
B. Agonism of the nicotinic acetylcholine (nAChR) receptor.
C. Agonism of the serotonin 5-HT_{2A} receptor.
D. Agonism of the μ receptor.
E. Agonism of the cannabinoid CB_1 receptor.

The correct response is option C: Agonism of the serotonin 5-HT_{2A} receptor.

Neurobiology of hallucinogens such as LSD is complex and involves many targets, including agonism of the serotonin 5-HT_2 receptor (option C). Caffeine is an antagonist at the adenosine A_{2A} receptor (option A), nicotine is an agonist at the nAChR receptor (option B), opioids are agonists at the μ receptor (option D), and cannabis is an agonist of the CB_1 receptor (option E). **(Hales RE, Yudofsky SC, Roberts LW [eds]: APP Textbook of Psychiatry, 6th Edition, Chapter 23, pp. 738–743 and Table 23–4, p. 740)**

39.2 What percentage of individuals with alcohol use disorder undergoing severe withdrawal exhibit seizures that require emergent hospital care?

A. Less than 5%.
B. 10%.
C. 15%.
D. 25%.
E. 50%.

The correct response is option A: Less than 5%.

Clinically significant withdrawal symptoms generally occur about 8 hours following cessation of heavy or prolonged drinking. Symptoms tend to reach maximal intensity on day 2 when blood alcohol content decreases but resolve considerably by days 4–5. Alcohol withdrawal symptoms are mediated in part by reduced central γ-aminobutyric acid (GABA) and increased glutamatergic neurotransmission. Less than 5% of individuals with alcohol use disorder undergoing severe withdrawal exhibit seizures that require emergent hospital care. Roughly the same percentage of individuals experience delirium tremens, characterized by agitation, auditory and visual hallucinations, and frank disorientation (Schuckit 2009). **(Hales RE, Yudofsky SC, Roberts LW [eds]: APP Textbook of Psychiatry, 6th Edition, Chapter 23, p. 746)**

39.3 You admit a 40-year-old patient with alcohol use disorder to your service. To manage his withdrawal, you would like to use a symptom-triggered approach (rather than fixed multiple daily dosing). Which one of the following should you use to assess the severity of alcohol withdrawal symptoms?

A. CAGE questions.
B. Clinical Institute Withdrawal Assessment for Alcohol Scale—Revised.
C. Alcohol Use Disorders Identification Test.
D. Michigan Alcoholism Screening Test.
E. TWEAK questionnaire.

The correct response is option B: Clinical Institute Withdrawal Assessment for Alcohol Scale—Revised.

The intensity of alcohol withdrawal can be closely monitored using the Clinical Institute Withdrawal Assessment for Alcohol Scale—Revised (Sullivan et al. 1989) (option B). This clinician-rated checklist, a 10-item scale used to monitor the clinical course of withdrawal symptoms, includes assessments of nausea; vomiting; tremor; sweating; anxiety; agitation; tactile, auditory, and visual disturbances; and clouding of sensorium. Higher total scores indicate more severe alcohol withdrawal symptoms and a greater risk of major withdrawal symptoms such as delirium tremens. The CAGE questions (option A), Alcohol Use Disorders Identification Test (option C), Michigan Alcoholism Screening Test (option D), and TWEAK questionnaire (option E) are all alcohol screening tools and are not designed to assess symptoms or severity of alcohol withdrawal. **(Hales RE, Yudofsky SC, Roberts LW [eds]: APP Textbook of Psychiatry, 6th Edition, Chapter 23, pp. 746–749 and Figure 23–2, pp. 747–748 and Tables 23–6, 23–7, p. 749)**

39.4 Which of the following medications has as its mechanism of action the inhibition of aldehyde dehydrogenase?

A. Acamprosate.
B. Diazepam.
C. Disulfiram.

D. Buprenorphine.

E. Naltrexone.

The correct response is option C: Disulfiram.

Disulfiram is believed to decrease alcohol use by blocking the enzyme aldehyde dehydrogenase (option C), thereby increasing acetaldehyde responsible for the so-called disulfiram reaction, which is aversive; however, disulfiram also blocks dopamine β-hydroxylase, the enzyme responsible for the conversion of dopamine to norepinephrine centrally. Decreases in norepinephrine neurotransmission have also been linked to the therapeutic effects of disulfiram.

Although the precise mechanisms remain to be elucidated, the glutamate modulator acamprosate (option A) is hypothesized to normalize glutamatergic/GABA dysregulation associated with chronic alcohol consumption and withdrawal. Diazepam (option B), a benzodiazepine, can be used for alcohol detoxification. Naltrexone (option E) blocks μ opioid receptors, preventing alcohol-induced increases in central dopamine linked to the pleasant or positive subjective effects of the drug. This mechanism may be responsible for the ability of naltrexone to reduce craving and heavy drinking (Rösner et al. 2010). Buprenorphine (option D) is a partial agonist of μ opioid receptors and is used to treat opioid use disorders, not alcohol use disorders. **(Hales RE, Yudofsky SC, Roberts LW [eds]: APP Textbook of Psychiatry, 6th Edition, Chapter 23, pp. 751–754 and Table 23–11, p. 753)**

39.5 Which of the following is a true statement about the epidemiology of alcohol use disorders?

A. Females have higher rates of drinking than males.

B. The association of heavy alcohol use with death from hepatocellular carcinoma is greater for females than for males.

C. Individuals with preexisting schizophrenia or bipolar disorder, blunted response to alcohol, and impulsivity are at low risk for developing alcohol use disorders.

D. Family history of alcohol use disorder poses no significant risk for development of the condition.

E. The prevalence of binge drinking is highest in Asian populations.

The correct response is option B: The association of heavy alcohol use and death from hepatocellular carcinoma is greater for females than for males.

Alcohol use disorders are influenced by numerous factors. Males have higher rates of drinking and related disorders than females (option A); however, due to physiological factors, women develop higher blood alcohol content levels per drink compared with men, which may predispose women to develop alcohol-induced diseases. Indeed, the association of heavy alcohol use and death from hepatocellular carcinoma is stronger for females than males (option B). Similarly, underage women are at a greater risk of being in an alcohol-related automobile crash compared with men. Women, however, are more likely to seek professional help for alcohol use disorder. Individuals with preexisting schizophrenia or bipolar disorder, blunted response (low sensitivity) to alcohol, and impulsivity are at high risk for developing alcohol use disorders (option C) (Schuckit et al. 2011; Yip et al. 2012). A family history of alcohol use disorder (option D) is also well known to impose significant risk of developing the condition. Evidence also reveals the importance of ethnicity in alcohol use disorders. Alcohol withdrawal severity is greater and mortality secondary to alcohol-induced liver disease is higher among non-Hispanic whites. A large study including individuals ages 60 years and older found that the prevalence of binge drinking was highest among non-Hispanic whites and lowest among Asians (option E) (Bryant and Kim 2012). **(Hales RE, Yudofsky SC, Roberts LW [eds]: APP Textbook of Psychiatry, 6th Edition, Chapter 23, pp. 756–757)**

39.6 Which of the following is a true statement about opioid intoxication?

A. Respiratory depression leading to overdose is due to opiate receptors located in the locus coeruleus.
B. The "high" from opioids occurs only when the rate of change in brain dopamine is slow.
C. Route of administration is not associated with the clinical aspects of opioid abuse.
D. The burst of locus coeruleus activity is associated with the "high" of all abused drugs.
E. Large, rapidly administered doses of opiates block GABA release.

The correct response is option A: Respiratory depression leading to overdose is due to opiate receptors located in the locus coeruleus.

The clinical aspects of opioid abuse are tied to route of administration and the rapidity with which an opiate bolus reaches the brain. The "high" from opioids occurs only when the *rate of change* in brain dopamine is fast (option B). Large, rapidly administered doses of opiates block GABA inhibition (not GABA release; option E) and produce the burst of nucleus accumbens (not locus coeruleus; option D) activity that is associated with the "high" of all abused drugs. Therefore, routes of administration that slowly increase opiate blood and brain levels, such as oral and transdermal routes, are effective for analgesia and sedation but do not produce an opiate "high" as occurs via smoking and intravenous routes (option C). Other acute effects, such as analgesia and respiratory depression leading to overdose, are due to opiate receptors located in other areas such as the locus coeruleus (option A). **(Hales RE, Yudofsky SC, Roberts LW [eds]: APP Textbook of Psychiatry, 6th Edition, Chapter 23, pp. 776–777)**

39.7 Which of the following antidepressants has approval from the U.S. Food and Drug Administration (FDA) as pharmacotherapy for smoking cessation?

A. Fluoxetine.
B. Venlafaxine.
C. Nortriptyline.
D. Bupropion.
E. Phenelzine.

The correct response is option D: Bupropion.

Most smokers report wanting to quit smoking and most try to quit on their own. However, only 3%–5% of smokers who try to quit unaided maintain their quit attempts 1 year later, and the majority relapse within the first 8 days of the quit attempt. First-line pharmacotherapies for nicotine dependence include nicotine-replacement therapy, bupropion (option D), and varenicline. These treatments generally double the chance of quitting smoking. Notwithstanding, rates of absti-nence are still only 20%–33% at 6 months (Fiore et al. 2008), suggesting an impor-tant role for behavior-based treatments for smoking cessation. The following are all antidepressants that are not FDA approved for smoking cessation: fluoxetine, (option A), a selective serotonin reuptake inhibitor; venlafaxine (option B), a sero-tonin-norepinephrine reuptake inhibitor; nortriptyline (option C), a tricyclic anti-depressant; and phenelzine (option E), a monoamine oxidase inhibitor. **(Hales RE, Yudofsky SC, Roberts LW [eds]: APP Textbook of Psychiatry, 6th Edition, Chapter 23, p. 796 and Table 23–18, p. 798)**

39.8 Which of the following statements about the epidemiology of cannabis use is true?

A. The number of daily users in the 12- to 17-year-old age group rose sharply from 2009 to 2011.
B. Less than half of new users of cannabis in 2010 were younger than 18 years.
C. Use of cannabis among adolescents plateaued over the decade 2001–2011.
D. In the decade prior to 2009, the number of youths who were daily users dra-matically increased.
E. The numbers of treatment admissions for cannabis use disorders in the United States have stayed the same over the past decade.

The correct response is option A: The number of daily users in the 12- to 17-year-old age group rose sharply from 2009 to 2011.

According to the 2011 National Survey on Drug Use and Health, 29.3% of persons ages 12 years and older used cannabis at least once in the prior year, and 4.5 million persons were classified as dependent on or abusing marijuana (Substance Abuse and Mental Health Services Administration 2012a). In 2010, there were 2.4 million recent cannabis initiates, 58.5% of whom were younger than 18 years (option B) (Substance Abuse and Mental Health Services Administration 2012a). Marijuana produces dependence (i.e., cannabis use disorder) in 9% of those who try it (National Institute on Drug Abuse 2012). Distressingly, data showed that 1.4 million youths ages 12–17 were current cannabis users in 2011, and the number of daily users among this age group rose sharply from 2009 to 2011 (option A), which is in contrast to the considerable decline of use during the preceding decade (Substance Abuse and Mental Health Services Administration 2012a) (options C, D). In addition, the recent availability of so-called synthetic cannabinoid-like compounds (e.g., "K2" and "spice"), which are associated with psychosis and adverse cardiovascular events in young individuals, has highlighted the urgency of addressing cannabis use disorders (Mir et al. 2011). Although systematic research on treatments for cannabis use disorders began approximately 20 years ago, treatment admissions for cannabis use disorders in the United States have increased twofold during the past decade, and both the absolute number (1 million) and the percentage of total treatment admissions for all illicit drugs (32%) were greater for marijuana than for any other illicit drug in 2010 (option E) (Substance Abuse and Mental Health Services Administration 2012b). **(Hales RE, Yudofsky SC, Roberts LW [eds]: APP Textbook of Psychiatry, 6th Edition, Chapter 23, pp. 761, 763)**

39.9   Which of the following is an FDA-approved pharmacotherapy for stimulant dependence?

A. Modafinil.
B. Acamprosate.
C. Disulfiram.
D. Buprenorphine.
E. There are no FDA-approved pharmacotherapies for stimulant dependence.

The correct response is option E: There are no FDA-approved pharmacotherapies for stimulant dependence.

Although some behavioral therapeutic strategies show promise, there are currently no indicated pharmacotherapies for stimulant dependence (option E) (Haile et al. 2012b; Kosten et al. 2011). Several medications have been assessed with limited success. A number of studies have shown that disulfiram, a medication indicated for alcohol use disorder, decreases cocaine use in a variety of patient populations; however, the therapeutic effects of disulfiram appear to depend on genetic profile (Kosten et al. 2013) and dose (Haile et al. 2012a). A promising line of research has found that antihypertensive medications such as doxazosin (Newton et al. 2012) and perindopril (Newton et al. 2010) block the positive subjective effects and desire for cocaine and methamphetamine. These medications have a number of advantages; namely, they have no abuse liability and they confer protection from adverse cardiovascular effects of stimulants. Recent studies indicate that the cholinesterase inhibitor rivastigmine also decreases the likelihood of methamphetamine use in individuals with methamphetamine use disorder (De La Garza et al. 2012). Modafinil (option A), a medication indicated for the treatment of narcolepsy, and N-acetylcysteine, the treatment for acetaminophen toxicity, have both shown promising therapeutic potential for cocaine dependence in select populations (Haile et al. 2012b). Clinical trials are ongoing. There are currently four medications with FDA approval for the maintenance treatment of alcohol dependence: disulfiram (option C), oral naltrexone, a long-acting intramuscular formulation of naltrexone, and acamprosate (option B). The use of buprenorphine for detoxification or maintenance treatment in opioid dependence is increasingly common, in part because buprenorphine (option D) can be prescribed in a physician's office with up to 1 month's prescription at a time. Recent evidence from randomized clinical trials has demonstrated the efficacy of behavioral therapies for stimulant use disorder. Two approaches most extensively investigated are cognitive-behavioral therapy and contingency management. These therapies are associated with modest increases in treatment retention and reductions in cocaine and methamphetamine use. **(Hales RE, Yudofsky SC, Roberts LW [eds]: APP Textbook of Psychiatry, 6th Edition, Chapter 23, pp. 792–793, 806 and Table 23–17, p. 793)**

39.10 Which of the following is a symptom of acute benzodiazepine toxicity?

A. Agitation.
B. Sweating.
C. Seizures.
D. Tachycardia.
E. Anterograde amnesia.

The correct response is option E: Anterograde amnesia.

Symptoms of acute toxicity of benzodiazepines include sedation, psychomotor impairment, and memory problems. It is well established that acute doses of benzodiazepines produce anterograde amnesia (option E), difficulty acquiring new learning, and sedation that may affect attention and concentration.

A withdrawal syndrome after high-dose chronic administration of chlordiazepoxide or diazepam can include grand mal seizures and psychosis. When one of these drugs is administered for short periods and at therapeutic doses, the withdrawal syndrome is usually mild, consisting of anxiety, headache, insomnia, dysphoria, tremor, and muscle twitching. After long-term treatment with therapeutic doses, the withdrawal syndrome increases in severity and may include autonomic dysfunction such as sweating (option B) or tachycardia (option D), nausea, vomiting, depersonalization, derealization, delirium, hallucinations, illusions, agitation (option A), and grand mal seizures (option C). **(Hales RE, Yudofsky SC, Roberts LW [eds]: APP Textbook of Psychiatry, 6th Edition, Chapter 23, p. 786)**

References

Bryant AN, Kim G: Racial/ethnic differences in prevalence and correlates of binge drinking among older adults. Aging Ment Health 16(2):208–217, 2012 22224754

De La Garza R 2nd, Newton TF, Haile CN, et al: Rivastigmine reduces "Likely to use methamphetamine" in methamphetamine-dependent volunteers. Prog Neuropsychopharmacol Biol Psychiatry 37(1):141–146, 2012 22230648

Fiore M, Jaen C, Baker T, et al; Clinical Practice Guideline Treating Tobacco Use and Dependence 2008 Update Panel, Liaisons, and Staff: A clinical practice guideline for treating tobacco use and dependence: 2008 update. A U.S. Public Health Service report. Am J Prev Med 35(2):158–176, 2008 18617085

Haile CN, De La Garza R 2nd, Mahoney JJ 3rd: The impact of disulfiram treatment on the reinforcing effects of cocaine. PloS One 7(11):e47702, 2012a 23144826

Haile CN, Mahoney JJ 3rd, Newton TF, De La Garza R 2nd: Pharmacotherapeutics directed at deficiencies associated with cocaine dependence: focus on dopamine, norepinephrine and glutamate. Pharmacol Ther 134(2):260–277, 2012b 22327234

Kosten TR, Newton TF 2nd, De La Garza R 2nd, Haile CN: Cocaine and Methamphetamine Dependence: Advances in Treatment. Washington, DC, American Psychiatric Publishing, 2011

Kosten TR, Wu G, Huang W, et al: Pharmacogenetic randomized trial for cocaine abuse: disulfiram and dopamine β-hydroxylase. Biol Psychiatry 73(3):219–224, 2013 22906516

Mir A, Obafemi A, Young A, et al: Myocardial infarction associated with use of the synthetic cannabinoid K2. Pediatrics 128:e1622-e1627, 2011

National Institute on Drug Abuse: Drug Facts: Marijuana. December 2012. Available at: http://www.drugabuse.gov/sites/default/files/marijuana_0.pdf. Accessed September 13, 2013.

Newton TF, De La Garza R 2nd, Grasing K: The angiotensin-converting enzyme inhibitor perindopril treatment alters cardiovascular and subjective effects of methamphetamine in humans. Psychiatry Res 179(1):96–100, 2010 20493549

Newton TF, De La Garza R 2nd, Brown G, et al: Noradrenergic α_1 receptor antagonist treatment attenuates positive subjective effects of cocaine in humans: a randomized trial. PLoS ONE 7(2):e30854, 2012 22319592

Rösner S, Hackl-Herrwerth A, Leucht S, et al: Opioid antagonists for alcohol dependence. Cochrane Database Syst Rev (12):CD001867, 2010 21154349

Schuckit MA: Alcohol-use disorders. Lancet 373(9662):492–501, 2009 19168210

Schuckit MA, Smith TL, Trim RS, et al: A prospective evaluation of how a low level of response to alcohol predicts later heavy drinking and alcohol problems. Am J Drug Alcohol Abuse 37(6):479–486, 2011 21797810

Substance Abuse and Mental Health Services Administration: Results from the 2011 National Survey on Drug Use and Health: Summary of National Findings (NSDUH Series H-44, HHS Publ No SMA 12–4713). Rockville, MD, Substance Abuse and Mental Health Services Administration, 2012a. Available at: http://www.samhsa.gov/data/nsduh/2k11results/nsduhresults2011.htm. Accessed September 13, 2013.

Substance Abuse and Mental Health Services Administration: The TEDS [Treatment Entry Data Set] Report: Marijuana Admissions Reporting Daily Use at Treatment Entry. Rockville, MD, Center for Behavioral Health Statistics and Quality, Substance Abuse and Mental Health Services Administration, February 2, 2012b. Available at: http://www.samhsa.gov/data/2k12/TEDS_SR_029_Marijuana_2012/TEDS_Short_Report_029_Marijuana_2012.pdf. Accessed September 13, 2013.

Sullivan JT, Sykora K, Schneiderman J, et al: Assessment of alcohol withdrawal: the revised clinical institute withdrawal assessment for alcohol scale (CIWA-Ar). Br J Addict 84(11):1353–1357, 1989 2597811

Yip SW, Doherty J, Wakeley J, et al: Reduced subjective response to acute ethanol administration among young men with a broad bipolar phenotype. Neuropsychopharmacology 37(8):1808–1815, 2012 22491350

CHAPTER 40

Suicidality

40.1 A patient at risk for suicide signs a safety contract, promising to call for help rather than act on suicidal impulses. This contract is most likely to accomplish which of the following?

    A. Reduce the need for hospitalization.
    B. Reduce the patient's suicide risk.
    C. Protect the psychiatrist from a malpractice lawsuit.
    D. Substitute for a detailed risk assessment.
    E. Help foster a therapeutic alliance.

The correct response is option E: Help foster a therapeutic alliance.

Suicide prevention contracts created between the clinician and the patient attempt to develop an expressed understanding that the patient will call for help rather than act out suicidal thoughts or impulses. These contracts have no legal authority, so are unable to protect the psychiatrist from a malpractice lawsuit (option C). Although they may be helpful in solidifying the therapeutic alliance (option E), contracts may falsely reassure the psychiatrist. They do not reduce the need for hospitalization (option A) or reduce the patient's suicide risk (option B). Suicide prevention agreements between psychiatrists and patients must not be used in place of adequate suicide assessment (Simon 1999) (option D). **(Hales RE, Yudofsky SC, Roberts LW [eds]: APP Textbook of Psychiatry, 6th Edition, Chapter 6, p. 185)**

40.2 Which of the following is true regarding passive suicidal ideation?

    A. It is relatively uncommon.
    B. It frequently leads to involuntary hospitalization.
    C. Discussion of such thoughts often damages the therapeutic alliance.
    D. It requires no further evaluation on the Beck Scale for Suicide Ideation.
    E. It is integral to the evaluation of thought content.

The correct response is option E: It is integral to the evaluation of thought content.

Suicidality and homicidality are integral to the evaluation of thought content (option E). Passive suicidal thoughts are common (option A), and discussion can often lead to a deepening of the alliance (option C). Most such thoughts do not lead to involuntary treatment (option B). The Beck Scale for Suicide Ideation (Beck et al. 1979) is a 21-item rating scale that consists of five screening items related to the wish to live or die and the desire to commit suicide. If the respondent reports any active or passive desire to attempt suicide, then an additional 14 items are administered (option D). **(Hales RE, Yudofsky SC, Roberts LW [eds]: APP Textbook of Psychiatry, 6th Edition, Chapter 1, pp. 24–25; Chapter 3, p. 71)**

40.3   Which of the following is the most consistently described risk factor for a completed suicide?

A. Past history of suicide attempts.
B. Female sex.
C. Increased age.
D. Living in a group home.
E. Being married.

The correct response is option A: Past history of suicide attempts.

The possibility of suicidal behavior exists at all times during major depressive episodes. Although the most consistently described risk factor is a past history of suicide attempts or threats (option A), most completed suicides are *not* preceded by unsuccessful attempts. Risks for suicide attempts are higher in women; however, risks for completion of suicides in women are lower (option B). The likelihood of suicide attempts lessens in middle and late life, although the risk of completed suicide does not (option C). Other features associated with an increased risk for completed suicide include being single or living alone (options D, E) and prominent feelings of hopelessness. The presence of borderline personality disorder (BPD) markedly increases risks for future suicide attempts. **(Hales RE, Yudofsky SC, Roberts LW [eds]: APP Textbook of Psychiatry, 6th Edition, Chapter 11, p. 368)**

40.4   Beck and coworkers have proposed that people with depression are prone to cognitive distortions in three major areas—self, world, and future (i.e., the "negative cognitive triad"). Which of the following dysphoric perspectives deriving from cognitive distortions about the *future* has been found to be highly associated with suicide risk?

A. Pessimism.
B. Suspiciousness.
C. Hopelessness.
D. Fear of harm.
E. Self-criticism.

The correct response is option C: Hopelessness.

Substantial evidence has been collected to support the concept of the negative cognitive triad of self, world, and future (Clark et al. 1999), and a large group of investigations has established that one of the elements of this triad, a view of the future as hopeless, is highly associated with suicide risk (option C). For example, Beck et al. (1985) found that hopelessness was the strongest predictor of eventual suicide in a sample of depressed inpatients followed for 10 years after discharge. Cognitive-behavioral therapy (CBT) has been demonstrated to be an effective treatment approach for reducing hopelessness and suicide attempts (Brown et al. 2005). While other negative cognitions (options A, B, D, E) may be present, they have not been found to have the same predictive value for suicide risks. **(Hales RE, Yudofsky SC, Roberts LW [eds]: APP Textbook of Psychiatry, 6th Edition, Chapter 32, p. 1124)**

40.5   What is the topic of the U.S. Food and Drug Administration (FDA) black box warning carried by all antidepressants?

A. Increased risk of suicidality in pediatric patients.
B. Increased risk of violence in pediatric patients.
C. Increased risk of cerebrovascular accidents in pediatric patients.
D. Increased risk of sudden death in pediatric patients.
E. Increased risk of hepatic disease in pediatric patients.

The correct response is option A: Increased risk of suicidality in pediatric patients.

In 2004, the FDA issued an advisory requiring that all antidepressant medications carry a black box warning regarding an increased risk of suicidality in pediatric patients. It is important to note that no completed suicides occurred in the more than 4,000 children included in the studies of selective serotonin reuptake inhibitor (SSRI) use. In addition, methodological limitations in the studies made drawing conclusions regarding efficacy and side effects difficult (Brent and Birmaher 2004). Furthermore, studies of SSRI use in children with anxiety disorders have not shown any increase in suicidal ideation or behavior. The clinical consensus is that SSRIs are clearly beneficial for children with anxiety disorders and probably so for depression, but monitoring for suicidal ideation is important, especially in the first few weeks of treatment. Since the black box warning, prescriptions of SSRIs for children have decreased. The adolescent suicide rate, which had been declining for about 15 years, began to rise. A reanalysis at the person level of longitudinal data from all of the controlled trials of fluoxetine for pediatric depression found no evidence of increased suicidal thoughts and behaviors in youth randomly assigned to medication versus placebo (Gibbons et al. 2012). **(Hales RE, Yudofsky SC, Roberts LW [eds]: APP Textbook of Psychiatry, 6th Edition, Chapter 34, p. 1204)**

40.6   Therapist effects were found to be significant in the Borderline Personality Disorder Study of Cognitive Therapy, a well-designed randomized clinical trial to test efficacy of CBT (Davidson et al. 2006). With which of the following provided by the therapists did patients have two to three times greater improvement in suicide-related outcomes?

A. Emergency services and medication management.
B. Cognitive techniques to modify core beliefs and schemas.
C. Behavioral strategies to promote adaptive functioning.
D. Higher quantity and more competent delivery of CBT.
E. Exposure to situations that triggered emotional distress.

The correct response is option D: Higher quantity and more competent delivery of CBT.

Because the active treatment group did not show improvements in number of psychiatric hospitalizations or emergency department admissions compared with the treatment-as-usual group, therapist effects were analyzed and found to impact treatment efficacy. Specifically, patients receiving a higher quantity of sessions and more competent delivery (option D), as assessed by a competence rating scale, had greater improvement in suicide-related outcomes (Norrie et al. 2013). In the active treatment group, all therapists provided cognitive techniques to modify core beliefs and schemas (option B) and behavioral strategies to promote adaptive functioning (option C). Therapists may have provided exposure to situations that triggered emotional distress (option E), which is a component of CBT treatment, but this specific technique was not a standard part of this protocol. In the treatment-as-usual group, only emergency services and medication management were provided (option A). **(Oldham JM, Skodol AE, Bender DS [eds]: APP Textbook of Personality Disorders, 2nd Edition, Chapter 12, p. 263)**

40.7   What are the findings of studies defining the structural, metabolic, and functional biology of brain circuits mediating personality traits in subjects at high risk for suicidal behavior?

A. Hippocampal volume gain in structural magnetic resonance imaging (MRI) studies of patients with BPD.
B. Increase of gray matter concentrations in insular cortex of those who attempt suicide compared with those who do not attempt it.
C. Improved executive cognitive functioning in subjects with BPD under stress leading to suicidal behavior.
D. Excessive cortical inhibition in functional MRI (fMRI) studies of subjects with BPD.
E. Hyperarousal of the amygdala and other limbic structures in fMRI studies of subjects with BPD.

The correct response is option E: Hyperarousal of the amygdala and other limbic structures in fMRI studies of subjects with BPD.

Neuroimaging and other studies have begun to define the structural, metabolic, and functional biology of brain circuits that mediate personality traits such as impulsive aggression and emotion dysregulation in subjects at high risk for suicidal behavior. fMRI research with subjects with BPD has found excessive "bottom-up" activation of the amygdala especially in response to negative emotion (option E) (Silbersweig et al. 2007). In structural MRI studies, hippocampal volume loss (option A), with and without diminished volume in the amygdala, is the most widely replicated finding in morphometric studies of BPD (Brambilla et al. 2004; Driessen et al. 2000; Irle et al. 2005; Schmahl et al. 2003) though not all (Zetzsche et al. 2007). In a study utilizing voxel-based morphometry (Soloff et al. 2012), compared to nonattempters, those who attempted suicide had diminished, not increased, gray-matter concentrations in insular cortex (option B), a limbic integration area that is activated in tasks involving social interaction, trust, cooperation, and also social exclusion (rejection). Among patients with BPD, impairment (not improvement; option C) of executive cognitive function under stress has been shown to contribute to suicidal behavior, as well as affective instability and impulsive aggression (Fertuck et al. 2006). The fMRI study results suggest that diminished cognitive function during affective arousal may result from the relative failure of "top-down" cortical inhibition from prefrontal and anterior cingulate functions (option D) (Silbersweig et al. 2007). **(Oldham JM, Skodol AE, Bender DS [eds]: APP Textbook of Personality Disorders, 2nd Edition, Chapter 18, pp. 396–398)**

40.8   In the acute-on-chronic risk model for suicidality in patients with personality disorders (PDs), which of the following is considered an acute risk?

A. Childhood sexual abuse.
B. Poor employment history.
C. Multiple prior treaters.
D. Discharge from the hospital.
E. Low socioeconomic status.

The correct response is option D: Discharge from the hospital.

The acute-on-chronic risk assessment model is a clinically relevant tool used to distinguish between nonmodifiable and potentially modifiable risk factors for suicide and suicidal behavior in patients with PDs. Chronic risk factors for suicide relate to those factors that have existed for many months or years, such as childhood sexual abuse (option A), poor employment history (option B), multiple prior treaters (option C), or low socioeconomic status (option E). A recent discharge from the hospital (option D) is an example of an acute risk or one that has existed for days, weeks, or at most months and can be modified by clinical interventions. **(Oldham JM, Skodol AE, Bender DS [eds]: APP Textbook of Personality Disorders, 2nd Edition, Chapter 18, pp. 386, 398–399)**

40.9 Suicide mortality is lowest for which of the following groups?

A. Women ages 15–24.
B. Men ages 15–24.
C. Women ages 65 and older.
D. Men ages 65 and older.
E. Women ages 60–64.

The correct response is option A: Women ages 15–24.

Suicide mortality is positively correlated with age. Suicide mortality in the United States in 2010 was almost twice as high for men ages 65 years and older (29.0 per 100,000 men; option D) than for men ages 15–24 years (16.9 per 100,000 men; option B). Among women, suicide mortality has long been lower than among men. In 2010, the suicide rate was 3.9 per 100,000 women ages 15–24 years versus 4.2 per 100,000 women ages 65 years and older (option A) (National Center for Health Statistics 2012). The rate for women ages 65 and older is higher than that for women ages 15–24 (option C). One trend causing concern, however, is the increase in suicide deaths among middle-aged adults in the United States between 1999 and 2010 (Centers for Disease Control and Prevention 2013). From 1999 to 2010, the age-adjusted suicide rate for persons ages 35–64 years increased by 28.4%, from 13.7 per 100,000 population to 17.6 ($P<0.001$). Among men, the greatest increases were observed among those ages 50–54 (49.4%, from 20.6 to 30.7) and those ages 55–59 (47.8%, from 20.3 to 30.0). Among women, the greatest increase was among those ages 60–64 (59.7%, from 4.4 to 7.0). The rate for women of this age is higher than that of women ages 18–24 (option E). The rise in suicide rate among those approaching late life may be due in part to the economic downtown during the period from 1999 to 2010, to a cohort effect in that baby boomers had higher suicide rates during adolescence and may represent a cohort at greater risk, and to a rising incidence of opioid overdose associated with increased availability (Centers for Disease Control and Prevention 2013). **(Steffens DC, Blazer DG, Thakur ME [eds]: APP Textbook of Geriatric Psychiatry, 5th Edition, Chapter 1, p. 20)**

40.10 Research on suicidality in patients with BPD has indicated the possibility of two patient groups with distinct patterns over time: a group with repeated high-lethality attempts and a group with repeated low-lethality attempts. The group with repeated low-lethality attempts is notable for which of the following?

A. Older age.
B. More psychiatric hospitalizations.
C. Comorbid histrionic or narcissistic PDs.
D. Poor baseline psychosocial functioning.
E. Recruitment for studies from inpatient populations.

The correct response is option C: Comorbid histrionic or narcissistic PDs.

Prospective studies of BPD have demonstrated that the vast majority of patients can expect significant symptom relief over time (Gunderson et al. 2011; Shea et al. 2002, 2009; Zanarini et al. 2012). In an effort to identify the clinical characteristics predicting higher-lethality suicide attempts over time in the subgroup that does not experience symptom relief, one prospective study (Soloff and Chiappetta 2012) identified predictors of continued high-lethality suicide attempts. The low-lethality group was notable for comorbid narcissistic or histrionic PD diagnoses (option C), whereas the high-lethality group was notable for older, not younger, age (option A); more, not fewer, inpatient psychiatric hospitalizations (option B); higher, not lower, baseline functioning (option D); and recruitment from outpatient, not inpatient, samples (option E). **(Oldham JM, Skodol AE, Bender DS [eds]: APP Textbook of Personality Disorders, 2nd Edition, Chapter 18, pp. 392–393)**

40.11 Which of the following is the best description of the stress-diathesis causal model of suicidal behavior?

A. A model suggesting an underlying neurobiological vulnerability to suicidal behavior in times of stress.
B. Another way to assess and communicate risk of suicide in clinical situations in the acute-on-chronic model.
C. A theory specifically discounting a patient's core personality traits.
D. A model for suicidal behavior developed exclusively for patients with PDs.
E. A model for suicide to be assessed only in retrospective studies.

The correct response is option A: A model suggesting an underlying neurobiological vulnerability to suicidal behavior in times of stress.

The stress-diathesis causal model of suicidal behavior suggests that specific personality traits may constitute a vulnerability to suicidal behavior at times of stress (option A). The likelihood of suicidal behavior increases when acute stressors are experienced by patients with personality traits such as emotion dysregulation or impulsive aggression, as in patients with BPD (option D), or a chronic tendency toward pessimism, as in patients with depression (Mann et al. 1999; Oquendo et al. 2004). The stress-diathesis causal model for suicidal behavior should not be confused with the acute-on-chronic risk model, which assists clinicians in assessing and communicating suicidality in patients with PD typically at a chronically elevated suicide risk (option B). The stress-diathesis model suggests that specific personality traits may constitute a vulnerability to suicidal behavior at times of stress, not that those traits should be discounted (option C). Prospective studies of patients with BPD have found that episodes of depression and negative life events predict suicidal behavior at 1 year (Soloff and Chiappetta 2012) and at 3 years (Yen et al. 2005), suggesting that the stress-diathesis model can be studied prospectively (option E). **(Oldham JM, Skodol AE, Bender DS [eds]: APP Textbook of Personality Disorders, 2nd Edition, Chapter 18, p. 386, 395–396)**

References

Beck AT, Kovacs M, Weissman A: Assessment of suicidal intention: the Scale for Suicide Ideation. J Consult Clin Psychol 47(2):343–352, 1979 469082

Beck AT, Steer RA, Kovacs M, Garrison B: Hopelessness and eventual suicide: a 10-year prospective study of patients hospitalized with suicidal ideation. Am J Psychiatry 142(5):559–563, 1985 3985195

Brambilla P, Soloff PH, Sala M, et al: Anatomical MRI study of borderline personality disorder patients. Psychiatry Res 131(2):125–133, 2004 15313519

Brent DA, Birmaher B: British warnings on SSRIs questioned. J Am Acad Child Adolesc Psychiatry 43(4):379–380, 2004 15187795

Brown GK, Ten Have T, Henriques GR, et al: Cognitive therapy for the prevention of suicide attempts: a randomized controlled trial. JAMA 294(5):563–570, 2005 16077050

Centers for Disease Control and Prevention (CDC): Suicide among adults aged 35–64 years—United States, 1999–2010. MMWR Morb Mortal Wkly Rep 62(17):321–325, 2013 23636024

Clark DA, Beck AT, Alford BA: Scientific Foundations of Cognitive Theory and Therapy of Depression. New York, Wiley, 1999

Davidson K, Norrie J, Tyrer P, et al: The effectiveness of cognitive behavior therapy for borderline personality disorder: results from the borderline personality disorder study of cognitive therapy (BOSCOT) trial. J Pers Disord 20(5):450–465, 2006 17032158

Driessen M, Herrmann J, Stahl K, et al: Magnetic resonance imaging volumes of the hippocampus and the amygdala in women with borderline personality disorder and early traumatization. Arch Gen Psychiatry 57(12):1115–1122, 2000 11115325

Fertuck EA, Lenzenweger MF, Clarkin JF, et al: Executive neurocognition, memory systems, and borderline personality disorder. Clin Psychol Rev 26(3):346–375, 2006 15992977

Gibbons RD, Brown CH, Hur K, et al: Suicidal thoughts and behavior with antidepressant treatment: reanalysis of the randomized placebo-controlled studies of fluoxetine and venlafaxine. Arch Gen Psychiatry 69(6):580–587, 2012 22309973

Gunderson JG, Zanarini MC, Choi-Kain LW, et al: Family study of borderline personality disorder and its sectors of psychopathology. Arch Gen Psychiatry 68(7):753–762, 2011 21727257

Irle E, Lange C, Sachsse U: Reduced size and abnormal asymmetry of parietal cortex in women with borderline personality disorder. Biol Psychiatry 57(2):173–182, 2005 15652877

Mann JJ, Waternaux C, Haas GL, Malone KM: Toward a clinical model of suicidal behavior in psychiatric patients. Am J Psychiatry 156(2):181–189, 1999 9989552

National Center for Health Statistics: Health, United States, 2012: With Special Feature on Emergency Care. Hyattsville, MD, U.S. Government Printing Office, 2012

Norrie J, Davidson K, Tata P, Gumley A: Influence of therapist competence and quantity of cognitive behavioural therapy on suicidal behaviour and inpatient hospitalisation in a randomised controlled trial in borderline personality disorder: further analyses of treatment effects in the BOSCOT study. Psychol Psychother 86(3):280–293, 2013 23420622

Oquendo MA, Galfalvy H, Russo S, et al: Prospective study of clinical predictors of suicidal acts after a major depressive episode in patients with major depressive disorder or bipolar disorder. Am J Psychiatry 161(8):1433–1441, 2004 15285970

Schmahl CG, Vermetten E, Elzinga BM, Douglas Bremner J: Magnetic resonance imaging of hippocampal and amygdala volume in women with childhood abuse and borderline personality disorder. Psychiatry Res 122(3):193–198, 2003 12694893

Shea MT, Stout R, Gunderson J, et al: Short-term diagnostic stability of schizotypal, borderline, avoidant, and obsessive-compulsive personality disorders. Am J Psychiatry 159(12):2036–2041, 2002 12450953

Shea MT, Edelen MO, Pinto A, et al: Improvement in borderline personality disorder in relationship to age. Acta Psychiatr Scand 119(2):143–148, 2009 18851719

Silbersweig D, Clarkin JF, Goldstein M, et al: Failure of frontolimbic inhibitory function in the context of negative emotion in borderline personality disorder. Am J Psychiatry 164(12):1832–1841, 2007 18056238

Simon RI: The suicide prevention contract: clinical, legal, and risk management issues. J Am Acad Psychiatry Law 27(3):445–450, 1999 10509943

Soloff PH, Chiappetta L: Prospective predictors of suicidal behavior in borderline personality disorder at 6-year follow-up. Am J Psychiatry 169(5):484–490, 2012 22549208

Soloff PH, Pruitt P, Sharma M, et al: Structural brain abnormalities and suicidal behavior in borderline personality disorder. J Psychiatr Res 46(4):516–525, 2012 22336640

Yen S, Pagano ME, Shea MT, et al: Recent life events preceding suicide attempts in a personality disorder sample: findings from the collaborative longitudinal personality disorders study. J Consult Clin Psychol 73(1):99–105, 2005 15709836

Zanarini MC, Frankenburg FR, Reich DB, Fitzmaurice G: Attainment and stability of sustained symptomatic remission and recovery among patients with borderline personality disorder and axis II comparison subjects: a 16-year prospective follow-up study. Am J Psychiatry 169(5):476–483, 2012 22737693

Zetzsche T, Preuss UW, Frodl T, et al: Hippocampal volume reduction and history of aggressive behaviour in patients with borderline personality disorder. Psychiatry Res 154(2):157–170, 2007 17306512

CHAPTER 41

Trauma- and Stressor-
Related Disorders

41.1 Which class of medication has been shown to be effective in reducing the full range of symptoms in adults with posttraumatic stress disorder (PTSD)?

A. Benzodiazepines.
B. Second-generation antipsychotic medications.
C. Selective serotonin reuptake inhibitors (SSRIs).
D. Anticonvulsants.
E. α_1-Adrenergic receptor antagonists.

The correct response is option C: Selective serotonin reuptake inhibitors (SSRIs).

SSRIs (option C) are the only medications shown to be effective in reducing the full range of PTSD symptoms (Brady et al. 2000; Davidson et al. 1996; van der Kolk et al. 1994). Some clinicians caution against the use of benzodiazepines in treating PTSD because of theoretical risks of interference with extinction learning, based on animal and very little human research. There is a lack of evidence for benzodiazepine (option A) efficacy as monotherapy, as well as risk of abuse in a population already at elevated risk for alcohol and substance use disorders. Second-generation antipsychotic agents such as olanzapine, quetiapine, and risperidone (option B) have been studied as monotherapy and/or augmentation therapy for PTSD (with mixed results) as well as for specific symptoms such as sleep disturbance. One large randomized controlled study of risperidone in chronic military-related PTSD failed to show efficacy (Krystal et al. 2011). A range of anticonvulsants (option D) have been studied for PTSD but have not shown strong evidence of efficacy, and none are first-line treatments. Prazosin (option E), an α_1-adrenergic receptor antagonist, has been investigated in the treatment of posttraumatic stress nightmares, and a systematic review found that three of four randomized controlled trials and several other studies demonstrated its benefit for this indication (Kung et al. 2012), although not for all symptoms of PTSD.

(Hales RE, Yudofsky SC, Roberts LW [eds]: APP Textbook of Psychiatry, 6th Edition, Chapter 14, pp. 477–479)

41.2   What is the most prominent focus of prolonged exposure therapy (PE) for the treatment of PTSD?

A. Targeted homework assignments designed to reshape dysfunctional cognitive beliefs that interfere with recovery.
B. Mindfulness exercises to enhance coping strategies.
C. Conjoint sessions to reduce the impact of the patient's PTSD symptoms on his or her intimate partner.
D. Repeated imaginal and in vivo exposures to enhance extinction of traumatic memories and decrease cue reactivity.
E. Intensive debriefing to prevent consolidation of traumatic memories.

The correct response is option D: Repeated imaginal and in vivo exposures to enhance extinction of traumatic memories and decrease cue reactivity.

The cognitive-behavioral therapy approaches with the greatest amount of evidence supporting efficacy include PE (Foa et al. 2005) and cognitive processing therapy (CPT; Resick et al. 2008); both have shown excellent treatment results across a range of populations with PTSD, including PTSD following sexual assault or combat trauma. PE focuses most prominently on 1) repeated imaginal exposure to the primary trauma memories to enhance extinction generally over the course of weekly 90-minute sessions and 2) in vivo exposures to decrease cue reactivity and avoidance (option D). In recent years, there has been growing interest in mindfulness- and acceptance-based approaches to managing PTSD (option B) (Schmertz et al. 2014), but these are separate from PE. CPT utilizes a written account of the traumatic experience but also focuses on reshaping dysfunctional cognitive beliefs that often interfere with recovery (option A). CPT is also designed to be delivered in the context of a couple, with conjoint sessions used to reduce the impact of a patient's PTSD symptoms on his or her intimate partner (option C). Intensive debriefing to prevent consolidation of traumatic memories (option E) is the key element of psychological critical incident stress debriefing, which although initially found to be useful has more recently been shown in group settings either to have no effect or to increase stress and PTSD symptoms (Rose et al. 2002; van Emmerik et al. 2002). **(Hales RE, Yudofsky SC, Roberts LW [eds]: APP Textbook of Psychiatry, 6th Edition, Chapter 14, pp. 474–475)**

41.3   In studies examining biological responses to trauma-related stimuli in subjects with PTSD, which of the following findings has been repeatedly confirmed?

A. Increased heart rate.
B. Decreased skin conductance.
C. Decreased facial electromyographic reactivity.
D. Decreased startle response.
E. Increased cortisol levels.

The correct response is option A: Increased heart rate.

One of the earliest and best replicated PTSD findings is heightened autonomic (options A, B) and facial electromyographic reactivity (option C) to external trauma-related stimuli, such as combat sounds and film clips, as well as to internal mental imagery of the traumatic event. Subjects with PTSD have also been found to show heightened electromyographic responses and more consistently heightened autonomic responses to startling stimuli (Pole 2007). Elevated startle responses (option D) suggest sensitization of the nervous system. Although substantial research has supported sympathetic overreactivity in PTSD (Southwick et al. 1999), a surprising finding has been that cortisol is not consistently elevated in PTSD (option E), as might be expected according to a classical stress model. This appears to be due to hypersensitivity of the hypothalamic-pituitary-adrenal axis to negative feedback. **(Hales RE, Yudofsky SC, Roberts LW [eds]: APP Textbook of Psychiatry, 6th Edition, Chapter 14, pp. 460–461)**

41.4 Which of the following statements regarding the DSM-5 criteria for acute stress disorder (ASD) is correct?

A. The diagnosis requires the presence of symptoms including marked avoidance, marked anxiety or increased arousal, at least one of six reexperiencing symptoms, and at least three of five dissociative symptoms.
B. The diagnosis requires at least two symptoms in each of the following five categories: intrusion symptoms, negative mood, dissociative symptoms, avoidance symptoms, and arousal symptoms.
C. The time course for ASD requires symptoms beginning and worsening after the traumatic event and persisting for 2 days until 1 month after the trauma.
D. The diagnosis includes but does not require dissociative symptoms.
E. The reexperiencing symptoms apply not only to directly experienced exposures but also to exposure through electronic media, television, movies, or pictures, regardless of whether the exposure was work related.

The correct response is option D: The diagnosis includes but does not require dissociative symptoms.

The diagnosis of ASD was introduced in DSM-IV (American Psychiatric Association 1994) because of the observation that certain symptoms appeared to predict the development of PTSD. In DSM-5 (American Psychiatric Association 2013), the ASD diagnosis still includes—but no longer requires—dissociative symptoms (option D). Dissociation has not been demonstrated to be a necessary independent predictor of PTSD diagnosis (option A), and the majority of people with PTSD did not meet criteria for ASD requiring dissociation (Bryant et al. 2011). In DSM-5, the ASD diagnosis requires the presence of at least 9 of 14 symptoms in *any* of five categories (intrusion symptoms, negative mood, dissociative symptoms, avoidance symptoms, and arousal symptoms; option B) beginning or worsening after the traumatic events and persisting for 3 days (instead of the 2 days required in DSM-IV) to 1 month after the trauma (option C). Experiencing repeated or extreme exposure to aversive details of the traumatic events does not apply to exposure through electronic media, television, movies, or pictures, unless this exposure is work related (option E). **(Hales RE, Yudofsky SC, Roberts LW [eds]: APP Textbook of Psychiatry, 6th Edition, Chapter 14, pp. 480, 482)**

41.5   Which of the following best describes the prevalence rates of suicidality in patients with adjustment disorders?

A. 0%.
B. 0–25%.
C. 25%–50%.
D. 50%–75%.
E. 75%–100%.

The correct response is option C: 25%–50%.

Adjustment disorders are associated with high levels of suicidality, with prevalence rates ranging from 25% to 50% (Kryzhanovskaya and Canterbury 2001; Pelkonen et al. 2005). Given that adjustment disorders have been associated with elevated risk for suicide, any patient with an adjustment disorder diagnosis should receive a careful safety assessment and treatment plan. Empirical support for the treatment of adjustment disorders is limited, however. Whereas some authors have argued that psychological interventions should be preferred over pharmacotherapy (Carta et al. 2009; Casey and Bailey 2011), others have advocated for antidepressant use (Stewart et al. 1992), especially if no improvement is seen from psychotherapy. Brief therapies are considered the most appropriate psychological interventions for adjustment disorders (Casey and Bailey 2011), despite the scarcity of controlled data. Very limited data are available on pharmacological agents for adjustment disorders; overall no empirical data support the use of one type of treatment over another. **(Hales RE, Yudofsky SC, Roberts LW [eds]: APP Textbook of Psychiatry, 6th Edition, Chapter 14, pp. 482–486)**

41.6   An 85-year-old woman who lost her husband to cancer more than a year ago is sent to you for consultation. Since her husband's death, she has experienced intense sorrow and longing for him. In addition, on most days she has difficulty accepting that he is dead and often blames herself for his death. She feels alone and desires "to be with him"; however, she has been eating and sleeping acceptably. She recently was able to enjoy attending the college graduation of one of her adult grandchildren. What is the most appropriate diagnosis?

A. Reactive attachment disorder.
B. Major depressive disorder.
C. Normal bereavement.
D. Adjustment disorder with depressed mood.
E. Other specified trauma- and stressor-related disorder.

The correct response is option E: Other specified trauma- and stressor-related disorder.

The severe and persistent grief and mourning reactions evident in this patient meet criteria for the proposed diagnosis persistent complex bereavement disorder, which appears in Section III ("Conditions for Further Study") of DSM-5. Because the proposed criteria sets in this section of DSM-5 are not intended for clinical use, the appropriate diagnosis in this case would be other specified trauma- and stressor-related disorder (persistent complex bereavement disorder) (option E). She does not meet criteria for major depressive disorder (option B), given her ability to eat and sleep normally, and her ability to enjoy some activities that are not associated with the deceased. The time course exceeds that for normal bereavement (option C). She does not meet criteria for an adjustment disorder, which does not include bereavement (option D). Reactive attachment disorder (option A) occurs in children, and its essential feature is an absent or grossly underdeveloped attachment between a child and putative caregiving adults. **(Hales RE, Yudofsky SC, Roberts LW [eds]: APP Textbook of Psychiatry, 6th Edition, Chapter 14, pp. 463, 488–489)**

References

American Psychiatric Association: Diagnostic and Statistical Manual of Mental Disorders, 4th Edition. Washington, DC, American Psychiatric Association, 1994

American Psychiatric Association: Diagnostic and Statistical Manual of Mental Disorders, 5th Edition. Arlington, VA, American Psychiatric Association, 2013

Brady K, Pearlstein T, Asnis GM, et al: Efficacy and safety of sertraline treatment of posttraumatic stress disorder: a randomized controlled trial. JAMA 283(14):1837–1844, 2000 10770145

Bryant RA, Friedman MJ, Spiegel D, et al: A review of acute stress disorder in DSM-5. Depress Anxiety 28(9):802–817, 2011 21910186

Carta MG, Balestrieri M, Murru A, Hardoy MC: Adjustment Disorder: epidemiology, diagnosis and treatment. Clin Pract Epidemiol Ment Health 5:15, 2009 19558652

Casey P, Bailey S: Adjustment disorders: the state of the art. World Psychiatry 10(1):11–18, 2011 21379346

Davidson JR, Malik ML, Sutherland SN: Response characteristics to antidepressants and placebo in post-traumatic stress disorder. Arch Gen Psychiatry 58:445–492, 1996

Foa EB, Hembree EA, Cahill SP, et al: Randomized trial of prolonged exposure for posttraumatic stress disorder with and without cognitive restructuring: outcome at academic and community clinics. J Consult Clin Psychol 73(5):953–964, 2005 16287395

Krystal JH, Rosenheck RA, Cramer JA, et al; Veterans Affairs Cooperative Study No. 504 Group: Adjunctive risperidone treatment for antidepressant-resistant symptoms of chronic military service-related PTSD: a randomized trial. JAMA 306(5):493–502, 2011 21813427

Kryzhanovskaya L, Canterbury R: Suicidal behavior in patients with adjustment disorders. Crisis 22(3):125–131, 2001 11831599

Kung S, Espinel Z, Lapid MI: Treatment of nightmares with prazosin: a systematic review. Mayo Clin Proc 87(9):890–900, 2012 22883741

Pelkonen M, Marttunen M, Henriksson M, et al: Suicidality in adjustment disorder: clinical characteristics of adolescent outpatients. Eur Child Adolesc Psychiatry 14(3):174–180, 2005 15959663

Pole N: The psychophysiology of posttraumatic stress disorder: a meta-analysis. Psychol Bull 133(5):725–746, 2007 17723027

Resick PA, Monson CM, Chard KM: Cognitive Processing Therapy Veteran/Military Version: Therapist's Manual. Washington, DC, Department of Veterans Affairs, 2008

Rose S, Bisson J, Churchill R, et al: Psychological debriefing for preventing post traumatic stress disorder (PTSD). Cochrane Database Syst Rev (2):CD000560, 2002 12076399

Schmertz SK, Gerardi M, Rothbaum BO: Posttraumatic stress disorder, in The Wiley Handbook of Cognitive Behavioral Therapy, Vol 3. Edited by Hofmann SG. Oxford, UK, Wiley, 2014

Southwick SM, Bremner JD, Rasmusson A, et al: Role of norepinephrine in the pathophysiology and treatment of posttraumatic stress disorder. Biol Psychiatry 46(9):1192–1204, 1999 10560025

Stewart JW, Quitkin FM, Klein DF: The pharmacotherapy of minor depression. Am J Psychother 46(1):23–36, 1992 1543251

van der Kolk BA, Dreyfuss D, Michaels M, et al: Fluoxetine in posttraumatic stress disorder. J Clin Psychiatry 55(12):517–522, 1994 7814344

van Emmerik AA, Kamphuis JH, Hulsbosch AM, et al: Single session debriefing after psychological trauma: a meta-analysis. Lancet 360(9335):766–771, 2002 12241834

Bibliography

American Psychiatric Association: Diagnostic and Statistical Manual of Mental Disorders, 5th Edition. Arlington, VA, American Psychiatric Association, 2013

Centers for Medicare and Medicaid Services: Health Homes for Enrollees with Chronic Conditions (Letter to State Medicaid Directors and State Health Officials, SMDL# 10-024, ACA# 12). Baltimore, MD. Department of Health and Human Services, November 16, 2010. Available at: http://www.cms.gov/smdl/downloads/SMD10024.pdf. Accessed December 2015.

Chew RH, Hales RE, Yudofsky SC: What Your Patients Need to Know About Psychiatric Medications, 2nd Edition. Washington, DC, American Psychiatric Publishing, 2009

Comai S, Tau M, Pavlovic Z, Gobbi G: The psychopharmacology of aggressive behavior: a translational approach: part 2: clinical studies using atypical antipsychotics, anticonvulsants, and lithium. J Clin Psychopharmacol 32(2):237–260, 2012 22367663

Dulcan MK (ed): Dulcan's Textbook of Child and Adolescent Psychiatry, Washington, DC, American Psychiatric Publishing, 2010

Dulcan MK (ed): Dulcan's Textbook of Child and Adolescent Psychiatry, 2nd Edition. Arlington, VA, American Psychiatric Association Publishing, 2016

Galanter M, Kleber HD, Brady KT (eds): The American Psychiatric Publishing Textbook of Substance Abuse Treatment, 5th Edition. Washington, DC, American Psychiatric Publishing, 2015

Hales RE, Yudofsky SC, Gabbard GO (eds): The American Psychiatric Publishing Textbook of Psychiatry, 5th Edition. Washington, DC, American Psychiatric Publishing, 2008

Hales RE, Yudofsky SC, Roberts LW (eds): The American Psychiatric Publishing Textbook of Psychiatry, 6th Edition. Washington, DC, American Psychiatric Publishing, 2014

Hodge SE, Subaran RL, Weissman MM, Fyer AJ: Designing case-control studies: decisions about the controls. Am J Psychiatry 169(8):785–789, 2012 22854929

Javed A, Cohen B, Detyniecki K, et al: Rates and predictors of patient-reported cognitive side effects of antiepileptic drugs: An extended follow-up. Seizure 29:34-40, 2015 26076842

Leo RJ: Clinical Manual of Pain Management in Psychiatry. Washington, DC, American Psychiatric Publishing, 2007

Levenson JL (ed): The American Psychiatric Publishing Textbook of Psychosomatic Medicine: Psychiatric Care of the Medically Ill, 2nd Edition. Washington, DC, American Psychiatric Publishing, 2011

Mitchell JE, Crosby RD, Wonderlich SA, Adson DE: Elements of Clinical Research in Psychiatry. Washington, DC, American Psychiatric Publishing, 2000

Oldham JM, Skodol AE, Bender DS (eds): The American Psychiatric Publishing Textbook of Personality Disorders, 2nd Edition. Washington, DC, American Psychiatric Publishing, 2014

Quitkin FM: Placebos, drug effects, and study design: a clinician's guide. Am J Psychiatry 156(6):829–836, 1999 10360119

Raney LE (ed): Integrated Care: Working at the Interface of Primary Care and Behavioral Health. Washington, DC, American Psychiatric Publishing, 2015

Schatzberg AF, Nemeroff CB (eds): The American Psychiatric Publishing Textbook of Psychopharmacology, 4th Edition. Washington, DC, American Psychiatric Publishing, 2009

Schatzberg AF, Nemeroff CB (eds): Essentials of Clinical Psychopharmacology, 3rd Edition. Washington, DC, American Psychiatric Publishing, 2013

Spiegel D: Neurophysiological correlates of hypnosis and dissociation. J Neuropsychiatry Clin Neurosci 3(4):440–445, 1991 1821268

Spiegel H, Spiegel D: Trance and Treatment: Clinical Uses of Hypnosis, 2nd Edition. Washington, DC, American Psychiatric Publishing, 2004

Steffens DC, Blazer DG, Thakur ME (eds): The American Psychiatric Publishing Textbook of Geriatric Psychiatry, 5th Edition. Washington, DC, American Psychiatric Publishing, 2015

Verma A, Anand V, Verma NP: Sleep disorders in chronic traumatic brain injury. J Clin Sleep Med 3(4):357–362, 2007 17694723

Yudofsky SC, Hales RE (eds): The American Psychiatric Publishing Textbook of Neuropsychiatry and Behavioral Neurosciences, 5th Edition. Washington, DC, American Psychiatric Publishing, 2008

CPSIA information can be obtained
at www.ICGtesting.com
Printed in the USA
FSOW03n0012090117
29285FS